Today and Tomorrow of Oncological Medicine

Today and Tomorrow of Oncological Medicine

Edited by Faith Gibbs

hayle medical

New York

Hayle Medical,
750 Third Avenue, 9th Floor,
New York, NY 10017, USA

Visit us on the World Wide Web at:
www.haylemedical.com

ISBN: 978-1-63241-842-5

Cataloging-in-Publication Data

Today and tomorrow of oncological medicine / edited by Faith Gibbs.
p. cm.
Includes bibliographical references and index.
ISBN 978-1-63241-842-5
1. Oncology. 2. Cancer. 3. Cancer--Treatment. 4. Tumors--Treatment. I. Gibbs, Faith.
RC254 .T63 2020
616.994--dc23

Table of Contents

Preface

There have been remarkable strides made in the treatment of cancer as the understanding of the underlying biological processes of the disease has evolved. The traditional approaches to oncological medicine consisted of tumor removal surgeries, radiation therapy and hormone therapy, until the late 19th century. In the past years, other modalities such as chemotherapy, immunotherapy and targeted therapies have emerged. With continuing research in the biology of cancer, therapies continue to be developed with increased precision, efficacy, survivability and better quality of life. The ideal goal of cancer therapy is the complete eradication of the cancer without any adverse effects on the body. The other objectives include the suppression of the cancer to a subclinical state, provision of palliative care without curative intent and provision of a good quality of life. Clinical trials are an important aspect in the development of oncological medicine. These test new drugs, combinations of treatments, new approaches to surgery or radiation therapy and gene therapy. This book provides comprehensive insights into the field of oncological medicine. It unfolds the present and future of oncological medicine. It aims to equip students and experts with the advanced topics and upcoming concepts in this area of study.

This book is a comprehensive compilation of works of different researchers from varied parts of the world. It includes valuable experiences of the researchers with the sole objective of providing the readers (learners) with a proper knowledge of the concerned field. This book will be beneficial in evoking inspiration and enhancing the knowledge of the interested readers.

In the end, I would like to extend my heartiest thanks to the authors who worked with great determination on their chapters. I also appreciate the publisher's support in the course of the book. I would also like to deeply acknowledge my family who stood by me as a source of inspiration during the project.

Editor

1

Denileukin Diftitox (Ontak) as Maintenance Therapy for Peripheral T-Cell Lymphomas: Three Cases with Sustained Remission

Alejandra C. Fuentes,[1] Ellen Szwed,[2] Cathy D. Spears,[2] Sandeep Thaper,[3] Long H. Dang,[2] and Nam H. Dang[2]

[1]*Department of Internal Medicine, University of Florida, Gainesville, FL 32610, USA*
[2]*Division of Hematology/Oncology, Department of Internal Medicine, University of Florida, Gainesville, FL 32610, USA*
[3]*Florida Cancer Specialists and Research Institute, Leesburg, FL 34748, USA*

Correspondence should be addressed to Nam H. Dang; nam.dang@medicine.ufl.edu

Academic Editor: Guido Fadda

Peripheral T-cell lymphomas (PTCL) are rare but markedly aggressive forms of non-Hodgkin's lymphoma (NHL). They carry a poor prognosis, with current therapeutic approach being generally ineffective. The most employed first-line treatment is CHOP (cyclophosphamide, doxorubicin, vincristine, and prednisone), which still results in high rates of relapses. Denileukin diftitox is a fusion protein combining the cytotoxic portion of the diphtheria toxin and the receptor-binding domain of the interleukin-2 (IL-2) molecule, thereby targeting cells expressing the IL-2 receptor, including both T-cell and B-cell lymphomas. It has been approved for the treatment of cutaneous T-cell lymphomas, and it has documented activity in PTCL both as a single agent and as part of combination therapy. This report documents three cases of PTCL where denileukin diftitox has been used as long-term maintenance therapy after complete remission was achieved. While the overall survival rate of patients with advanced stage, refractory PTCL is generally poor (with median overall survival of 5.5 months), the three patients described in this report are all experiencing an ongoing complete remission for more than four years.

1. Introduction

Non-Hodgkin's lymphomas (NHL) are a heterogeneous group of lymphoproliferative disorders. Approximately 71,850 new cases of NHL and 19,790 deaths are projected for 2015, accounting for 4% of new cases and 3% of cancer deaths [1]. Although only about 15–20% of NHL cases originate from the T-cell lineage, T-cell non-Hodgkin's lymphomas are generally more aggressive and have a poorer prognosis than their B-cell counterpart, with decreased short-term survival and frequent relapses.

Peripheral T-cell lymphomas (PTCL) comprise most of the cases of T-cell NHL. The classification and treatment options for PTCL have advanced since the REAL Classification recognized PTCL as a specific entity independent from the B-Cell lineage in 1994 [2]. Due to the rarity of PTCL and lack of randomized controlled trials, there is no consensus on first-line therapy. CHOP (cyclophosphamide, doxorubicin, vincristine, and prednisone) has been widely used, largely based on results extrapolated from studies on aggressive B-cell lymphomas. However, CHOP has failed to improve survival and often culminates with frequent relapses, with a 5-year overall survival rates ranging around 32–35% [3, 4]. Studies comparing intensive therapies to CHOP have not demonstrated improved overall survival [5]. These findings highlight the crucial need for improved treatment strategies. In the past few years, advances in molecular biology have identified different cell surface molecular markers, leading to promising novel therapies that are currently under ongoing investigation and are being used as salvage therapy for relapsed disease [3, 4].

Denileukin diftitox (DD) is a recombinant cytotoxic fusion protein that binds the enzymatically active portion of the diphtheria toxin to the receptor-binding domain of the interleukin-2 molecule, thereby targeting cells producing the IL-2 receptor. These cells can derive from multiple lineages, including B and T lymphocytes, macrophages, and natural killer cells. Previous work has demonstrated that DD exhibited significant single-agent activity and was well tolerated in both T-cell and B-cell malignancies, as well as CD25+ and CD25− tumors [6–8].

In 2008 we reported the first case of prolonged remission with long-term maintenance therapy with DD in a patient with advanced stage, relapsed/refractory PTCL [9]. This patient is presently experiencing an ongoing complete remission of more than 9 years (ND, personal communications). To date, no other such cases had been described. This current report describes three additional cases of patients with advanced stage PTCL in which DD was used successfully as long-term maintenance therapy to maintain ongoing remission, hence illustrating the exciting potential of this novel drug as an agent that can be used as maintenance therapy in selected cases of PTCL.

2. Case 1

The patient is a 51-year-old African-American female with past medical history significant for Hepatitis B and with relapsed/refractory Stage IVB subcutaneous panniculitis gamma delta T-cell lymphoma. In November 2004 she first came to local medical attention with a firm, nontender 4 × 2 cm growth in her forehead and a smaller one in her left anterior shoulder. Biopsy of the forehead nodule revealed atypical T-cell proliferation with necrosis, and flow cytometry studies demonstrated the presence of a population of CD3+, CD4+, CD8+, CD5+, and CD56− cells.

Her complete blood count at that time revealed WBC 4,200 per mm^3 (normal differential), Hgb. 10.5 g/dL, Hct. 32.2%, and platelets 297 K/mm^3. Bone marrow studies showed normal aspirate and core biopsy, with no evidence of abnormal cells. She was diagnosed with an inflammatory reaction of unclear etiology and was placed on a prednisone taper for 6 months, which resulted in clinical improvement and resolution of her nodules by April 2005. Her local dermatologist prescribed Plaquenil after the prednisone taper, based on a presumed diagnosis of lymphoid dermatitis.

In November 2006, she experienced a recurrence of subcutaneous nodules in her right eye, left forearm, and left chest area, each measuring approximately 1 cm in size. Her WBC was 4,900 per mm^3 with predominant lymphocytosis at 41%, Hgb. 12.2 g/dL, Hct. 36.9%, and platelets 349 K/mm^3. Computed tomography (CT) scan also revealed a new subcutaneous soft tissue density measuring 3.8 × 2.3 cm in the left anterior abdomen. Biopsy of the abdominal mass showed morphologically atypical lymphocytes that appeared to rim adipocytes in a manner described for panniculitis-like T-cell lymphoproliferative disorders, with Ki-67 proliferation marker expressed in many of the cells. Immunohistochemical stains showed a predominance of CD3+/CD5+ T-cells, comprised of a mixture of CD4+ and CD8+ cells, with a few background CD20+ B-cells. CD56, CD57, CD30, ALK-1, and CD10 markers were negative. CD25 was not tested. However, a clonal population was not identified by flow cytometry and T-cell gene rearrangement analysis was negative. By January 2007, her nodules were increasing in size and in light of her clinical picture she was treated for presumed lymphoma with 6 cycles of CVP (cytoxan, vincristine, and prednisone) every 3 weeks. She tolerated the treatment well and her nodules resolved. Follow-up PET scan in July 2007 showed abnormal FDG activity in the head of the pancreas, and all labs were otherwise normal. Patient was thereafter lost to follow-up.

In May 2010, she presented to the emergency department with bilateral lower extremity swelling, upper extremity nodules, fevers, night sweats, abdominal pain, vomiting, and diarrhea for one month. CT imaging revealed recurrent multiple indurated lesions in the left flank. Biopsy of a right arm nodule showed lobular panniculitis and focal fat necrosis with involvement by an atypical T-cell infiltrate. Molecular studies were positive for a monoclonal rearranged band of T-cell receptor gamma gene and flow cytometry revealed increased level of gamma/delta T-cells at approximately 40%, consistent with subcutaneous panniculitis-like T-cell lymphoma. Bone marrow biopsy showed normal cellularity (80–90%) with multilinear hematopoiesis and no evidence of lymphoma. She received 3 cycles of ICE (ifosfamide, carboplatin, and etoposide) combination therapy, but her disease continued to progress with increasing number of subcutaneous nodules and continuing constitutional symptoms. She then received two cycles of ESHAP (etoposide, methylprednisolone, cytarabine, and cisplatin) with mixed response based on CT scan with no evidence of adenopathy but increase in nodularity and size of the anterior abdomen subcutaneous nodule. She was evaluated for stem cell transplantation, but she needed to attain at least partial remission before being a candidate.

Since she had multiple relapses despite treatment with CVP, ICE, and ESHAP combination therapies, she was started on treatment with DD in December 2010. The treatment was administered intravenously at 18 μg/kg daily for 5 days every 4 weeks, with steroid premedication. After a total of 8 cycles, CT imaging confirmed resolution of her subcutaneous nodules (Figure 1). Due to the clinical and radiological response, she then received an additional 8 cycles of DD as maintenance therapy, given at 18 μg/kg daily for 5 days every 8 weeks, which she continued to tolerate well without side effects. Her performance status remained zero throughout the entirety of her disease course and treatment, and the patient has now achieved ongoing complete remission of more than 4 years, as documented by periodic surveillance scans, physical exams, and routine blood tests.

3. Case 2

The patient is a 71-year-old Caucasian male with past medical history of type-2 diabetes mellitus, deep vein thrombosis with inferior vena cava filter placement in 2010, and newly diagnosed stage IVB peripheral T-cell lymphoma.

He first presented to an outside institution in April 2010 with complaints of progressive groin adenopathy, leg swelling, and fatigue for several months. His CBC at that

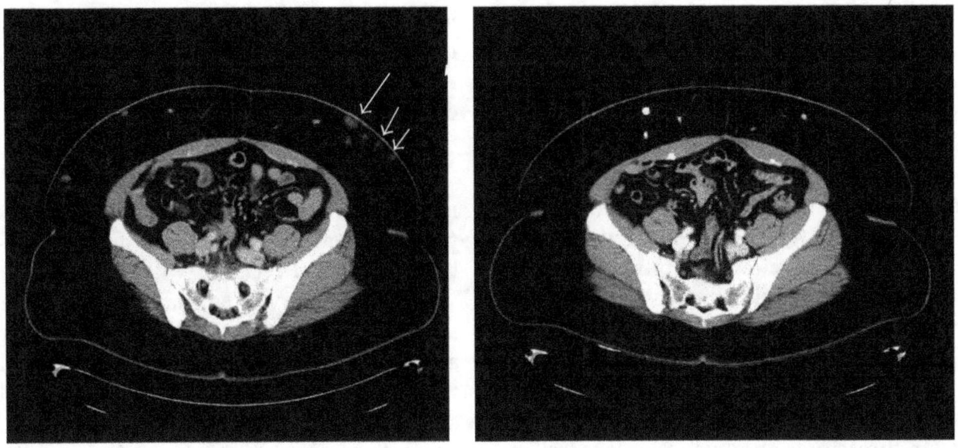

(a) (b)

Figure 1: Case 1: CTs of the abdomen illustrating (a) subcutaneous nodules prior to initiation of denileukin diftitox and (b) resolution of the subcutaneous nodules after treatment with denileukin diftitox.

time revealed WBC 6,300 per mm^3 (with 77.0% neutrophils and 9.6% lymphocytes), Hgb. 13.8 g/dL, Hct. 44.3%, and platelets 252 K/mm^3. CT imaging demonstrated disease on both sides of the diaphragm with a 1.5 cm left axillary node and subcarinal node, as well as diffuse lymphadenopathy in the retroperitoneum, pelvis, and left groin. A lymph node biopsy was positive for peripheral T-cell lymphoma, NOS. Bone marrow biopsy did not show definitive morphologic involvement with a T-cell lymphoproliferative disorder, but T-cell clonality analysis was positive for a clonal T-cell receptor beta gene rearrangement. Flow cytometric analysis of the bone marrow detected a small population of T-cells (5%), which had an inverted CD4 : CD8 ratio at 0.3 : 1; otherwise no aberrant antigen expression was detected. CD25 was not tested.

He was started on treatment with CHOP combination chemotherapy and achieved complete remission after 6 cycles by August 2010, as documented by end-of-treatment CT scans showing complete resolution of adenopathy and repeat bone marrow biopsy indicating complete clearance of tumor cells. CBC at this time revealed WBC 3,000 per mm^3 (with 70.3% neutrophils and 15.5% lymphocytes), Hgb. 14.9 g/dL, Hct. 43.6%, and platelets 138 K/mm^3.

He was not a candidate for consolidation with stem cell transplantation due to his age. In view of the high risk of relapse and poor prognosis associated with stage IVB PTCL, the patient opted for maintenance therapy with DD, starting with the first cycle in December 2010. DD was administered intravenously at 18 μg/kg daily for 5 days every 4 weeks, for the first eight cycles, and then additional 8 cycles were given at 18 μg/kg daily for 5 days every 8 weeks. He completed a total of 16 cycles without any side effects. He experienced decreased fatigue and improved performance status from 1 to 0. The patient has now maintained an ongoing complete remission of greater than 4 years as documented by periodic surveillance scans, bone marrow biopsies, physical exams, and routine blood tests.

4. Case 3

The patient is a 27-year-old Hispanic female with past medical history of coarctation of the aorta, with Stage IIIA CD30+ anaplastic large cell lymphoma, null type, positive for ALK-1 (anaplastic lymphoma kinase-1).

She first presented in August 2010 to an outside institution with fevers, night sweats, paresthesias, 15 lb weight loss, and bilateral supraclavicular adenopathy with mild swelling in her groin. CT scans revealed extensive mediastinal, pelvic, and retroperitoneal lymphadenopathy with accompanying ascites and mild splenomegaly. The largest nodes were a mesenteric lymph node measured 2.3 cm and a right inguinal lymph node 3 cm. Right inguinal lymph node biopsy revealed anaplastic large cell lymphoma of null type, ALK-1 positive. Immunohistochemical stain was strongly positive for ALK-1, CD4, CD30, CD25, and epithelial membrane antigen (EMA) at 60%, mildly positive for CD45, and negative for CD3, CD20, and CD8. The pattern of ALK-1 immunostain was diffuse cytoplasmic with peripheral intensification, suggesting ALK partner with TPM3 (t(1; 2)(q25; p23)). Bone marrow studies showed a normal aspirate and core biopsy, without evidence of abnormal cells. Her WBC was 9,700/mm^3, Hgb. 11.2 g/dL, Hct. 33.4%, and platelets 285 K/mm^3.

She received CHOP combination chemotherapy with initial response and resolution of palpable lymphadenopathy after three cycles. However, two weeks after her third cycle in October 2010, she noted increasing cervical adenopathy. A repeat CT scan revealed left cervical, left supraclavicular and right inguinal lymphadenopathy, with the largest inguinal node measuring 1.7 cm with heterogenous appearance. Cervical lymph node biopsy revealed persistent anaplastic large cell lymphoma with the same immunophenotype. Her CBC showed WBC 3,400/mm^3, Hgb. 11.5 g/dL, Hct. 35.9%, and platelets 218 K/mm^3. She was referred to our institution in November 2010, where she received four cycles of ICE (ifosfamide, carboplatin, and etoposide) salvage chemotherapy, finishing in December 2010. Follow-up CBC in January 2011 showed WBC 3,900/mm^3, Hgb. 9.1 g/dL, Hct. 25.5%, and platelets 72 K/mm^3, and CT scan at that time demonstrated remission with no evidence of nodal disease.

She declined consolidation with stem cell transplantation and opted for maintenance therapy with DD, which was initiated in February 2011. She received 6 cycles administered intravenously at 18 μg/kg daily for 5 days every 4 weeks, and then additional 4 cycles were administered intravenously at 18 μg/kg daily for 5 days every 8 weeks. She received a total of 10 cycles by March 2012 and was then lost to follow-up. CT imaging after cycles 3, 6, and 10 were negative for recurrence of disease. Associated side effects included fatigue and weight gain after the first cycle and bilateral leg swelling after the fifth cycle (improved with furosemide administration), as well as anasarca and lower extremity deep vein thrombosis (DVT) after the tenth cycle.

She returned in January 2013 to reestablish care and has continued to show no recurrence of disease. The patient has now maintained an ongoing complete remission of greater than 4 years as documented by periodic surveillance scans, physical exams, and routine blood tests.

5. Discussion

Although PTCL only account for 6% of NHLs and are relatively rare when compared to their B-cell counterparts, they tend to be aggressive and are associated with higher international prognostic index (IPI) scores. Relapses after treatment with CHOP, the most employed therapy, are common, leading to poor prognosis and short-term survival, with 5-year overall survival (OS) rates ranging around 32–35% [3, 4]. Patients with relapsed or refractory PTCL have a reported median progression-free survival of 3.1 months and a median OS of 5.5 months [10]. In contrast, after using DD as maintenance therapy, the cases presented in this report have achieved ongoing sustained remission for over 4 years. DD as maintenance therapy has only been reported in one prior case [9], and this patient is presently experiencing sustained remission for 9+ years (ND, personal communications). To our knowledge, these are the only four patients who have received DD as maintenance therapy, and all four of them have achieved remarkable results. As exemplified in these cases, this novel targeted therapy may provide an alternative to stem cell transplantation (SCT), whose role as consolidation therapy in PTCL remains controversial, with some studies supporting its efficacy and others suggesting lack of improved outcomes [11–14]. Additionally, as evidenced in this report, not all patients meet criteria for SCT.

The efficacy of DD as salvage therapy in otherwise refractory PTCL has already been well documented in a phase II trial [6]. It has also been demonstrated that combination therapy with DD and CHOP is effective, with OS rate of 63.3% and median duration of response of 30 months, as opposed to historical data of 32–35% and 12 months, respectively, with CHOP alone [15]. However, it is important to note that previous publications on DD have studied its activity with limited cycles of treatment (a maximum of 8 cycles), with disease eventually recurring. In contrast, the cases presented here demonstrate the efficacy of DD when it is used as maintenance therapy (over a span of 1-2 years), which can result in long-term remission, even long after DD has been discontinued.

In our first case, although stage IVB subcutaneous panniculitis gamma delta T-cell lymphoma typically results in poor survival, DD was successful as salvage therapy after the disease had relapsed with CVP, ICE, and ESHAP and subsequently served as maintenance therapy, resulting in sustained remission. Maintenance therapy in our second case also resulted in sustained remission, despite the fact that the patient had stage IVB PTCL, NOS, which is typically associated with poor prognosis. Although ALK-1 positive anaplastic large cell lymphoma is generally associated with improved prognosis due to superior response rates to CHOP-like regimens [5, 16], our patient in the third case had stage III disease that was refractory to CHOP, rendering a poor prognosis. However, she also has experienced continuing sustained remission for more than four years following long-term therapy with DD. Our first two cases tolerated the drug exceedingly well and case 3 exhibited some adverse events (anasarca and DVT). While DD can be associated with adverse reactions including capillary leak syndrome, infusion reactions, and visual changes, among others, it is not associated with cumulative toxicity or clinically significant myelosuppression [6].

Although a specific mechanism remains unclear, it is our hypothesis that the activity of DD as long-term maintenance therapy involves its ability to potentially regulate the immune system. Specifically, T-regulatory cell population is CD25+ and long-term DD therapy may depress the level of CD25+ T regulatory cell populations, resulting in increased immune activity against the cancer cells and long-term remission. Such immune-surveillance activity by anti-CD25 agents has been described in prior studies [17–20]. This may explain how DD is effective against a heterogeneous group of lineages, including T-cell and B-cell malignancies, and both CD25+ and CD25− tumors [6–8].

Given the demonstrated efficacy of DD as maintenance therapy and its general tolerability in advanced stage PTCL with generally poor prognosis, our findings can have significant implications. Additional studies would need to be conducted in a formal clinical trial setting to firmly establish the role of DD as potential maintenance therapy in PTCL.

Consent

Written informed consent was obtained from the patient for publication of this case report and accompanying images. A copy of the written consent is available for review.

Authors' Contribution

All authors contributed, read, and approved the final paper.

Acknowledgment

The authors would like their patients for their willingness to share their experiences with their medical community.

References

[1] American Cancer Society, *Cancer Facts and Figures 2015*, American Cancer Society, Atlanta, Ga, USA, 2015, http://www.cancer.org/research/cancerfactsstatistics/cancerfactsfigures2015/index.

[2] N. L. Harris, E. S. Jaffe, H. Stein et al., "A revised European-American classification of lymphoid neoplasms: a proposal from the International Lymphoma Study Group," *Blood*, vol. 84, no. 5, pp. 1361–1392, 1994.

[3] L. Karlin and B. Coiffier, "The changing landscape of peripheral T-cell lymphoma in the era of novel therapies," *Seminars in Hematology*, vol. 51, no. 1, pp. 25–34, 2014.

[4] N. M. Reddy and A. M. Evens, "Chemotherapeutic advancements in peripheral T-cell lymphoma," *Seminars in Hematology*, vol. 51, no. 1, pp. 17–24, 2014.

[5] M. P. Escalón, N. S. Liu, Y. Yang et al., "Prognostic factors and treatment of patients with T-cell non-Hodgkin lymphoma: the M. D. Anderson Cancer Center experience," *Cancer*, vol. 103, no. 10, pp. 2091–2098, 2005.

[6] N. H. Dang, B. Pro, F. B. Hagemeister et al., "Phase II trial of denileukin diftitox for relapsed/refractory T-cell non-Hodgkin lymphoma," *British Journal of Haematology*, vol. 136, no. 3, pp. 439–447, 2007.

[7] B. Y. Wong, S. A. Gregory, and N. H. Dang, "Denileukin diftitox as novel targeted therapy for lymphoid malignancies," *Cancer Investigation*, vol. 25, no. 6, pp. 495–501, 2007.

[8] N. H. Dang, F. B. Hagemeister, B. Pro et al., "Phase II study of denileukin diftitox for relapsed/refractory B-cell non-Hodgkin's lymphoma," *Journal of Clinical Oncology*, vol. 22, no. 20, pp. 4095–4102, 2004.

[9] B. Y. Wong, Y. Ma, R. Fitzwilson, and N. H. Dang, "De novo maintenance therapy with denileukin diftitox (Ontak) in a patient with peripheral T-cell lymphoma is associated with prolonged remission," *American Journal of Hematology*, vol. 83, no. 7, pp. 596–598, 2008.

[10] V. Mak, J. Hamm, M. Chhanabhai et al., "Survival of patients with peripheral T-cell lymphoma after first relapse or progression: spectrum of disease and rare long-term survivors," *Journal of Clinical Oncology*, vol. 31, no. 16, pp. 1970–1976, 2013.

[11] C. E. Dearden and F. M. Foss, "Peripheral T-cell lymphomas: diagnosis and management," *Hematology/Oncology Clinics of North America*, vol. 17, no. 6, pp. 1351–1366, 2003.

[12] M. Jagasia, D. Morgan, S. Goodman et al., "Histology impacts the outcome of peripheral T-cell lymphomas after high dose chemotherapy and stem cell transplant," *Leukemia and Lymphoma*, vol. 45, no. 11, pp. 2261–2267, 2004.

[13] N. Mounier, C. Gisselbrecht, J. Briere et al., "All aggressive lymphoma subtypes do not share similar outcome after front-line autotransplantation: A matched-control analysis by the Groupe d'Etude des Lymphomes de l'Adulte (GELA)," *Annals of Oncology*, vol. 15, no. 12, pp. 1790–1797, 2004.

[14] K. W. Zamkoff, M. D. Matulis, A. C. Mehta, M. W. Beaty, R. E. Hutchison, and T. C. Gentile, "High-dose therapy and autologous stem cell transplant does not result in long-term disease-free survival in patients with recurrent chemotherapy-sensitive ALK-negative anaplastic large-cell lymphoma," *Bone Marrow Transplantation*, vol. 33, no. 6, pp. 635–638, 2004.

[15] F. M. Foss, N. Sjak-Shie, A. Goy et al., "A multicenter phase II trial to determine the safety and efficacy of combination therapy with denileukin diftitox and cyclophosphamide, doxorubicin, vincristine and prednisone in untreated peripheral T-cell lymphoma: the CONCEPT study," *Leukemia and Lymphoma*, vol. 54, no. 7, pp. 1373–1379, 2013.

[16] J. O. Armitage, "The aggressive peripheral T-cell lymphomas: 2013," *American Journal of Hematology*, vol. 88, no. 10, pp. 910–918, 2013.

[17] S. Spranger and T. Gajewski, "Rational combinations of immunotherapeutics that target discrete pathways," *Journal for ImmunoTherapy of Cancer*, vol. 1, article 16, 2013.

[18] J. Kline, I. E. Brown, Y.-Y. Zha et al., "Homeostatic proliferation plus regulatory T-cell depletion promotes potent rejection of B16 melanoma," *Clinical Cancer Research*, vol. 14, no. 10, pp. 3156–3167, 2008.

[19] A. J. Rech and R. H. Vonderheide, "Clinical use of anti-CD25 antibody daclizumab to enhance immune responses to tumor antigen vaccination by targeting regulatory T cells," *Annals of the New York Academy of Sciences*, vol. 1174, pp. 99–106, 2009.

[20] R. P. M. Sutmuller, L. M. van Duivenvoorde, A. van Elsas et al., "Synergism of cytotoxic T lymphocyte-associated antigen 4 blockade and depletion of $CD25^+$ regulatory T cells in antitumor therapy reveals alternative pathways for suppression of autoreactive cytotoxic T lymphocyte responses," *The Journal of Experimental Medicine*, vol. 194, no. 6, pp. 823–832, 2001.

2

Synchronous Multicentric Giant Cell Tumour of Distal Radius and Sacrum with Pulmonary Metastases

Varun Sharma Tandra, Krishna Mohan Reddy Kotha, Moorthy Gadisetti Venkata Satyanarayana, Kali Varaprasad Vadlamani, and Vyjayanthi Yerravalli

Department of Orthopaedics and Traumatology, Osmania Medical College, Osmania General Hospital, Afzalgunj, Hyderabad, Andhra Pradesh 500012, India

Correspondence should be addressed to Krishna Mohan Reddy Kotha; kisna.kmc04@gmail.com

Academic Editor: Yoshihito Yokoyama

Giant cell tumour (GCT) is an uncommon primary bone tumour, and its multicentric presentation is exceedingly rare. We report a case of a 45-year-old female who presented to us with GCT of left distal radius. On the skeletal survey, osteolytic lesion was noted in her right sacral ala. Biopsy confirmed both lesions as GCT. Pulmonary metastasis was also present. Resection-reconstruction arthroplasty for distal radius and thorough curettage and bone grafting of the sacral lesion were done. Multicentric GCT involving distal radius and sacrum with primary sacral involvement is not reported so far to our knowledge.

1. Introduction

Giant cell tumour (GCT) of bone accounts for about 5% of all primary bone tumours in adults. It occurs most commonly in third to fifth decades of life and affects both males and females with slight female preponderance [1, 2]. Giant cell tumours usually occur as a solitary lytic lesion in the ends of long bones, often extending to subarticular location. Multicentric presentation accounts for less than 1% of GCTs of bone [2]. Sacrum is the commonest site in the axial skeleton for solitary GCTs but its involvement in multicentric GCT (MCGCT) is extremely rare [3, 4]. GCTs are generally considered as benign tumours; less than 2% of cases have pulmonary metastases, which are benign in nature [2].

2. Case Report

We report a case of a 45-year-old female who presented to us with a swelling in her left wrist of about one-year duration. The plain radiograph showed a subarticular expansile lytic lesion with "*soap-bubble*" appearance involving distal radius epiphysis with metaphyseal extension and with well-defined margins, suggestive of GCT (Figures 1(a) and 1(b)). Further on the skeletal survey an osteolytic lesion was noted in her right sacral ala. Biopsy of both lesions was performed, and it revealed both lesions as GCT (Figure 4(b)). Only lesion in her wrist was operated on initially, and the sacral lesion was left untreated as the patient was unwilling to undergo major surgery on her back.

"Resection-reconstruction arthroplasty" of distal radius was done using autogenous nonvascularized proximal fibula (Figures 1(c) and 1(d)). The graft was fixed to radius proximally with narrow dynamic compression plate and distally to the ulna with K-wires. In the follow-up, K-wires were removed and the patient was doing well for six months after which she was lost to follow-up.

Twelve months later, she came back to us with complaints of low back pain for three months. Pain was disabling at the time of presentation. There was no history of motor weakness or paraesthesias in her lower limbs, bladder bowel disturbances, or any fever. She could sit and walk with the help of support with difficulty.

On physical examination, no swelling or local signs of inflammation were noted in her low back. Tenderness was

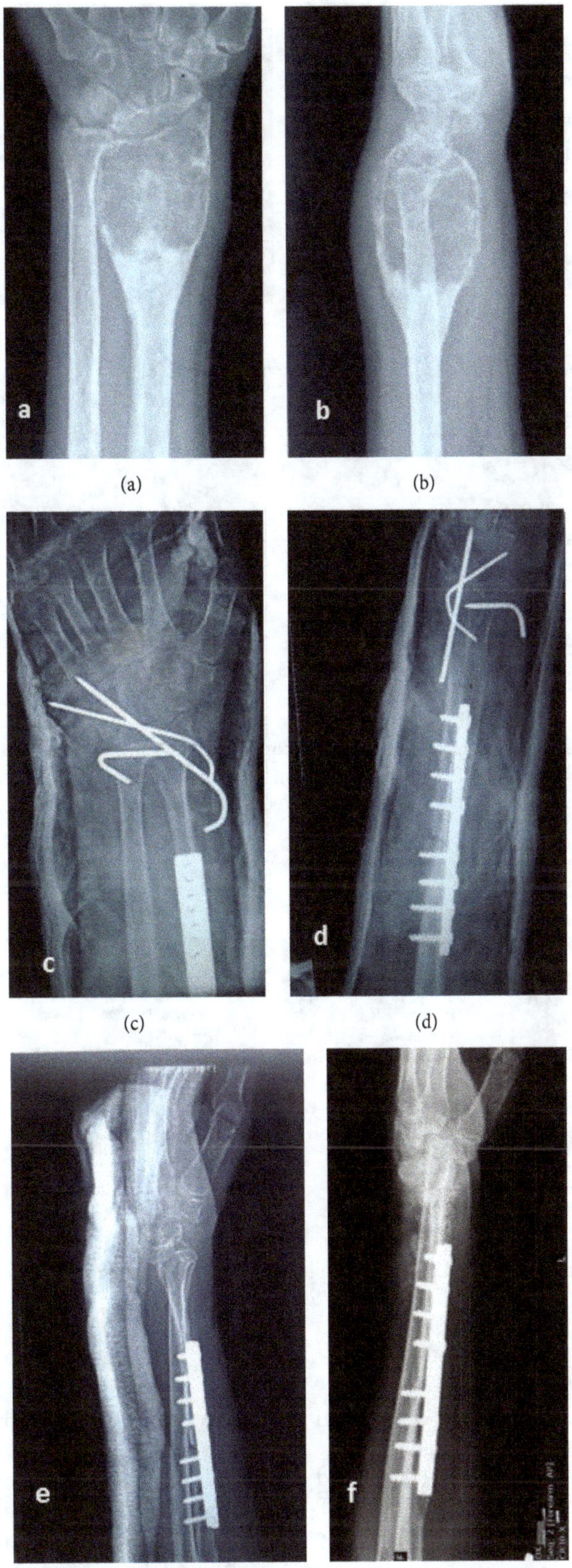

(a) (b)

(c) (d)

(e) (f)

Figure 1: (a and b) Preop plain radiograph of left wrist showing expansile solitary lytic lesion involving left distal radius; (c and d) postoperative radiographs after resection and reconstruction arthroplasty of left wrist; (e) radiographs of her left wrist showing wrist subluxation following k-wire removal; (f) 1 year follow-up radiograph of her left wrist with gross subluxation of wrist.

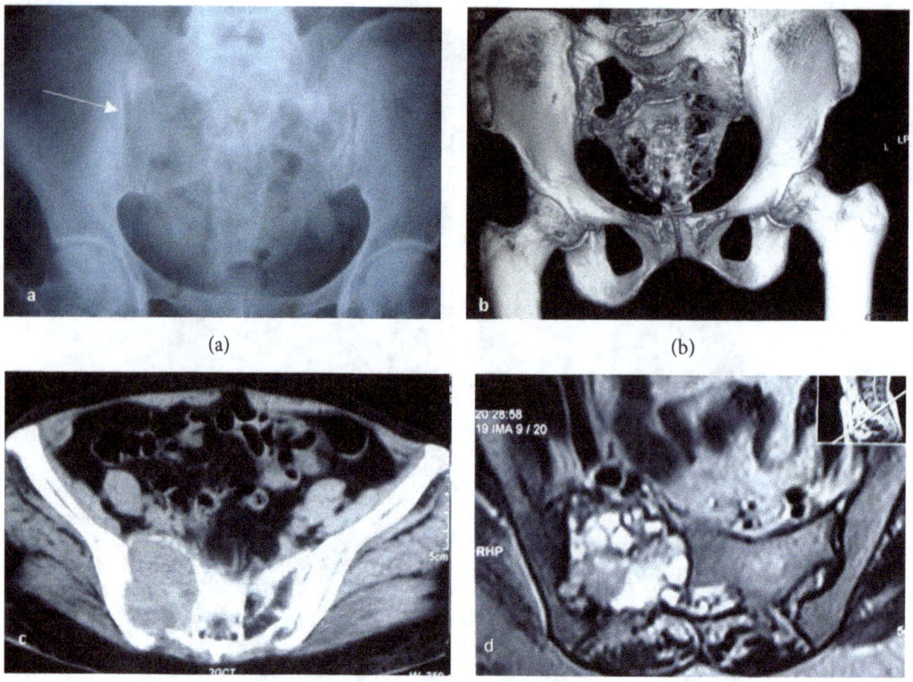

(a) (b) (c) (d)

Figure 2: (a) Radiograph of the pelvis AP view; (b) 3D reconstruction and (c) axial section of CT showing expansile lytic lesion involving the right sacral ala with cortical break and surrounding soft-tissue component extending into right SI joint space and pelvis measuring 5.2 × 5.7 × 6.3 cm eroding the adjacent iliac bone. Mass extending into the sacral canal. (d) MRI showing large expansile heterogeneous lobulated lesion with few septations involving right sacroiliac joint. Predominantly lytic lesion with cortical destruction features suggestive of GCT.

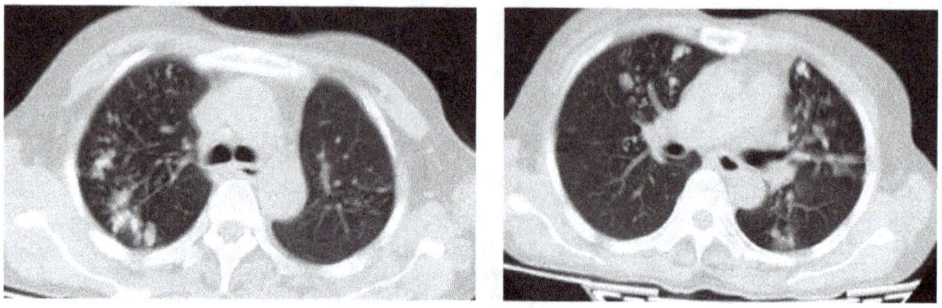

(a) (b)

Figure 3: Multiple irregular opacities in apical segments of right upper lobe and left lingular superior segment, anterobasal and posterobasal segments suggestive of metastasis.

noted in the sacrum and right sacroiliac joint. We ordered for a radiograph of pelvis in which we found a large expansile lytic lesion involving body of sacrum and right sacral ala and breach of sacroiliac joint was noted (Figure 2(a)). Further CT with three-dimensional reconstruction was done to delineate the lesion (Figure 2(b)).

The review radiographs of her left forearm showed wrist subluxation (Figures 1(e) and 1(f)), though the patient had no complaints in her wrist. Skeletal survey and screening radiographs showed suspicious lesions in her lung fields which turned out to be pulmonary metastases on Contrast Enhanced CT (CECT) of chest (Figure 3). CECT of brain and abdomen were normal. Technetium[99] whole body bone scan showed hotspots in the sacrum and both lungs; there was no evidence of recurrence at distal radius.

After optimizing the patient, sacral lesion was treated by thorough intralesional curettage and bone grafting (Figure 4(a)). The procedure relieved patient of severe episodic pain. The patient developed superficial surgical site infection which later went on to heal with regular dressings and antibiotics. Patient is clinically asymptomatic at one-year follow-up. Pulmonary metastases could not be evaluated

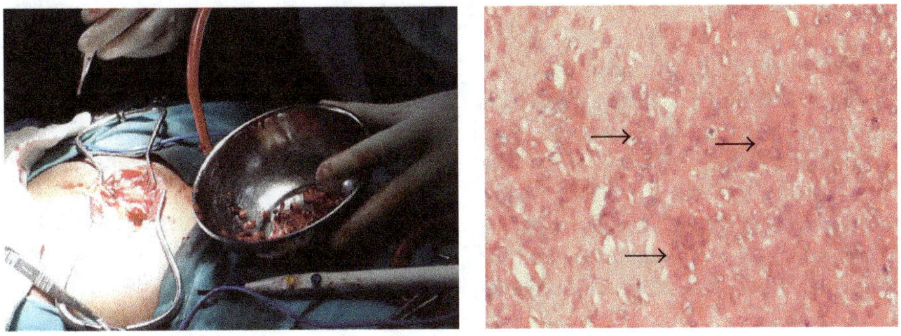

(a) (b)

FIGURE 4: (a) Intraoperative photograph of curettage and bone grafting of the sacral lesion; (b) histopathology slide showing characteristic osteoclast like giant cells (arrows) in the background of mononuclear cells.

further or treated as the patient was unwilling for any intervention.

3. Discussion

Less than 1% of cases of GCT are multicentric in origin [1, 4–10]. Most of the cases of MCGCT are reported as single case or as small series [2, 5–15]. Hoch et al. published the largest known series of 30 cases of MCGCT in 2006 [2]. Dhillon and Prasad [4] in 2007 published a comprehensive review on "Multicentric giant-cell tumor of bone" where a total of 101 cases reported so far worldwide were described.

Hoch et al. classified tumours as being "synchronous" when multiple tumours had been discovered at the initial presentation or when a second tumour had been diagnosed within six months after the first. If the second tumour developed more than six months after the first lesion, the lesions were considered to be "metachronous" [1, 2, 16]. In our patient, sacral lesion was found incidentally on the skeletal survey at the initial presentation and is hence classified as synchronous.

Most of the case series reported occurrence of MCGCT at a younger age when compared to solitary GCT [8, 14, 16]. The mean age of multicentric GCT was found to be 22.5 years [4]. Distal radius and sacrum are among the common sites for solitary GCT in the appendicular and axial skeletons, respectively. The age of our patient and the sites of tumor are typical of solitary giant cell tumour, which typically presents in third to fifth decades of life [2].

Though the commonest site of occurrence for the MCGCT is long bones around the knee [2, 4], it was found that they tend to develop more frequently in atypical sites like the small bones of hands and feet and at atypical locations like metaphyseal and metadiaphyseal regions in the bone [2, 4]. Though sacrum happens to be the most common site in the axial skeleton for solitary GCT [3], curiously, the bones of pelvis and spine above the sacrum were reported to be involved frequently in MCGCT, and sacral involvement was found to be extremely rare.

To our knowledge, only a few cases are reported so far worldwide where the sacrum was involved in a case of MCGCT [6, 11, 15]. In none of the cases reported, sacral involvement was noted in the first presentation. Sacral GCT is asymptomatic initially, slow growing, and often diagnosed late when it attains a huge size [17]. Sacral GCT though was incidental finding at initial presentation.

The differences in predilection for age and site for multicentric GCT from solitary GCT suggest that probably a different pathogenetic mechanism of origin is involved in multicentric GCT when compared to solitary GCT. The possible mechanisms of multicentricity suggested include direct extension to contiguous bone, metastasis, and multiple independent foci of disease; the last of them might be true in our case.

The histological appearance of lesions of multicentric GCT is similar to that of solitary GCT of bone [2, 5]. The differential diagnosis for such polyostotic lesions includes brown tumours (hyperparathyroidism), multifocal osteomyelitis (cystic type of tuberculosis), metastasis, multiple myeloma, and some other primary osseous tumours with a giant cell component, such as fibrosarcoma, osteosarcoma, angiosarcoma, and chondroblastoma. The possibility of pre-existing systemic conditions in which GCT of bone is known to arrive, such as Paget's disease, must also be considered. Biopsy is considered essential for the diagnosis of GCT.

GCT of the sacrum has higher local recurrence rate than in any other skeletal location; it is found to be as high as 33.9% [17]. *En bloc* resection, though effective at preventing recurrence, is associated with greater morbidity to patient [17]. Intralesional curettage followed by intracavitary inactivation of the lesion is chosen rather than *en bloc* resection, which has several complications. Medical management with denosumab or bisphosphonates were not considered as they are largely experimental, though evidence in their favour is building up their optimal dosing schedule and duration of treatment is yet to be established.

Tumour recurrence is a common problem with GCT when compared to pulmonary metastasis [1, 2, 5]. Recurrence is dependent on the type of treatment given to GCT [2]. Pulmonary metastasis is reported only rarely in case of multicentric GCT [2]. Pulmonary metastasis was not found in the case series of sacral GCT reported by Balke et al. [3].

4. Conclusion

In summary, GCT of multicentric origin is uncommon and sacral involvement in a case of MCGCT is extremely rare and is reported only a few times in the literature. Ours is the first case of MCGCT where sacral involvement is noted in the first presentation. MCGCTs are known to occur in young females, at atypical sites in the body and at atypical locations in the bone. Presentation in the age group and location typical for solitary GCT cannot rule out chance of another synchronous or metachronous focus of GCT.

References

[1] J. J. Eckardt and T. J. Grogan, "Giant cell tumor of bone," *Clinical Orthopaedics and Related Research*, vol. 204, pp. 45–58, 1986.

[2] B. Hoch, C. Inwards, M. Sundaram, and A. E. Rosenberg, "Multicentric giant cell tumor of bone: clinicopathologic analysis of thirty cases," *The Journal of Bone and Joint Surgery—Series A*, vol. 88, no. 9, pp. 1998–2008, 2006.

[3] M. Balke, M. P. Henrichs, G. Gosheger et al., "Giant cell tumors of the axial skeleton," *Sarcoma*, vol. 2012, Article ID 410973, 10 pages, 2012.

[4] M. S. Dhillon and P. Prasad, "Multicentric giant cell tumour of bone," *Acta Orthopaedica Belgica*, vol. 73, no. 3, pp. 289–299, 2007.

[5] I.-H. Park and I.-H. Jeon, "Multicentric giant cell tumor of bone: ten lesions at presentation," *Skeletal Radiology*, vol. 32, no. 9, pp. 526–529, 2003.

[6] M.-A. Rousseau, B. Ilharreborde, F. Larousserie, A. Babinet, B. Tomeno, and P. Anract, "Multicentric giant-cell tumor," *Revue de Chirurgie Orthopedique et Reparatrice de l'Appareil Moteur*, vol. 93, no. 8, pp. 848–853, 2007.

[7] P. Bacchini, F. Bertoni, P. Ruggieri, and M. Campanacci, "Multicentric giant cell tumour of the skeleton," *Skeletal Radiology*, vol. 24, no. 5, pp. 371–374, 1995.

[8] C. A. Cummins, M. T. Scarborough, and W. F. Enneking, "Multicentric giant cell tumour of bone," *Clinical Orthopaedics and Related Research*, no. 322, pp. 245–252, 1996.

[9] K. Dumford, T. E. Moore, C. W. Walker, and J. Jaksha, "Multifocal, metachronous, giant cell tumor of the lower limb," *Skeletal Radiology*, vol. 32, no. 3, pp. 147–150, 2003.

[10] A. Haskell, O. Wodowoz, and J. O. Johnston, "Metachronous multicentric giant cell tumor: a case report and literature review," *Clinical Orthopaedics and Related Research*, no. 412, pp. 162–168, 2003.

[11] C. B. Kos, W. K. Taconis, M. W. Fidler, and J. J. A. M. Ten Velden, "Multifocal giant cell tumors in the spine: a case report," *Spine*, vol. 22, no. 7, pp. 821–822, 1997.

[12] A. Mondal, B. Kundu, R. Kundu, and M. K. Bhattacharya, "Multifocal giant cell tumour of bone in a skeletally immature patient—a case report," *Indian Journal of Pathology and Microbiology*, vol. 44, no. 4, pp. 479–481, 2001.

[13] Y.-K. Park, K. N. Ryu, C.-S. Han, and D. K. Bae, "Multifocal, metachronous giant-cell tumor of the ulna—a case report," *The Journal of Bone and Joint Surgery - American Volume*, vol. 81, no. 3, pp. 409–413, 1999.

[14] F. H. Sim, D. C. Dahlin, and J. W. Beabout, "Multicentric giant-cell tumor of bone," *Journal of Bone and Joint Surgery—Series A*, vol. 59, no. 8, pp. 1052–1060, 1977.

[15] P. G. Stratil and G. S. Stacy, "Multifocal metachronous giant cell tumour in a 15-year-old boy," *Pediatric Radiology*, vol. 35, no. 4, pp. 444–448, 2005.

[16] C. A. Peimer, A. L. Schiller, H. J. Mankin, and R. J. Smith, "Multicentric giant-cell tumor of bone," *The Journal of Bone & Joint Surgery—American Volume*, vol. 62, no. 4, pp. 652–656, 1980.

[17] Z. M. Yang, C. C. Shen, H. Li, Z. L. Shi, and H. M. Tao, "Current treatment of sacral giant cell tumour of bone: a review," *Journal of International Medical Research*, vol. 40, no. 2, pp. 415–425, 2012.

3

Endometrioid Paraovarian Borderline Cystic Tumor in an Infant with Proteus Syndrome

Liliana Vasquez,[1] Mariela Tello,[1] Ivan Maza,[1] Monica Oscanoa,[1] Milagros Dueñas,[2] Haydee Castro,[3] and Alan Latorre[4]

[1]*Department of Oncology and Radiotherapy, Rebagliati Hospital, Lima, Peru*
[2]*Department of Genetics, Rebagliati Hospital, Lima, Peru*
[3]*Department of Gynecology-Oncology, Rebagliati Hospital, Lima, Peru*
[4]*Department of Pathology, Rebagliati Hospital, Lima, Peru*

Correspondence should be addressed to Liliana Vasquez; lilianavasq@gmail.com

Academic Editor: Yoshihito Yokoyama

Ovarian and paraovarian neoplasms are uncommon in children, mainly originating from germ cell tumors and, least frequently, epithelial tumors. There is an association between genital tract tumors and Proteus syndrome, a rare, sporadic, and progressive entity, characterized by a postnatal overgrowth in several tissues caused by a mosaic mutation in the AKT1 gene. We describe a 20-month-old asymptomatic infant with Proteus syndrome who developed an endometrioid paraovarian borderline cystic tumor. This is the youngest patient so far reported in the literature with this rare syndrome and an adnexal tumor of borderline malignancy. A total of nine patients have been described with female tract tumors and associated Proteus syndrome, which includes bilateral ovarian cystadenomas and other benign masses. A paraovarian neoplasm is extremely rare in children and could be considered a criterion for Proteus syndrome. Standardized staging and treatment of these tumors are not well established; however, most authors conclude that these neoplasms must be treated as their ovarian counterparts.

1. Introduction

Ovarian and paraovarian neoplasms are rare in children and represent less than 5% of solid tumors [1–3]. The most common age at presentation is the second decade of life and usually older girls are at greatest risk of malignancy [4]. Incidence of ovarian neoplasms in the pediatric age group is unknown, but it is estimated at 2.6 cases per 100,000 girls per year [2]. The most common histological subtype of pediatric ovarian cancer is derived from germ cells [5–7], followed by epithelial tumors, such as cystadenomas or adenocarcinomas. Primary malignant paraovarian epithelial tumors are even more rare, previously described in literature as cystadenocarcinomas with low malignant potential [8, 9].

Proteus syndrome (PS) is a rare and sporadic disorder that causes postnatal overgrowth of multiple tissues in a mosaic pattern [10].

Cohen Jr. and Hayden first described it in 1979 as "a new hamartomatous syndrome" [11]. Wiedemann et al. further explained the syndrome and named it Proteus syndrome [12]. Since its first description until today, there have only been approximately 200 diagnosed cases in developed countries. PS is a progressive disorder that most commonly affects the skeleton, skin, adipose, and central nervous systems, causing severe overgrowth and disfigurement, physical disability, and a decline in the patient's quality of life [13]. It is associated with a range of tumors, pulmonary complications, and a striking predisposition to deep vein thrombosis and pulmonary embolism [14]. Among such tumors are those derived from lymphatic tissue and ovarian tumors, which are also included in the diagnostic criteria for this syndrome.

We report an infant with PS, who developed an endometrioid borderline paraovarian cystic tumor. This is the tenth case reported worldwide presenting an adnexal mass

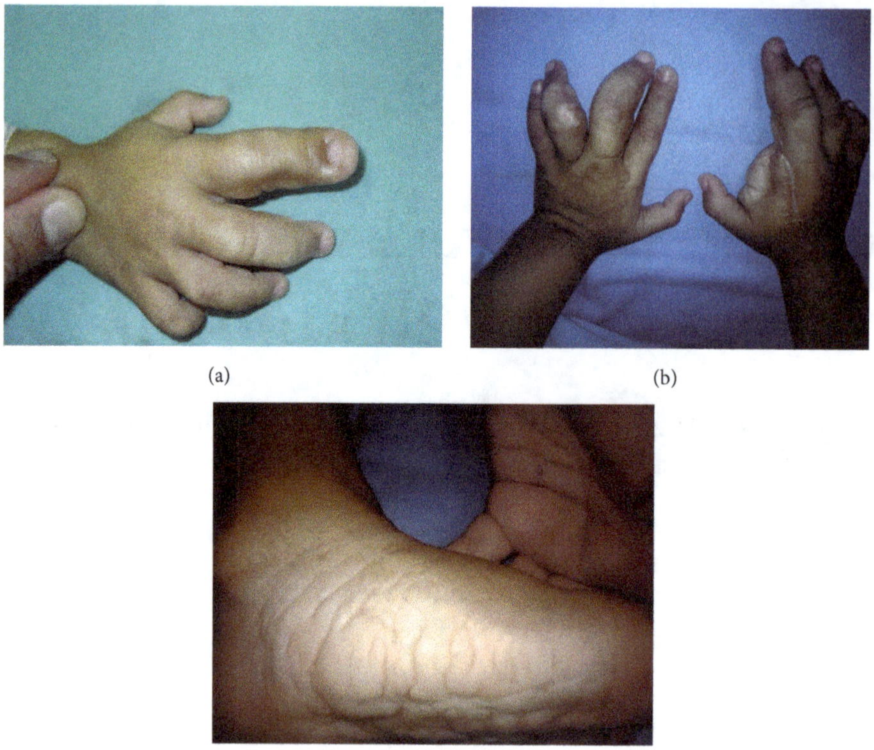

FIGURE 1: (a) Asymmetric overgrowth of the second finger of right hand. (b) After finger amputation. (c) Cerebriform connective tissue nevus of foot.

associated with this rare syndrome and the first case reported in our region.

2. Case Report

A female patient, originated from a third pregnancy and nonconsanguineous marriage, is described. Her mother was hospitalized during the second and third trimester of pregnancy, due to preterm labor and oligohydramnios. She was delivered vaginally at 36 weeks of gestation, with a birth weight of 3098 g. Upon birth, she presented normal anthropometric parameters and had no family history of any disease. At five months of age, she was noted to have abnormal augmentation of the size of her inferior limbs and asymmetric finger growth, especially involving the second finger on the right hand (Figures 1(a) and 1(b)) that required amputation at 12 months of age. Also, the patient showed several soft tissue and epidermic nevi (Figure 1(c)).

According to the clinical criteria for diagnosis of PS, our patient had the three general criteria and also had specific criteria from categories A and B (Table 1) [15, 16]. A genetic study was performed in two affected tissues, looking for the c.49G>A mutation in the AKT1 gene, but it could not been found.

At 20 months of age, the patient presented painless vaginal bleeding and gynecomastia; no pain or size augmentation in the abdominal region was noted. An ultrasound image showed a right solid paraovarian mass, measuring 29 × 25 × 27 mm, with scarce peripheral vascularization on Doppler imaging. The uterus and both ovaries presented no alterations. At first, CA 125 level was elevated (164 UI). A pelvic contrast-enhanced computed tomography (CT) showed a heterogeneously enhanced round mass next to the right ovary (Figure 2). No metastases were found. The patient underwent a laparotomy, where a right 2 × 2 cm violaceous paraovarian tumor was found. Excision of the tumor (tumorectomy) was completed with no evidence of rupture (Figures 3(a) and 3(b)). Omentum, peritoneal surface, and ascitic fluid samples were taken; but as fluid was scarce, peritoneal lavage was performed. Pathology was described as a well-differentiated endometrioid borderline tumor with villoglandular pattern

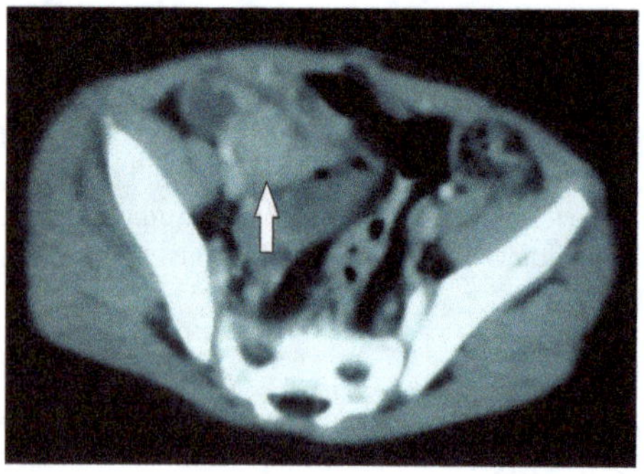

FIGURE 2: Preoperative axial contrast-enhanced CT scan showing a mass growing next to the right ovary (white arrow).

Table 1: Revised Proteus syndrome diagnostic criteria (Turner et al., 2004) [15].

To make a diagnosis of PS, one must have all the general criteria and various specific criteria	
General criteria	All of the following: (i) Mosaic distribution of lesions (ii) Sporadic occurrence (iii) Progressive course
Specific criteria	Either (i) category A, (ii) two from category B, or (iii) three from category C
Specific criteria categories	(A) Cerebriform connective tissue nevus[a] (B) (1) Linear epidermal nevus (2) Asymmetric, disproportionate overgrowth[b] One or more: (a) Limbs: Arms/legs Hands/feet/digits Extremities (b) Hyperostoses of the skull (c) External auditory meatus (d) Megaspondylodysplasia (e) Viscera: spleen/thymus (3) Specific tumors before 2nd decade One of the following: (a) Ovarian cystadenoma (b) Parotid monomorphic adenoma (C) (1) Dysregulated adipose tissue Either one: (a) Lipomas (b) Regional absence of fat (2) Vascular malformations One or more: (a) Capillary malformation (b) Venous malformation (c) Lymphatic malformation (3) Lung cysts (4) Facial phenotype[c] All: (a) Dolichocephaly (b) Long face (c) Down slanting palpebral fissures and/or minor ptosis (d) Low nasal bridge (e) Wide or anteverted nares (f) Open mouth at rest

[a]Cerebriform connective tissue nevi are skin lesions characterized by deep grooves and gyrations as seen on the surface of the brain.
[b]Asymmetric, disproportionate overgrowth should be carefully distinguished from asymmetric, proportionate overgrowth (see Discussion for recommended methods of distinction).
[c]The facial phenotype has been found, to date, only in PS in patients who have mental deficiency and, in some cases, seizures and/or brain malformations.

G1 (Figures 4(a) and 4(b)); peritoneal lavage tested positive for tumoral cells, (Figure 4(c)) but no other abnormal pathological findings were made.

The patient presented a favorable postoperatory evolution and received 3 cycles of adjuvant chemotherapy administered every 21 days; a 3-hour infusion of paclitaxel 175 mg/m^2 on days 1, 8, and 15; and carboplatin AUC 6 during day 1. At the time of this report, the patient is alive and well at 2 years of follow-up with no evidence of disease.

3. Discussion

Ovarian and paraovarian masses are infrequent among girls, representing less than 5% of solid tumors among children and less than 1.5% of malignant tumors [2]. Clinically, presenting symptoms are abdominal pain, a palpable tumor on a routine examination, or the presence of endocrine alterations, such as precocious puberty [17]. Diagnosis of malignant lesions generally occurs late, because of low levels of suspicion or unspecific symptoms.

According to the World Health Organization (WHO), ovarian tumors are classified into major 3 groups (surface epithelial tumors, germ cell tumors, and sex-cord stromal tumors) and other minor tumors. The most common histological group at pediatric age is the one originating from germ cells [5–7], with a great variety of histological subgroups [18]. Epithelial tumors are very rare among young girls; moreover, the finding of an endometrioid subtype, typically seen among older women [7], is even more infrequent. Also, most papers refer mainly to ovarian pathology; there is very little information regarding fallopian tubes and paratubal/paraovarian masses, this being restricted to small series and reports on clinical cases.

PS is a rare disorder, characterized by an abnormal overgrowth of several tissues, caused by a mosaic activating mutation in the AKT1 gene (c.49G>A, p.Glu17Lys) [10, 19]. Clinical diagnosis includes congenital morphological criteria, typical skin lesions, and association with tumors in postnatal life [10, 20]. This gene is in charge of sporadically activating growth of various tissues (epidermal, connective, osseous, fat, and endothelial) during embryonic development and it is characterized by partial gigantism of hands and feet, skin hemihypertrophy, epidermal nevi, subcutaneous hamartomas, macrocephaly, cranial anomalies, and connective tissue nevi. The latter is almost pathognomonic [15, 21]. Our patient met the established criteria for clinical diagnosis of PS showed in Table 1; however, the genetic testing performed could not find the target mutation in AKT1 gene.

Several benign and malignant tumors are associated with PS [10, 22], such as lipomas, haemangiomas, and lymphangiomas and, less frequently, genital tract tumors. These neoplasia cases usually occur in the second decade of life, most commonly bilateral ovarian cystadenomas or salivary gland monomorphic adenomas [15], which have an important role in establishing diagnosis for PS. Gordon et al. [23] reported a girl with PS and bilateral mucinous cystadenomas of the ovary. Furthermore, Babovic et al. [24] described the association among microdeletion of gene 10q23

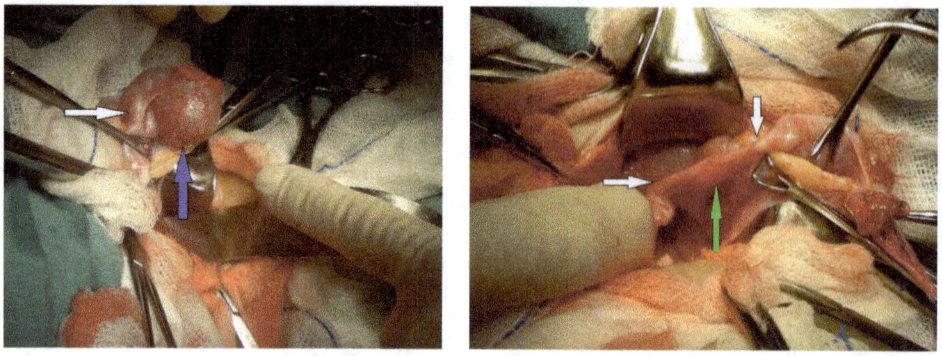

(a) (b)

FIGURE 3: Intraoperative findings of laparotomy. (a) Paraovarian mass (blue arrow) and right tube (white arrow). Right ovary is located behind tumor. (b) After tumor excision, left and right tubes (white arrows) and normal uterus (green arrow) are shown.

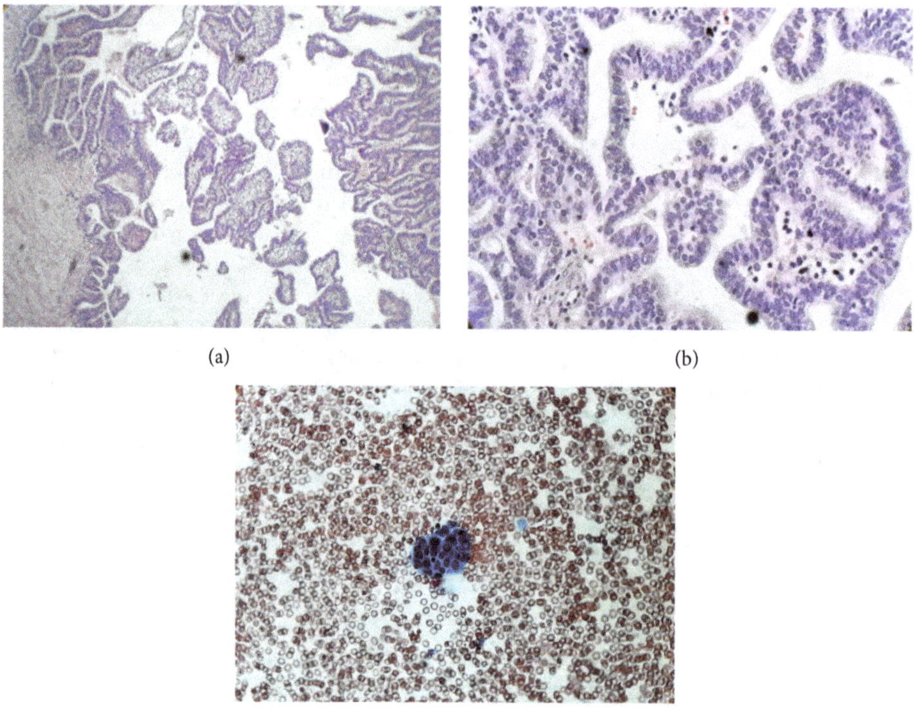

(a) (b) (c)

FIGURE 4: H&E stain, microscopic image. (a) 10x magnification. Architecture of paraovarian endometrioid borderline cystic tumor with villoglandular pattern. (b) 40x magnification. (c) 40x peritoneal wash. Pleomorphic, well-differentiated endometrioid groups of tumor cells, found in a peritoneal fluid.

and bilateral cystadenoma of the ovary and young polyposis in a teenager. Reports of patients with adnexal tumors and PS are rare and mainly describe benign tumors [25–27]. When conducting a revision of reported cases worldwide, we found only 9 cases, and one of them, reported by Raju et al. [28], belongs to a 3-year-old girl with PS, who developed a low-or-borderline malignant endometrioid cystadenoma lesion with villoglandular pattern. Development of a borderline ovarian neoplasia at a very young age supports the genetic mechanism of overgrowth seen in this syndrome and also represents the youngest patient suffering from endometrioid paraovarian cystic tumor.

Staging and treatment of epithelial paraovarian tumors among adult women are not adequately described [29] and there is even less evidence regarding the pediatric population. Its rarity in children has not allowed publishing multicentric prospective series; therefore, management is mainly based on studies involving adult patients. The majority of authors defend the fact that these tumors must be handled like their ovarian counterparts [8], that is, performing an adequate surgical staging, whether it is conservative or radical. In the present case, conservative surgery (tumorectomy) was performed due to the patient's young age, desired future fertility, and lack of unfavorable intraoperative findings, such as tumoral adherences or rupture. Surgical treatment is vital and could be curative; chemotherapy is only used in cases of patients with inoperable disease or a microscopic or macroscopic residual disease but remains controversial. Due to the presence of ascitic fluid (testing positive for tumoral cells), stage IC was established, employing adjuvant chemotherapy. Due to the fact that this disorder is rare, there is no consensus on follow-up [30], although it is accepted worldwide that this should be frequent and based on tumoral markers and pelvic imaging.

In conclusion, the finding of a paraovarian neoplasm is extremely rare in children and could be considered a clinical criterion for PS. Standardized staging and treatment of these tumors are not well established; however, most authors conclude that these neoplasms must be treated as their ovarian counterparts.

Consent

Written informed consent was obtained from the patient's parents for publication of this case report and accompanying images. A copy of the written consent is available for review.

References

[1] E. Gonzalo, I. Merino, A. Fdez-Teijeiro, and A. Navajas, "Tumores ováricos en la infancia: a propósito de una revisión casuística," *Anales Españoles de Pediatría*, vol. 49, no. 5, pp. 491–494, 1998.

[2] K. A. P. Schultz, S. F. Sencer, Y. Messinger, J. P. Neglia, and M. E. Steiner, "Pediatric ovarian tumors: a review of 67 cases," *Pediatric Blood and Cancer*, vol. 44, no. 2, pp. 167–173, 2005.

[3] D. L. Cass, E. Hawkins, M. L. Brandt et al., "Surgery for ovarian masses in infants, children, and adolescents: 102 consecutive patients treated in a 15-year period," *Journal of Pediatric Surgery*, vol. 36, no. 5, pp. 693–699, 2001.

[4] M. F. Brown, A. Hebra, K. McGeehin, and A. J. Ross III, "Ovarian masses in children: a review of 91 cases of malignant and benign masses," *Journal of Pediatric Surgery*, vol. 28, no. 7, pp. 930–932, 1993.

[5] M. H. Malogolowkin, G. H. Mahour, M. Krailo, and J. A. Ortega, "Germ cell tumors in infancy and childhood: a 45-year experience," *Fetal and Pediatric Pathology*, vol. 10, no. 1-2, pp. 231–241, 1990.

[6] M. Gribbon, S. H. Ein, and K. Mancer, "Pediatric malignant ovarian tumors: a 43-year review," *Journal of Pediatric Surgery*, vol. 27, no. 4, pp. 480–484, 1992.

[7] A. López Saiz, M. S. Fernández, V. Segarra et al., "Solid ovarian tumors in childhood," *Cirugía Pediátrica*, vol. 10, no. 3, pp. 104–107, 1997.

[8] M. M. Altaras, R. Jaffe, M. Corduba, M. Holtzinger, and C. Bahary, "Primary paraovarian cystadenocarcinoma: clinical and management aspects and literature review," *Gynecologic Oncology*, vol. 38, no. 2, pp. 268–272, 1990.

[9] K. Kaur, S. Gopalan, S. K. Gupta, and L. K. Dhaliwal, "Parovarian cystadenocarcinoma: a case report," *Asia-Oceania Journal of Obstetrics and Gynaecology*, vol. 16, no. 2, pp. 131–135, 1990.

[10] L. G. Biesecker, "The multifaceted challenges of Proteus syndrome," *Journal of the American Medical Association*, vol. 285, no. 17, pp. 2240–2243, 2001.

[11] M. M. Cohen Jr. and P. W. Hayden, "A newly recognized hamartomatous syndrome," *Birth Defects: Original Article Series*, vol. 15, no. 5, pp. 291–296, 1979.

[12] H.-R. Wiedemann, G. R. Burgio, P. Aldenhoff, J. Kunze, H. J. Kaufmann, and E. Schirg, "The proteus syndrome," *European Journal of Pediatrics*, vol. 140, no. 1, pp. 5–12, 1983.

[13] M. M. Cohen Jr., "Overgrowth syndromes: an update," *Advances in Pediatrics*, vol. 46, pp. 441–491, 1999.

[14] L. G. Biesecker and J. C. Sapp, "Proteus Syndrome," in *GeneReviews*, R. A. Pagon, M. P. Adam, H. H. Ardinger et al., Eds., University of Washington, Seattle, Wash, USA, 2012, http://www.ncbi.nlm.nih.gov/books/NBK99495/.

[15] J. T. Turner, M. M. Cohen Jr., and L. G. Biesecker, "Reassessment of the Proteus syndrome literature: application of diagnostic criteria to published cases," *American Journal of Medical Genetics*, vol. 130, no. 2, pp. 111–122, 2004.

[16] M. M. Cohen Jr., "Proteus syndrome," in *Overgrowth Syndromes*, M. M. Cohen Jr., G. Neri, and R. Weksberg, Eds., chapter 9, pp. 75–110, Oxford University Press, New York, NY, USA, 2002.

[17] K. S. H. de Silva, S. Kanumakala, S. R. Grover, C. W. Chow, and G. L. Warne, "Ovarian lesions in children and adolescents—an 11-year review," *Journal of Pediatric Endocrinology and Metabolism*, vol. 17, no. 7, pp. 951–957, 2004.

[18] C. R. Pinkerton, "Malignant germ cell tumours in childhood," *European Journal of Cancer Part A*, vol. 33, no. 6, pp. 895–901, 1997.

[19] M. J. Lindhurst, J. C. Sapp, J. K. Teer et al., "A mosaic activating mutation in AKT1 associated with the proteus syndrome," *The New England Journal of Medicine*, vol. 365, no. 7, pp. 611–619, 2011.

[20] L. G. Biesecker, R. Happle, J. B. Mulliken et al., "Proteus syndrome: diagnostic criteria, differential diagnosis, and patient evaluation," *American Journal of Medical Genetics*, vol. 84, no. 5, pp. 389–395, 1999.

[21] P. Redondo, "Malformaciones vasculares (I). Concepto, clasificación, fisiopatogenia y manifestaciones clínicas," *Actas Dermo-Sifiliográficas*, vol. 98, no. 3, pp. 141–158, 2007.

[22] M. M. Cohen Jr., "Proteus syndrome: clinical evidence for somatic mosaicism and selective review," *American Journal of Medical Genetics*, vol. 47, no. 5, pp. 645–652, 1993.

[23] P. L. Gordon, R. S. Wilroy, O. E. Lasater, and M. M. Cohen Jr., "Neoplasms in Proteus syndrome," *American Journal of Medical Genetics*, vol. 57, no. 1, pp. 74–78, 1995.

[24] N. Babovic, P. S. Simmons, C. Moir et al., "Mucinous cystadenoma of ovary in a patient with juvenile polyposis due to 10q23 microdeletion: expansion of phenotype," *American Journal of Medical Genetics Part A*, vol. 152, no. 10, pp. 2623–2627, 2010.

[25] Š. Smrkolj, L. Sorč, J. Šinkovec, and S. Rakar, "Müllerian papilloma in a patient with Proteus syndrome: case report and review of the literature," *European Journal of Gynaecological Oncology*, vol. 33, no. 4, pp. 428–432, 2012.

[26] K. M. Ezzeldin, A. A. Ezzeldin, A. J. Zahrani, and M. M. Al-Zaiem, "Precocious puberty in a female with Proteus syndrome," *Saudi Medical Journal*, vol. 23, no. 3, pp. 332–334, 2002.

[27] J. H. Hong, J. K. Lee, S. H. Song et al., "Unilateral ovarian dermoid cyst accompanied by an ipsilateralparatubal cyst in a girl with Proteus Syndrome discovered by laparoscopic surgery," *Journal of Pediatric and Adolescent Gynecology*, vol. 23, no. 3, pp. e107–e110, 2010.

[28] R. R. Raju, W. R. Hart, D. K. Magnuson, J. R. Reid, and D. G. Rogers, "Genital tract tumors in Proteus syndrome: report of a case of bilateral paraovarian endometrioid cystic tumors of borderline malignancy and review of the literature," *Modern Pathology*, vol. 15, no. 2, pp. 172–180, 2002.

[29] A. L. F. A. De Areia, C. Frutuoso, N. Amaral, I. Dias, and C. De Oliveira, "Paraovarian tumor of borderline malignancy—a case report," *International Journal of Gynecological Cancer*, vol. 14, no. 4, pp. 680–682, 2004.

[30] V. L. Seltzer, L. Molho, A. Fougner et al., "Parovarian cystadenocarcinoma of low-malignant potential," *Gynecologic Oncology*, vol. 30, no. 2, pp. 216–221, 1988.

4

Antiangiogenic Therapies and Extracranial Metastasis in Glioblastoma

Mohamed H. Khattab,[1] Ariel E. Marciscano,[1] Simon S. Lo,[2] Michael Lim,[1,3] John J. Laterra,[4] Lawrence R. Kleinberg,[1] and Kristin J. Redmond[1]

[1] *Department of Radiation Oncology & Molecular Radiation Sciences, Johns Hopkins University, 401 North Broadway, Suite 1440, Baltimore, MD 21231-5678, USA*
[2] *Department of Radiation Oncology, Case Western Reserve University, University Hospitals Seidman Cancer Center, Cleveland, OH 44106, USA*
[3] *Department of Neurosurgery, Johns Hopkins University, 600 N. Wolfe Street, Phipps Room 123, Baltimore, MD 21287, USA*
[4] *Department of Neurology/Neuro-Oncology, Johns Hopkins University, 601 N. Caroline Street, Baltimore, MD 21287, USA*

Correspondence should be addressed to Kristin J. Redmond; kjanson3@jhmi.edu

Academic Editor: Se-Hoon Lee

We present a case report of a patient with glioblastoma multiforme (GBM) complicated by extracranial metastasis (ECM) whose survival of nearly four years surpassed the anticipated life expectancy given numerous negative prognostic factors including EGFRvIII-mutation, unmethylated MGMT promoter status, and ECM. Interestingly, while this patient suffered from locally aggressive disease with multiple intracranial recurrences, the proximal cause of death was progressive extracranial disease and complications related to pulmonary metastases. Herein, we review potential mechanisms of ECM with an emphasis upon glioblastoma molecular and genetic profiles and the potential implications of targeted agents such as bevacizumab.

1. Introduction

Glioblastoma multiforme (GBM) is one of the most lethal human malignancies. The median survival of patients with newly diagnosed GBM treated with adjuvant radiation therapy (RT) with concurrent and adjuvant temozolomide (TMZ) remains dismal at 14.6 months. The majority of patients ultimately succumb to local recurrence in the central nervous system [1]. Extracranial metastasis (ECM) is a rare phenomenon of GBM, estimated to occur in less than 2% of diagnoses [2, 3]. However, a recent study from Europe reported that circulating glioblastoma cells were present in 20.6% of GBM patients [4].

Current literature suggests that the median time from initial diagnosis to detection of ECM is approximately 8.5 months and the interval of time between detection of distant metastasis and death is only 1.5 months, suggesting that development of ECM is a harbinger of morbidity and mortality [2, 3]. The factors that predispose GBM patients to the development ECM are currently not well understood.

2. Case Presentation

A previously healthy 51-year-old right-handed African American gentleman initially presented following an unwitnessed seizure. MRI revealed focal enhancement in the posterior temporal lobe measuring approximately 9 mm as well as T2 hyperintensity within the right insular cortex and right temporal lobe. He was empirically treated for HSV encephalitis until CSF HSV PCR assay returned negative. Given persistent mental status changes, MR imaging at 4 and 9 months after initial presentation revealed an enhancing temporoparietal mass with interval enlargement between scans. He underwent right temporal craniotomy with postoperative pathology consistent with WHO grade IV astrocytoma (GBM) with small cell features (Figure 1(a)). Specific histopathological findings of cellular atypia with variable morphology ranging from packed cells with relatively homogeneous ovoid nuclei to less cellular areas with a whorled configuration, foci of necrosis with scattered calcifications, numerous mitoses, and

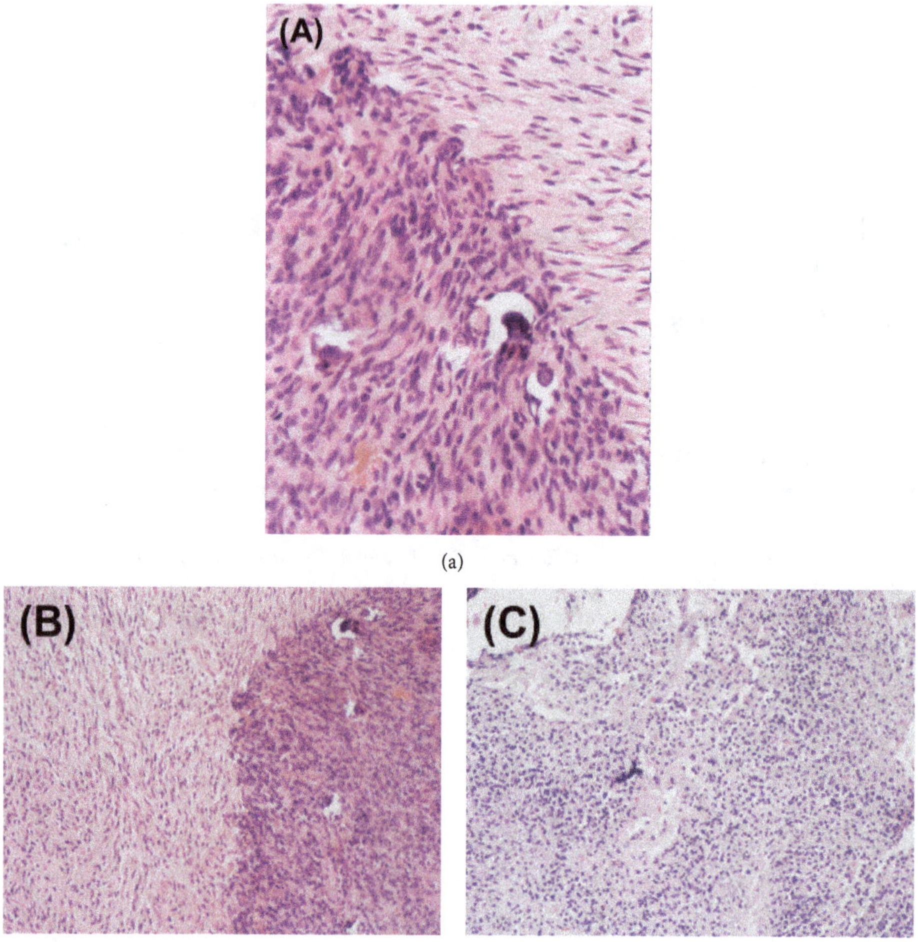

(a)

(b) (c)

FIGURE 1: Surgical pathological specimens from (a) initial craniotomy and (b-c) repeat craniotomy for recurrent intracranial disease. Histopathological analysis of the initial (a) right temporal lobe specimen demonstrated glioblastoma with small cell features. The pathological specimen after second resection (b) demonstrated active glioblastoma, almost entirely viable with <5% necrosis. Following the third and final (c) craniotomy for locally recurrent disease, predominantly viable (approximately 15% necrosis) active glioblastoma was identified. Molecular studies were negative for MGMT methylation and EGFR amplification was detected by FISH.

endothelial proliferation were noted. Immunohistochemical staining demonstrated strong staining for vimentin and negative staining for EMA. Additional tumor analysis revealed an unmethylated MGMT gene promoter and EGFR amplification, later confirmed to be EGFRvIII positive.

He was treated with adjuvant radiotherapy (RT) delivered (6000 cGy in 30 fractions) with concurrent daily temozolomide (TMZ, 75 mg/m^2/day) followed by adjuvant TMZ (150 mg/m^2/day × 5 days every 28 days). Follow-up MRI after two cycles of adjuvant TMZ revealed increased enhancement within the surgical cavity. TMZ was switched to metronomic scheduling (120 mg daily) during the third cycle due to concern of progression versus pseudoprogression for a total of 8 additional cycles. MR imaging a month later revealed marked progressive enhancement and the patient underwent repeat resection with postoperative imaging indicating gross total resection and pathologic confirmation of recurrent GBM (Figure 1(b)).

At 27 months following his initial diagnosis, the patient initiated bevacizumab monotherapy which was discontinued after four cycles due to radiographic progression with development of a mildly enhancing intracavitary nodule. A third craniotomy was performed with pathology demonstrating mitotically active, recurrent GBM (Figure 1(c)). The patient did well postoperatively without radiographic evidence of disease. He was clinically stable without neurologic deficits and maintained an excellent performance status at this time. Surveillance MRI two months following surgery demonstrated nodular tumor recurrence with dural extension and he enrolled in a clinical trial investigating genetically modified T-cells expressing anti-EGFRvIII. The protocol consisted of apheresis, followed by cyclophosphamide, fludarabine, T-cell infusion, and eight infusions of IL-2 (this trial is registered with Clinical Trial: NCT01454596).

After two months of therapy in the aforementioned clinical trial he developed left homonymous hemianopia with

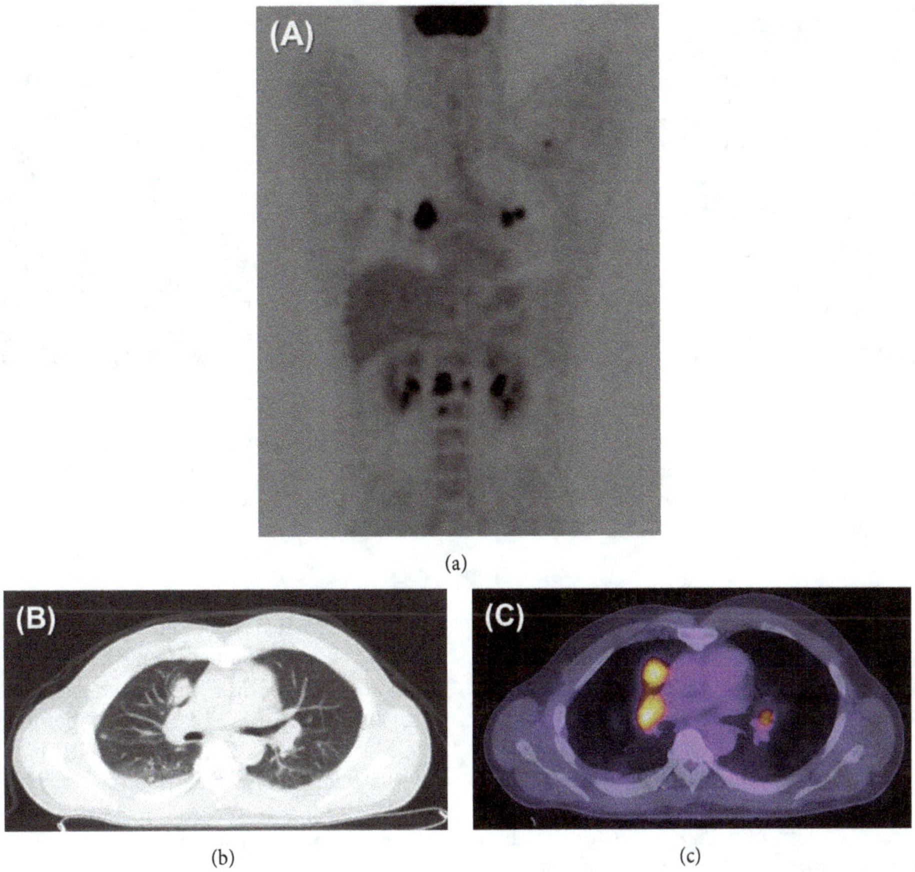

FIGURE 2: (a) Whole body FDG PET imaging demonstrating hypermetabolic osseous and visceral metastases including bilateral pulmonary nodules and hilar adenopathy. (b) CT imaging demonstrating mediastinal adenopathy, multiple pulmonary nodules, and right pleural effusion. (c) Coregistered PET/CT imaging demonstrating intense FDG uptake within GBM lung metastases.

brain MRI revealing infiltrative enhancement around the right temporal lobe surgical cavity and increased vasogenic edema throughout the right temporal and parietal lobes. He underwent reirradiation (3600 cGy in 20 fractions) with concurrent bevacizumab. He continued with adjuvant bevacizumab for an additional two cycles and maintained a good performance status throughout therapy.

The patient developed back pain and abdominal discomfort approximately 40 months following initial diagnosis and 3 months following reinitiation of bevacizumab therapy. CT imaging of the chest demonstrated multiple pulmonary nodules, including a 2.5 cm right middle lobe nodule and a 1.2 cm left lower lobe nodule along with bilateral hilar adenopathy. A staging fluorodeoxyglucose positron emission tomography (FDG PET) scan noted abnormal uptake within several right hilar lymph nodes and diffuse osseous FDG uptake within the sternum, thoracic, lumbar, and pelvic bones. The pulmonary nodules identified on CT imaging were also found to be FDG-avid, right middle lobe (SUV 11.5), two left upper lobe nodules (SUV 6.4 and 5.1), and right upper lobe (SUV 5.0) (Figure 2). Flexible bronchoscopy with biopsy was performed and demonstrated malignant spindle cell tumors with geographic necrosis consistent with metastatic GBM. The tumor cells were positive for GFAP, weakly positive for S100, and negative for synaptophysin, EMA, HHV-8, HMB-45, desmin, CD34, keratin, chromogranin, and CD117. MIB-1 proliferative index was approximately 40%. AFB and GMS stains were negative.

One month later, he resumed treatment with bevacizumab and, in the 43rd month, carboplatin. Restaging FDG PET imaging after 2 cycles revealed extracranial progression of disease with worsening pulmonary and skeletal metastases. Of note, synchronous brain MRI was stable at this time with no evidence of intracranial recurrence or progression (Figure 3). He continued with a third and final cycle of concurrent bevacizumab and carboplatin with continued decline of his respiratory status. 46 months from initial diagnosis, he ultimately passed away secondary to acute respiratory failure. At the time of his death, there was no clinical or radiographic evidence of disease within the central nervous system.

3. Discussion

It is currently unknown if the use of bevacizumab is implicated in the potentiation of ECM. It is notable that extracranial dissemination of this patient's disease coincided with administration of bevacizumab therapy.

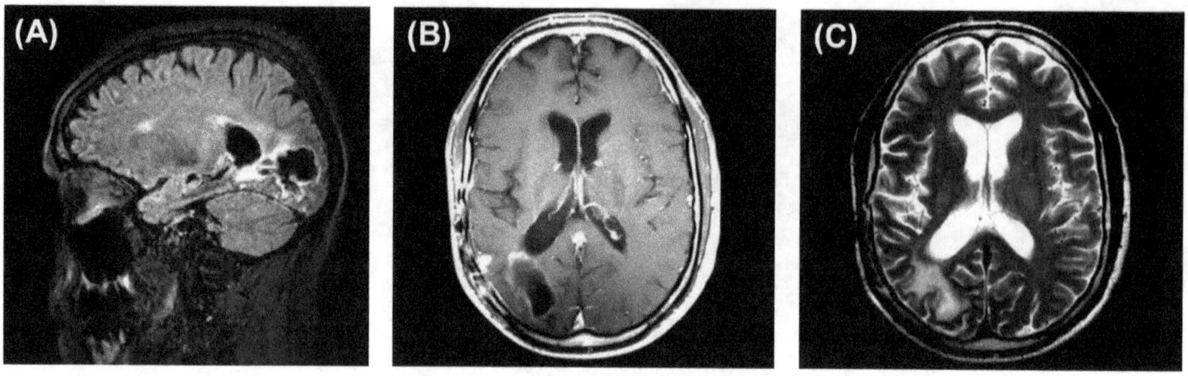

(a) (b) (c)

Figure 3: Intracranial imaging during final course of salvage therapy with bevacizumab and carboplatin. (a) FLAIR, (b) T1-weighted axial, and (c) T2-weighted axial magnetic resonance imaging demonstrating stable intracranial disease at time of respiratory decline. Postsurgical hyperintensity surrounds area of resection in the right temporal and occipital lobes communicating with the right occipital horn, unchanged with respect to prior imaging.

Concerns have been raised that anti-VEGF therapies, including bevacizumab, lead to transformation of primary and recurrent GBM into a more infiltrative phenotype [5, 6]. The withdrawal and reversal of VEGF inhibition have been observed to rapidly increase regrowth of tumor vasculature [7] and therapies administered after bevacizumab failure often only provide transient tumor control [8]. Potential mechanisms have recently been elucidated, illustrating that anti-VEGF inhibitors alter tumor programming and growth pattern of recurrent GBMs in a fashion that promotes resistance to antiangiogenic therapies as well as a more invasive phenotype [5]. It is also postulated that glioblastoma stem cells may differentiate directly into new vessels in the presence of VEGF blockade, yielding a conduit for additional tumor growth and dissemination [9].

The rationale for bevacizumab use in glioblastoma is that inhibition of VEGF normalizes tumor vasculature, thus decreasing tumor interstitial pressure. This improves access to chemotherapeutic drugs as well as oxygen delivery, thus improving efficacy of radiation therapy [10–12]. However, it has also been argued that normalization of the blood-brain barrier, as shown by other antiangiogenic agents when combined with TMZ, may yield less tumor kill, thus generating debate [10, 13].

It remains unknown if extracranial dissemination is impacted by the interaction of targeted treatments and biological factors such as MGMT methylation status or EGFR amplification [14]. A landmark study by Hegi et al. reported that GBM patients with methylated MGMT promoters derive significant benefit from the addition of adjuvant TMZ to RT in comparison to their unmethylated counterparts. Furthermore, MGMT promoter methylation was found to be an independent favorable prognostic factor [15].

Extrapolation from other disease sites may suggest a potential relationship between MGMT status and ECM [16–19]. Kohonen-Corish et al. reported that MGMT hypermethylation is present in up to one-third of patients with distant melanoma metastases and there is considerable heterogeneity of MGMT expression depending on the site of metastasis. Additionally, MGMT promoter methylation did correlate with resistance to TMZ therapy, reemphasizing the role of MGMT in modulating chemosensitivity [20]. With regard to extracranial metastasis among other primary brain tumors, MGMT promoter hypermethylation has been associated with ECM in oligodendrogliomas [16].

EGFR gene amplification is another biological factor potentially implicated in ECM of primary brain tumors [21]. EGFR gene amplification has been observed in pediatric low-grade gliomas that disseminate possibly through a mechanism of induced FABP7 nuclear translocation [16]. FABP7 is involved in glial-guided neuronal migration and EGFR-mediated nuclear translocation may be associated with a propensity for dissemination [22]; however, this relationship has yet to be established in GBM.

As we enter an era of emerging novel therapeutics including immunotherapies and targeted agents, there is potential for unforeseen side effects and unintended detrimental sequelae as a consequence of treatment. While unmethylated MGMT promoter status and amplified EGFR expression, as seen in our case report above, predict a poor prognosis, the relation of these biomarkers to success of targeted antiangiogenic therapies warrants further investigation.

References

[1] R. Stupp, W. P. Mason, M. J. van den Bent et al., "Radiotherapy plus concomitant and adjuvant temozolomide for glioblastoma," *The New England Journal of Medicine*, vol. 352, no. 10, pp. 987–996, 2005.

[2] M. Lun, E. Lok, S. Gautam, E. Wu, and E. T. Wong, "The natural history of extracranial metastasis from glioblastoma multiforme," *Journal of Neuro-Oncology*, vol. 105, no. 2, pp. 261–273, 2011.

[3] G. Kalokhe, S. A. Grimm, J. P. Chandler, I. Helenowski, A. Rademaker, and J. J. Raizer, "Metastatic glioblastoma: case presentations and a review of the literature," *Journal of Neuro-Oncology*, vol. 107, no. 1, pp. 21–27, 2012.

[4] C. Muller, J. Holtschmidt, M. Auer et al., "Hematogenous dissemination of glioblastoma multiforme," *Science Translational Medicine*, vol. 6, no. 247, p. 247ra101, 2014.

[5] E. di Tomaso, M. Snuderl, W. S. Kamoun et al., "Glioblastoma recurrence after cediranib therapy in patients: lack of 'rebound" revascularization as mode of escape," *Cancer Research*, vol. 71, no. 1, pp. 19–28, 2011.

[6] J. F. de Groot, G. Fuller, A. J. Kumar et al., "Tumor invasion after treatment of glioblastoma with bevacizumab: radiographic and pathologic correlation in humans and mice," *Neuro-Oncology*, vol. 12, no. 3, pp. 233–242, 2010.

[7] M. R. Mancuso, R. Davis, S. M. Norberg et al., "Rapid vascular regrowth in tumors after reversal of VEGF inhibition," *Journal of Clinical Investigation*, vol. 116, no. 10, pp. 2610–2621, 2006.

[8] F. M. Iwamoto, L. E. Abrey, K. Beal et al., "Patterns of relapse and prognosis after bevacizumab failure in recurrent glioblastoma," *Neurology*, vol. 73, no. 15, pp. 1200–1206, 2009.

[9] L. Ricci-Vitiani, R. Pallini, M. Biffoni et al., "Tumour vascularization via endothelial differentiation of glioblastoma stem-like cells," *Nature*, vol. 468, no. 7325, pp. 824–830, 2010.

[10] E. M. Thompson, E. P. Frenkel, and E. A. Neuwelt, "The paradoxical effect of bevacizumab in the therapy of malignant gliomas," *Neurology*, vol. 76, no. 1, pp. 87–93, 2011.

[11] D. Shweiki, A. Itin, D. Soffer, and E. Keshet, "Vascular endothelial growth factor induced by hypoxia may mediate hypoxia-initiated angiogenesis," *Nature*, vol. 359, no. 6398, pp. 843–845, 1992.

[12] B. Millauer, L. K. Shawver, K. H. Plate, W. Risau, and A. Ullrich, "Glioblastoma growth inhibited *in vivo* by a dominant-negative Flk-1 mutant," *Nature*, vol. 367, no. 6463, pp. 576–579, 1994.

[13] T. T. Batchelor, P. Mulholland, B. Neyns et al., "Phase III randomized trial comparing the efficacy of cediranib as monotherapy, and in combination with lomustine, versus lomustine alone in patients with recurrent glioblastoma," *Journal of Clinical Oncology*, vol. 31, no. 26, pp. 3212–3218, 2013.

[14] S. L. Gerson, "MGMT: its role in cancer aetiology and cancer therapeutics," *Nature Reviews Cancer*, vol. 4, no. 4, pp. 296–307, 2004.

[15] M. E. Hegi, A.-C. Diserens, T. Gorlia et al., "*MGMT* gene silencing and benefit from temozolomide in glioblastoma," *The New England Journal of Medicine*, vol. 352, no. 10, pp. 997–1003, 2005.

[16] G. Li, Z. Zhang, J. Zhang et al., "Occipital anaplastic oligodendroglioma with multiple organ metastases after a short clinical course: a case report and literature review," *Diagnostic Pathology*, vol. 9, no. 1, article 17, 2014.

[17] M. Esteller, S. R. Hamilton, P. C. Burger, S. B. Baylin, and J. G. Herman, "Inactivation of the DNA repair gene O6-methylguanine-DNA methyltransferase by promoter hypermethylation is a common event in primary human neoplasia," *Cancer Research*, vol. 59, pp. 793–797, 1999.

[18] V. Voelter, A.-C. Diserens, A. Moulin et al., "Infrequent promoter methylation of the MGMT gene in liver metastases from uveal melanoma," *International Journal of Cancer*, vol. 123, no. 5, pp. 1215–1218, 2008.

[19] J. Brabender, H. Usadel, R. Metzger et al., "Quantitative O^6-methylguanine DNA methyltransferase methylation analysis in curatively resected non-small cell lung cancer: associations with clinical outcome," *Clinical Cancer Research*, vol. 9, no. 1, pp. 223–227, 2003.

[20] M. R. J. Kohonen-Corish, W. A. Cooper, J. Saab, J. F. Thompson, R. J. A. Trent, and M. J. Millward, "Promoter hypermethylation of the O^6-methylguanine DNA methyltransferase gene and microsatellite instability in metastatic melanoma," *Journal of Investigative Dermatology*, vol. 126, no. 1, pp. 167–171, 2006.

[21] N. Shinojima, K. Tada, S. Shiraishi et al., "Prognostic value of epidermal growth factor receptor in patients with glioblastoma multiforme," *Cancer Research*, vol. 63, no. 20, pp. 6962–6970, 2003.

[22] U. Tabori, S. Rienstein, Y. Dromi et al., "Epidermal growth factor receptor gene amplification and expression in disseminated pediatric low-grade gliomas," *Journal of Neurosurgery*, vol. 103, no. 4, pp. 357–361, 2005.

5

Urothelial Superior Vena Cava Syndrome with Limited Response to Radiation Therapy

Nishan Bingham,[1] H. James Wallace III,[2] Joanne Monterroso,[3] Claire Verschraegen,[3] Brenda L. Waters,[4] and Christopher J. Anker[2]

[1]*University of Vermont College of Medicine, 89 Beaumont Avenue, Burlington, VT 05405, USA*
[2]*Division of Radiation Oncology, University of Vermont Cancer Center, 111 Colchester Avenue, Mailstop 301SH2, Burlington, VT 05401, USA*
[3]*Division of Hematology Oncology, University of Vermont Cancer Center, 89 Beaumont Avenue, Suite E-214, Burlington, VT 05405, USA*
[4]*Department of Pathology and Laboratory Medicine, University of Vermont Medical Center, 111 Colchester Avenue Main Campus, East Pavilion, Burlington, VT 05401, USA*

Correspondence should be addressed to Christopher J. Anker; chris.anker@UVMHealth.org

Academic Editor: Francesco A. Mauri

Radiation therapy (RT) is the standard of care for cases of superior vena cava (SVC) syndrome secondary to metastatic adenopathy. Histologies vary in radiosensitivity and response time, making alternative therapies such as chemotherapy and/or intravenous stenting preferable alternative options for certain diagnoses. Metastatic urothelial carcinoma is a particularly rare cause of SVC syndrome with only 3 cases reported in the literature. Consequently, optimal management remains challenging, particularly in cases of high tumor burden. Here we present a case of highly advanced metastatic urothelial cancer with SVC syndrome and tracheal compression. The patient started urgent RT but expired midway through her treatment course due to systemic progression of disease, requiring SVC and tracheal stenting. The authors review the literature including discussion of the few other known cases of SVC syndrome due to urothelial carcinoma and a review of this histology's response to RT. This experience suggests, that in cases of SVC syndrome with widespread advanced disease, stenting and chemotherapy with or without RT may be the most important initial treatment plan, depending on goals of care.

1. Introduction

Instances of metastatic urothelial carcinoma causing superior vena cava (SVC) syndrome are extremely rare. Average survival of SVC syndrome is six months but varies with histology [1]. For most cases, urgent treatment with radiation therapy (RT) with or without stenting is the standard of care, while some histologies are best treated with chemotherapy [2, 3]. Although RT has proven beneficial in symptom palliation and disease control for urothelial cancer, there remain very limited data regarding its utility in cases of high tumor burden. Here we report a patient with widely metastatic bladder cancer causing SVC syndrome and tracheal compression. The disease was unresponsive to RT and steroids and required stenting. However within 1.5 weeks the patient died from extensive systemic tumor burden. This case underscores the challenges of selecting therapy for urothelial SVC syndrome as well as the need for further characterization of the timeframe of urothelial carcinoma's response to RT.

2. Case Report

A 48-year-old woman presented to her primary care physician with dysuria and urinary frequency unresponsive to antibiotics. One month later she presented to the emergency room with worsening flank pain and new-onset dyspnea, cough, hoarseness, and fatigue. She had no history of smoking or chronic bladder irritation, nor did she report

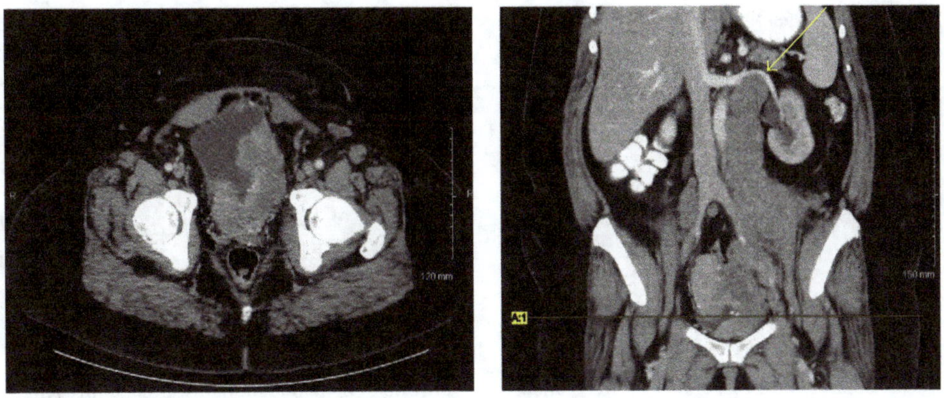

(a) (b)

Figure 1: Axial (a) and coronal (b) pelvic CT scan images showing bladder wall thickening and retroperitoneal masses displacing left renal vein (arrow). The axial image in (a) is at the level of the horizontal line noted in (b).

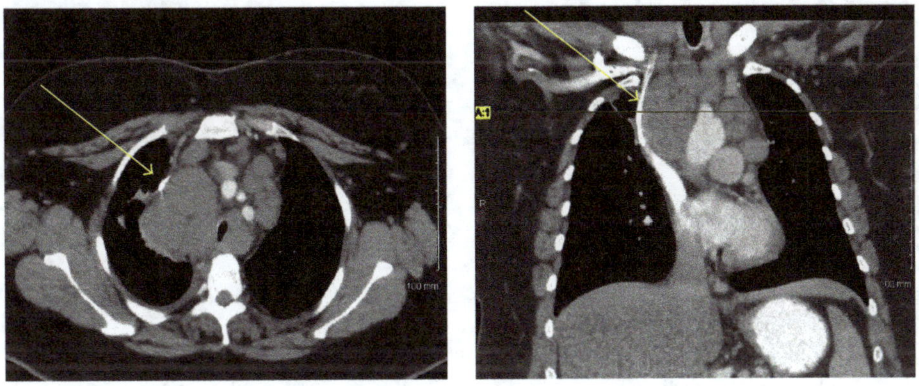

(a) (b)

Figure 2: Axial (a) and coronal (b) chest CT images showing mediastinal lymphadenopathy compressing the SVC (arrows) and trachea. The axial image in (a) is at the level of the horizontal line noted in (b).

any occupational exposure to known chemical carcinogens. Exam was notable for tachycardia, right eye ptosis and miosis, cervical edema, bilateral supraclavicular lymphadenopathy, and stridor. Urine cytology showed high grade malignant cells. Flexible cystoscopy showed a solid mass in the left mid-lateral wall. Pelvic (Figure 1) and chest (Figure 2) computed tomography (CT) scans showed widespread disease with a thickened, calcified bladder wall, bulky retroperitoneal masses, and extensive lymphadenopathy compressing the SVC and trachea. Supraclavicular node biopsy (Figure 3) supported the diagnosis of stage IV urothelial carcinoma with GATA3 positive, cytokeratin 7 (CK 7) positive, and cytokeratin 20 (CK 20) negative immunohistochemistry. She began dexamethasone (4 mg every 6 hours) and RT (30 Gy in 10 fractions planned) to the mediastinum for SVC and tracheal decompression. However, over several days, her dyspnea worsened, and she developed tumor lysis syndrome with hypertension and acute kidney injury. Persistent tracheal compression prompted stenting and ICU transfer. On the 7th day, respiratory decompensation required intubation with tracheostomy for bilateral vocal cord paralysis from nerve compression. RT was held after only 18 Gy and chemotherapy was not administered because of rapid deterioration. She died on hospital day 11 shortly after the family withdrew care. Autopsy showed a large, expansile tumor mass originating in the bladder wall (Figure 4), massive tumor adenopathy anterior to the trachea (Figure 5), along the aorta (Figure 6), and metastases to lung, liver, spleen, omentum, ovaries/uterus (Figure 7), and cervix/vagina (Figure 8).

3. Discussion

RT is considered standard of care in cases of malignancy causing compression of the SVC and trachea because it generally provides a prompt and durable response. Exceptions include small-cell lung cancer and lymphoma, which usually respond to chemotherapy within 72 hours. Newer techniques from interventional radiology such as stenting provide alternative management options, but there are no randomized trials comparing these techniques.

While 96–100% of ovarian adenocarcinomas are CK 7+/CK 20−, compared with only 11–63% of bladder cancers [4, 5], urothelial carcinomas display immunohistochemical GATA3 positivity whereas ovarian cells do not [6, 7]. GATA3

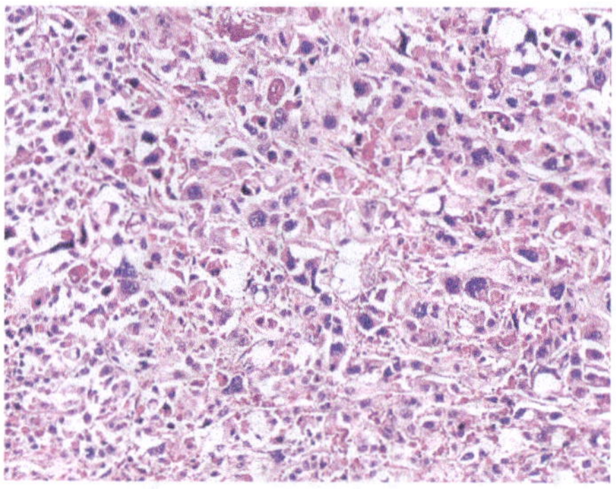

FIGURE 3: The supraclavicular lymph node was entirely effaced by sheets of highly pleomorphic epithelioid cells with enlarged hyperchromatic nuclei, focal cytoplasmic vacuolization, and areas (not pictured here) of necrosis.

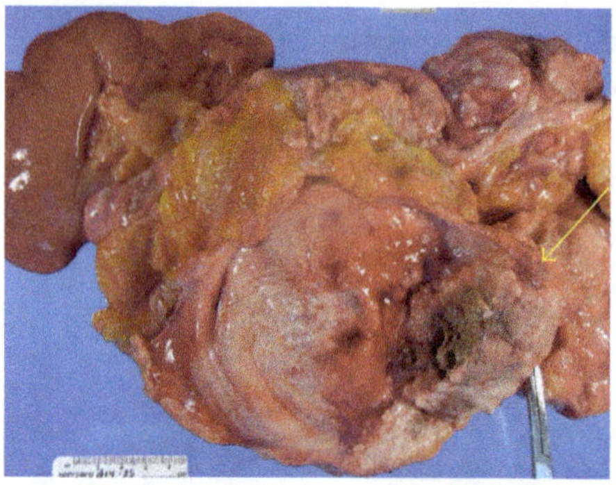

FIGURE 4: Tumor mass (arrow), left side of the bladder. Extensive metastases to lymph nodes with normal urothelium.

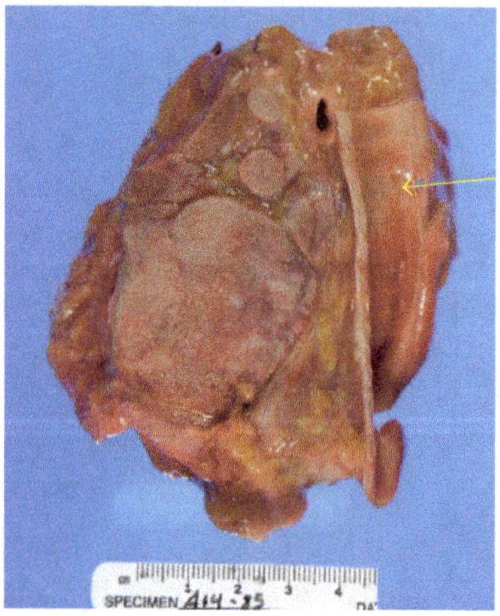

FIGURE 5: Massive adenopathy anterior to trachea (arrow).

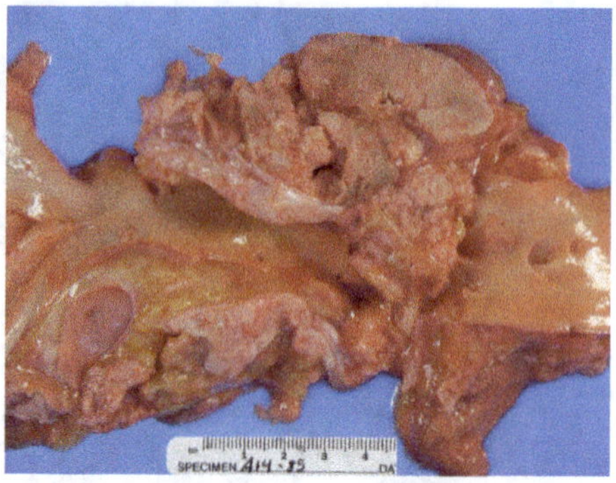

FIGURE 6: Lymphadenopathy along entire length of aorta by tumor.

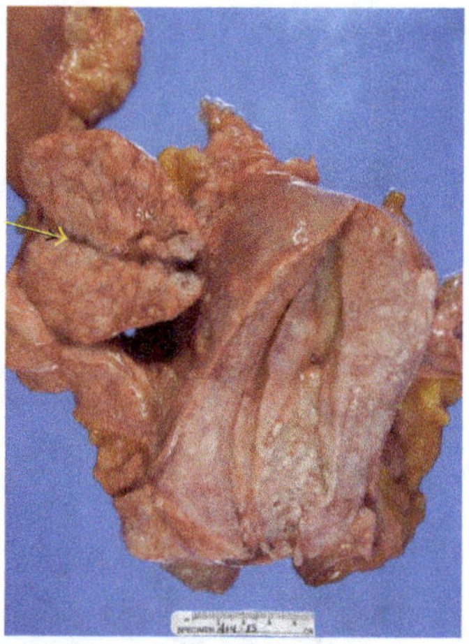

FIGURE 7: Massive enlargement of ovary (arrow) and uterus from extensive tumor infiltration.

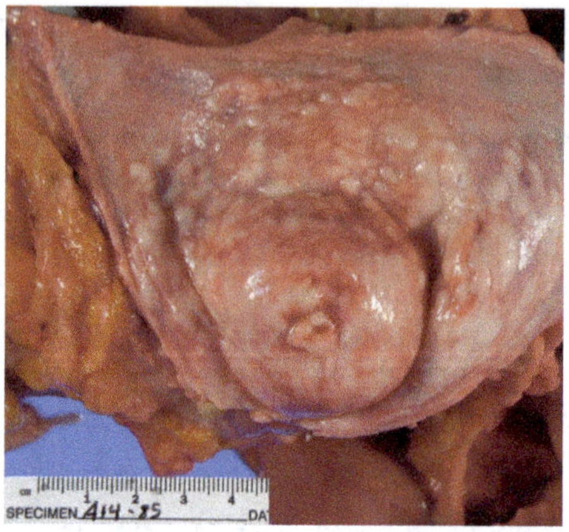

FIGURE 8: Tumor infiltrating surface of exocervix and vagina.

is a sensitive urothelial immunomarker staining in 86% of patients, and it is also specific as the only additional carcinomas it stains positive for are breast (94%) and to a much lower frequency endometrial (2%). Moreover, the finding at autopsy of tumor appearing to originate from the bladder was consistent with a primary urothelial carcinoma. SVC syndrome from a primary bladder cancer is extremely rare, with only three cases reported in the literature. One case was treated with 40 Gy of RT over 20 days causing grade 3 esophagitis, but no tumor response. Treatment was switched to paclitaxel, gemcitabine, and cisplatin which decreased the offending tumor size by 90%. The patient died 10 months later due to bleeding from a brain metastasis [8]. None of the other cases survived more than one month, although one had initial improvement with chemoradiation [9–11].

Currently, the standard of care for metastatic urothelial carcinoma is cisplatin-based combination chemotherapy. The combination of cisplatin and gemcitabine has shown improved tolerability compared to that of methotrexate, vincristine, adriamycin, and cisplatin [12]. Overall, poor performance status and the presence of bone or visceral metastases are the most reliable prognostic indicators of a poor response to treatment, with very few patients living beyond six years [12].

Experience with SVC syndrome from urothelial carcinoma remains extremely limited, with little to no follow-up. In rapidly progressive disease, immediate stenting followed by chemotherapy or chemoradiation may be reasonable treatment options. Palliative RT for bleeding has been shown to induce hemostasis within two weeks in 72% of patients with muscle-invasive disease who develop gross hematuria, suggesting that such a time frame may be necessary to observe significant benefit from RT [13]. Stereotactic hypofractionated techniques may present an alternative treatment strategy that could improve long-term local control. In a report detailing treatment outcomes for brain metastases from bladder cancer, the one patient treated with stereotactic radiosurgery survived over one year with good local control, while five of eleven patients receiving whole brain radiation died during treatment [14].

Targeted treatment decisions should be based on clinical signs and symptoms, as well as overall treatment goals. Local therapies may significantly improve quality of life and survival especially when SVC syndrome is a life threatening issue. For urothelial carcinoma, systemic therapy may also be necessary for treatment of SVC syndrome. Interestingly, in the future, further characterization of radio- and chemosensitivities for genomic subsets of urothelial carcinoma may provide rapid histologic and genomic characterization that could clarify optimal therapy in both acute and long-term settings [15–17].

References

[1] L. D. Wilson, F. C. Detterbeck, and J. Yahalom, “Clinical practice. Superior vena cava syndrome with malignant causes,” *The New England Journal of Medicine*, vol. 356, no. 18, pp. 1862–1869, 2007.

[2] N. Tanigawa, S. Sawada, K. Mishima et al., “Clinical outcome of stenting in superior vena cava syndrome associated with malignant tumors. Comparison with conventional treatment,” *Acta Radiologica*, vol. 39, no. 6, pp. 669–674, 1998.

[3] J. B. Yu, L. D. Wilson, and F. C. Detterbeck, “Superior vena cava syndrome-a proposed classification system and algorithm for management,” *Journal of Thoracic Oncology*, vol. 3, no. 8, pp. 811–814, 2008.

[4] N. P. Wang, S. Zee, R. J. Zarbo, C. E. Bacchi, and A. M. Gown, “Coordinate expression of cytokeratins 7 and 20 defines unique subsets of carcinomas,” *Applied Immunohistochemistry*, vol. 3, no. 2, pp. 99–107, 1995.

[5] P. Chu, E. Wu, and L. M. Weiss, “Cytokeratin 7 and cytokeratin 20 expression in epithelial neoplasms: a survey of 435 cases,” *Modern Pathology*, vol. 13, no. 9, pp. 962–972, 2000.

[6] J. P. T. Higgins, G. Kaygusuz, L. Wang et al., “Placental S100 (S100P) and GATA3: markers for transitional epithelium and urothelial carcinoma discovered by complementary DNA microarray,” *The American Journal of Surgical Pathology*, vol. 31, no. 5, pp. 673–680, 2007.

[7] H. Liu, J. Shi, M. L. Wilkerson, and F. Lin, “Immunohistochemical evaluation of GATA3 expression in tumors and normal tissues: a useful immunomarker for breast and urothelial carcinomas,” *American Journal of Clinical Pathology*, vol. 138, no. 1, pp. 57–64, 2012.

[8] H. Wakeda, R. Hamasuna, Y. Asada, and T. Kamoto, “Superior vena cava syndrome due to metastasis from urothelial cancer: a case report and literature review,” *Urology Annals*, vol. 5, no. 4, pp. 291–293, 2013.

[9] V. Lanteri, H. C. Park, G. E. Lopez et al., “Superior vena cava syndrome in a 56-year-old man,” *The Journal of Urology*, vol. 126, no. 5, pp. 665–669, 1981.

[10] N. D. Greyson and R. J. Howard, “Superior vena caval obstruction due to atrial metastasis,” *Clinical Nuclear Medicine*, vol. 14, no. 9, pp. 698–699, 1989.

[11] I. A. Voutsadakis, G. Masouris, K. Tsapakidis, and C. N. Papandreou, “Rapid fatal outcome from pulmonary arteries compression in transitional cell carcinoma,” *Journal of Oncology*, vol. 2009, Article ID 579407, 3 pages, 2009.

[12] H. Von der Maase, S. W. Hansen, J. T. Roberts et al., “Gemcitabine and cisplatin versus methotrexate, vinblastine, doxorubicin, and cisplatin in advanced or metastatic bladder cancer: results of a large, randomized, multinational, multicenter, phase III study,” *Journal of Clinical Oncology*, vol. 18, no. 17, pp. 3068–3077, 2000.

[13] E. Lacarrière, C. Smaali, A. Benyoucef, C. Pfister, and P. Grise, “The efficacy of hemostatic radiotherapy for bladder cancer-related hematuria in patients unfit for surgery,” *International Braz J Urol*, vol. 39, no. 6, pp. 808–816, 2013.

[14] A. S. Mahmoud-Ahmed, J. H. Suh, P. A. Kupelian et al., “Brain metastases from bladder carcinoma: presentation, treatment and survival,” *The Journal of Urology*, vol. 167, no. 6, pp. 2419–2422, 2002.

[15] W. Choi, S. Porten, S. Kim et al., “Identification of distinct basal and luminal subtypes of muscle-invasive bladder cancer with different sensitivities to frontline chemotherapy,” *Cancer Cell*, vol. 25, no. 2, pp. 152–165, 2014.

[16] The Cancer Genome Atlas Research Network, “Comprehensive molecular characterization of urothelial bladder carcinoma,” *Nature*, vol. 507, no. 7492, pp. 315–322, 2014.

[17] N. D. James, S. A. Hussain, E. Hall et al., “Radiotherapy with or without chemotherapy in muscle-invasive bladder cancer,” *The New England Journal of Medicine*, vol. 366, no. 16, pp. 1477–1488, 2012.

6

Progressive Multifocal Leukoencephalopathy with Negative JC Virus PCR following Treatment of Follicular Lymphoma: Implications for Biologics in the Era of Targeted Cancer Therapy

Kimberly A. Silverio[1] and Shyam A. Patel[2]

[1]*Department of Gynecologic Oncology, Helen Diller Family Comprehensive Cancer Center, University of California, San Francisco (UCSF), 550 16th Street, San Francisco, CA 94158, USA*
[2]*Department of Medicine, Stanford University Medical Center, 300 Pasteur Drive, Stanford, CA 94305, USA*

Correspondence should be addressed to Shyam A. Patel; shyam2@stanford.edu

Academic Editor: Jose I. Mayordomo

Anticancer therapy predisposes patients to infections by the immunosuppression that results from treatment. Although 85% of patients with progressive multifocal leukoencephalopathy (PML) have concurrent HIV/AIDS, PML can also develop in patients after they receive chemotherapy for cancer. The case herein describes a 69-year-old man with history of follicular lymphoma who presented with progressive dysarthria and right-sided paralysis. He received rituximab one year prior to presentation. PET scan suggested no recurrence of lymphoma. Cerebrospinal fluid (CSF) analysis was negative and showed fewer than 500 copies/mL of JC virus. However, brain biopsy showed chromatin margination and viropathic change within oligodendrocytes, confirming PML. He was started on mirtazapine and mefloquine with some clinical improvement. To our knowledge, this is the first case of rituximab-associated PML in a patient with negative JC virus PCR from the CSF. Recognition of PML in the differential of oncology patients with CNS symptoms is an important consideration as we enter the era of targeted therapy and personalized cancer medicine involving biologics. Furthermore, screening of patients for presence of subclinical JC viremia prior to the use of biologics may be an important component of assessing patient candidacy for these agents.

1. Introduction

Novel treatment modalities for cancer, including biologic agents such as monoclonal antibodies, have resulted in remarkable improvements in clinical outcomes for patients with cancer over the recent two decades. Targeted therapy and personalized cancer medicine have led to increased treatment efficacy with reduced toxicity. However, novel modalities of treatment do not remain without complications. As targeted therapy for cancer has only been on the market since approximately the 1990s, we do not have enough robust data on adverse effects and management of these complications. Some recent literature has underscored the potentially adverse effects of rituximab in treatment of non-Hodgkin's lymphoma, namely, PML. Complications such as these have significant implications as we approach an era of personalized cancer medicine, as the toxicity of novel agents typically presents with more subtle and elusive symptomatology compared to conventional chemotherapy. Such symptomatology is rooted in the specific mechanism of action of targeted agents. The clinical significance, however, is of utmost importance. This case describes a patient with a subacute presentation of a complication characterized by high mortality in the setting of treatment for follicular lymphoma with a biologic agent.

2. Case Description

A 69-year-old man with a history of stage IIIB follicular lymphoma, atrial fibrillation, and pulmonary sarcoidosis presented with progressive dysarthria and right-sided paralysis over a two-month period. The patient noticed increasing

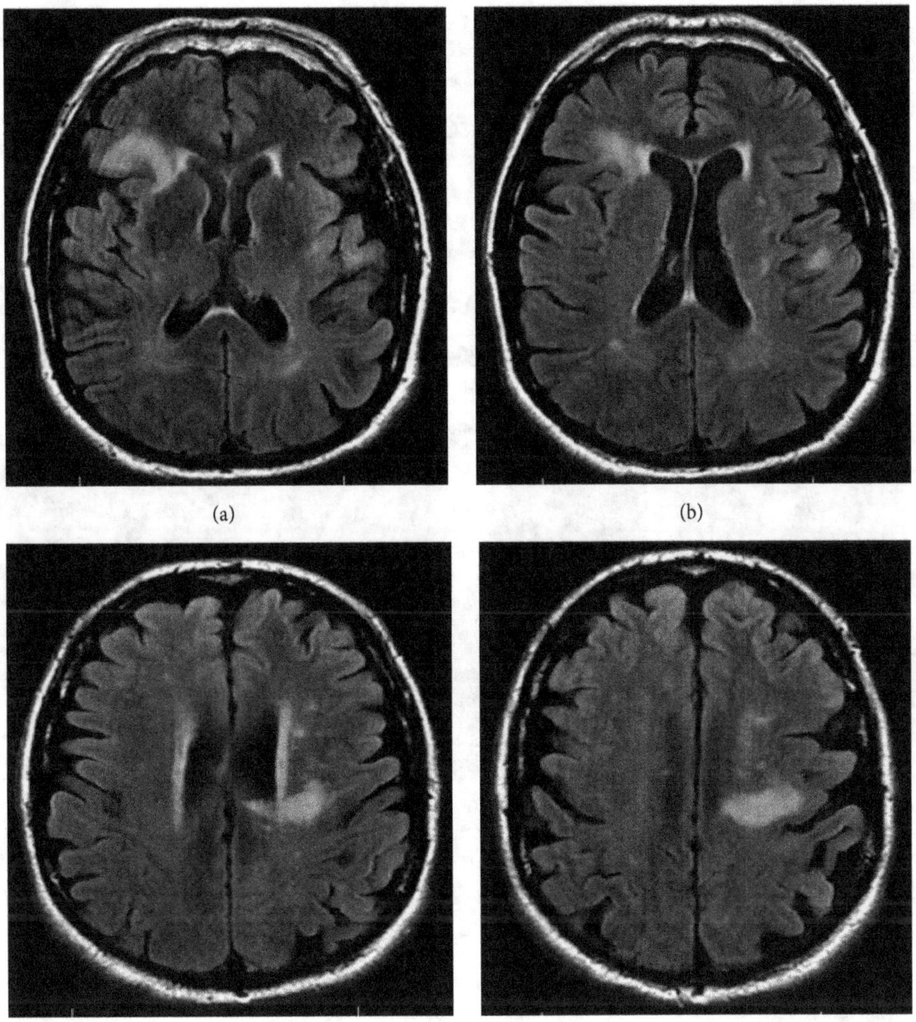

(a) (b) (c) (d)

FIGURE 1: Axial images of MRI of the brain showing multiple confluent foci of T2-weighted FLAIR hyperintensity involving the inferior right and left frontal lobes, as well as periventricular regions (a-b). Hyperintensities are also seen in the left corona radiata (c-d). These areas are representative CNS demyelination. Several foci had restricted diffusion. There was no flow-limiting stenosis, occlusion, or aneurysm in intracranial and extracranial circulations. Images progress superiorly to inferiorly from (a) through (d).

difficulty with speech and fine-motor function such as handwriting and finally decided to seek evaluation due to nonresolving symptoms. Regarding relevant past medical history, he was diagnosed with follicular lymphoma 20 years prior to presentation and had three recurrences in the interim. He completed six cycles of rituximab and bendamustine one year prior to presentation for his lymphoma. Upon admission to the hospital for progressive neurological symptoms, workup was initiated. There was high concern for cerebrovascular etiology versus recurrence of lymphoma with CNS involvement. MRI of the brain showed multiple confluent foci of T2-weighted FLAIR hyperintensity involving the inferior frontal lobes and left corona radiata, initially suggestive of an inflammatory, neoplastic, or vasculitic process. These hyperintensities were noted on axial images (Figure 1) and sagittal images (Figure 2). There was no flow-limiting stenosis, occlusion, or aneurysm. Corresponding T1-weighted sagittal images and DWI sequences are shown for comparison (Figure 3). His lab values (including CBC and metabolic panel) on admission were unremarkable. Rheumatologic workup was done: ANA was negative, ANCA titer was $< 1:20$, complement C3 was 104 mg/dL (within normal limits), and complement C4 was 23 mg/dL (within normal limits). Workup for inflammatory etiology showed CRP of 0.16 mg/dL and ESR of 17 mm/hr. Workup for neurosarcoidosis showed ACE level of 27 mcg/L (within normal limits). Workup for immunodeficiency showed nonreactive HIV screen, nonreactive HCV screen, IgA level of 270 mg/dL, IgG level of 836 mg/dL, and IgM level of 44 mg/dL (all within normal limits). Syphilis ELISA was < 0.8, and Lyme antibody screen was < 0.9. Workup for possible recurrence of lymphoma showed beta2-microglobulin of 2.28 mcg/mL and LDH of 109 U/L (within normal limits). PET scan revealed no hypermetabolic lesions in the brain to suggest recurrence

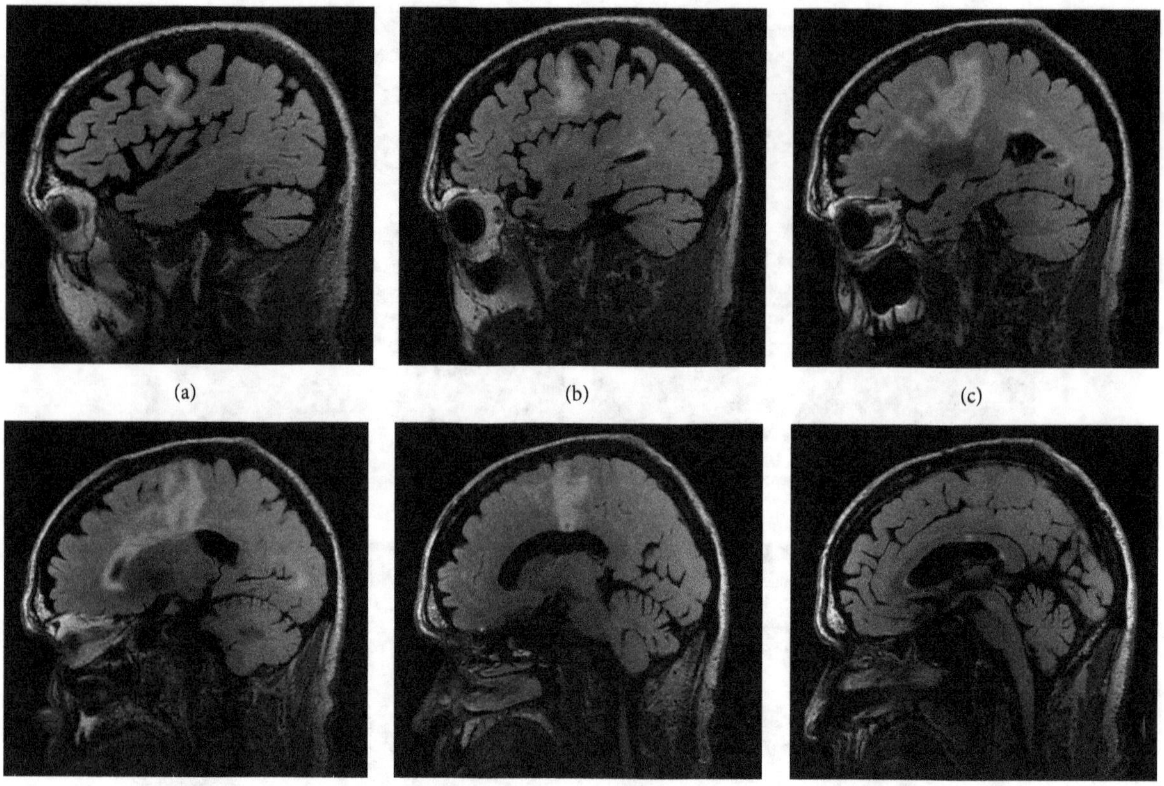

(a) (b) (c) (d) (e) (f)

Figure 2: Sagittal images of MRI of the brain with T2-weighted FLAIR hyperintensities. Images progress from left to right from (a) through (f). Areas of demyelination correspond anatomically with axial images from Figure 1.

of his lymphoma (Figure 4). Skin biopsy was done and was negative for intravascular lymphoma. Finally, lumbar puncture was pursued, and CSF was clear and colorless. Other studies of the CSF showed WBC, 0; RBC, 0; glucose, 57 mg/dL; protein, 38 mg/dL; no organisms; and VDRL, nonreactive. Blood cultures remained negative. CSF PCR was negative for JC virus PCR (<500 copies/mL). Due to concern for inflammatory etiology of his symptoms, he was started empirically on high-dose IV methylprednisolone, but there was no subsequent improvement. A repeat MRI of the brain showed mildly increased size of several nonenhancing confluent subcortical and periventricular T2/FLAIR signal hyperintensities mostly in left corona radiata and right temporal lobe with associated foci of restricted diffusion. There were scattered punctate foci of enhancement in the bilateral cerebral hemispheres not definitively seen on the prior MRI. Ultimately, a frontal lobe brain biopsy was performed given the elusive diagnosis. The brain biopsy revealed perivascular mixed chronic inflammation, chromatin margination with viropathic change within oligodendrocytes, demyelination, and SV40 stain positivity confirming JC virus infection (Figure 5). The patient was started in mefloquine and mirtazapine, given the recent data on this regimen in non-HIV/AIDS-related PML. He had clinical improvement and is currently being managed as an outpatient.

3. Discussion

PML is a demyelinating disease that affects oligodendrocytes and can lead to significant morbidity and mortality. The infectious agent is JC virus, which is a papovavirus first isolated by John Cunningham in 1971. JC virus is a lytic virus in oligodendrocytes [1]. PML was previously thought to occur exclusively in patients with HIV/AIDS (CD4 < 500/mcl), and approximately 85% of cases have coexisting HIV infection. PML is in fact an AIDS-defining illness. However, PML development is not exclusive to HIV/AIDS patients. Other risk factors include hematological and lymphoreticular malignancies (resulting in inherent immunosuppression) and receipt of agents such as cyclophosphamide, prednisone, and rituximab (resulting in medication-induced immunosuppression).

The pathophysiology of PML development in patients with cancer who have received rituximab involves reactivation of endemic JC virus [2]. The virus enters the body via the oral or respiratory route. It establishes latency in the kidneys and lymphoreticular tissues. Importantly, the virus can replicate without causing clinical manifestations, as was the case here. Immunosuppression causes reactivation and dissemination to the brain by B cells, which serve as reservoirs of the virus. Infected astrocytes acquire a bizarre shape and distortion of nuclei, and demyelination results in diverse neurological symptoms.

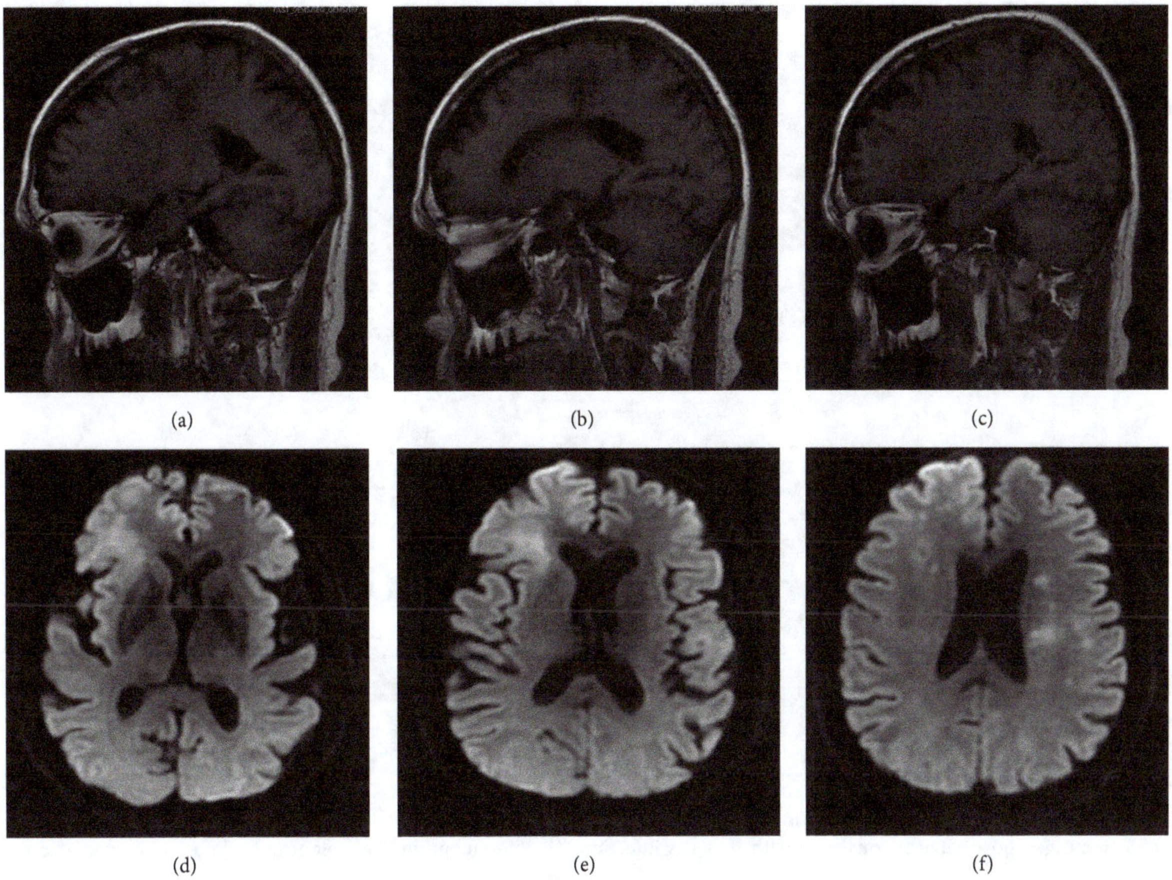

Figure 3: T1-weighted sagittal images (a–c) and diffusion-weighted images (DWI) (d–f). Images progress from right to left from (a) through (c). Images progress superiorly to inferiorly from (d) through (f).

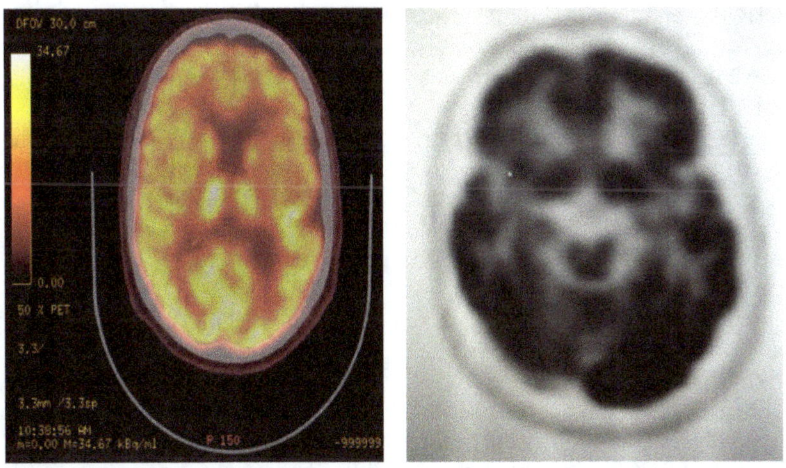

Figure 4: PET scan of the brain showing no hypermetabolic lesions in the brain to suggest lymphoma. Hypometabolism is seen in the right frontal operculum and left frontal vertex. There is a larger area of subtle asymmetric decreased FDG activity seen in posterior left frontal lobe and left parietal lobe.

Monoclonal antibody therapy has been linked to PML in the past decade. The integrin inhibitor natalizumab, for example, has been associated with PML via a mechanism that likely involves disruption of inflammatory T cell extravasation [3]. The link between PML and rituximab is less well characterized but has been described in some case reports. One of the first reports on PML development after rituximab treatment was in 2007 [4]. This was a case in which a 44-year-old female was diagnosed with PML two years after receiving rituximab and then died. PCR of JC virus from the CSF

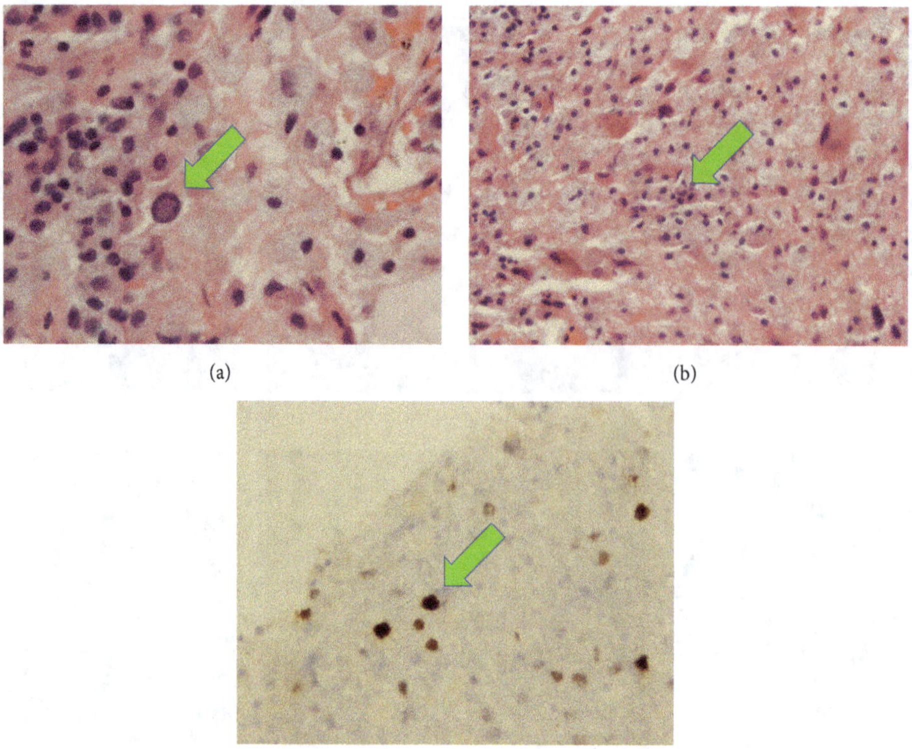

(a) (b) (c)

Figure 5: Frontal lobe biopsy of the brain showing chromatic margination in oligodendrocytes (a), perivascular mixed chronic inflammation (b), and SV40 antigen positivity (c) consistent with JC virus infection. The aforementioned histological findings are demarcated by green arrows.

was positive. In another case, a 48-year-old female developed PML after 5 cycles of R-CHOP chemotherapy, and JC virus testing by PCR of CSF was positive [5]. In a report of 57 cases of postrituximab PML, JC viral PCR of CSF was used as a confirmatory criterion for PML [6].

A striking and clinically significant aspect of the case described here was that the patient's JC virus PCR from CSF was negative. JC virus PCR from the CSF has a sensitivity of 74–93% and specificity of 92–99% for PML [7]. Potential etiologies for false negative PCR include low viral load in CSF, storage of specimen prior to testing, low volume specimen, or loss of DNA during concentration. The case herein highlights the concept that a diagnosis of PML can be made in the absence of CSF PCR positivity. Specifically, radiographic (i.e., MRI) and pathologic (i.e., brain biopsy) findings are sufficient for diagnosis. This is especially important because prior case studies have used JC virus CSF PCR as a confirmatory criterion for PML [6].

From a practical perspective, it is important to identify which subsets of patients may be at risk for PML after receiving biologics. JC viremia is common in the general population, but PML does not develop in healthy persons due to absence of immunosuppression. However, in patients who become immunosuppressed, the presence of JC viremia is a risk factor for PML because viral reactivation can occur. This underscores the importance of a secondary prevention strategy, namely, testing for JC viremia prior to starting biologics. For example, in patients who are candidates for natalizumab for multiple sclerosis, the potential for JC virus reactivation can be assessed by testing for JC virus exposure via antibody index or real-time PCR of plasma or urine [8]. In the same respect, for patients who are candidates for biologics for cancer, PCR of JC virus from the plasma may be a useful screening measure prior to initiation of immunosuppressive biologics, and these can divert adverse events.

Recent advances in the treatment options for non-HIV/AID-associated PML have been made in the past six years. The use of mefloquine and mirtazapine for non-HIV/AIDS-related PML came to the forefront after screening FDA-approved agents for activity against JC virus. Screening of approximately 2000 drugs showed that mefloquine, a known antimalarial agent, harbored the ability to inhibit JC virus infection by inhibiting viral replication after cell entry [9]. The use of mirtazapine, which has serotonin receptor inhibitory activity, came to attention when it was discovered that JC virus uses the serotonin receptor to gain cell entry [10]. The patient in this case showed improvement after starting this regimen.

In summary, this case report highlights the need to maintain a high index of suspicion for opportunistic infections in cancer patients without HIV/AIDS. Conventional chemotherapy, namely, antimetabolites and DNA-disrupting agents, has long been recognized to cause immunosuppression with resulting complications. However, novel anticancer agents have not been available for enough time to appreciate the potential complications. Novel agents that may have the potential to predispose patients to subacute infections or inflammatory complications include monoclonal antibody therapy that depletes immune cells, immune checkpoint inhibitors, and antigrowth factor therapy. This case emphasizes the need to recognize PML in the differential diagnosis of cancer patients with neurological symptoms, regardless of whether they had received conventional chemotherapy or novel agents. The case underscores the diagnostic limitations such as sensitivity of CSF viral PCR testing for JC virus; leptomeningeal detection JC virus is not a prerequisite for PML. Negative JC viral PCR testing should be followed by ultrasensitive PCR or by brain biopsy. Empiric treatment for PML should be considered given the minimal risks of regimens that have been proven effective, such as mirtazapine and mefloquine, and given that PML can be rapidly fatal once diagnosed [11, 12]. Finally, this case highlights the utility of screening for JC viremia in patients who may be candidates for novel biologics for cancer treatment.

Consent

Consent to publish has been obtained from the participant to report individual patient data.

Authors' Contribution

Kimberly A. Silverio and Shyam A. Patel wrote the paper. Shyam A. Patel conceptualized the paper and approved the final version.

References

[1] F. I. De-Simone, R. Sariyer, Y. Otalora et al., "IFN-gamma inhibits JC virus replication in Glial cells by suppressing T-antigen expression," *PLoS ONE*, vol. 10, no. 6, Article ID e0129694, 2015.

[2] P. Sudhakar, D. M. Bachman, A. S. Mark, J. R. Berger, and S. Kedar, "Progressive multifocal leukoencephalopathy," *Journal of Neuro-Ophthalmology*, vol. 35, no. 3, pp. 296–305, 2015.

[3] E. O. Major, "Progressive multifocal leukoencephalopathy in patients on immunomodulatory therapies," *Annual Review of Medicine*, vol. 61, no. 1, pp. 35–47, 2010.

[4] S. G. Freim Wahl, M. R. Folvik, and S. H. Torp, "Progressive multifocal leukoencephalopathy in a lymphoma patient with complete remission after treatment with cytostatics and rituximab: case report and review of the literature," *Clinical Neuropathology*, vol. 26, no. 2, pp. 68–73, 2007.

[5] H. Yokoyama, T. Watanabe, D. Maruyama, S.-W. Kim, Y. Kobayashi, and K. Tobinai, "Progressive multifocal leukoencephalopathy in a patient with B-cell lymphoma during rituximab-containing chemotherapy: case report and review of the literature," *International Journal of Hematology*, vol. 88, no. 4, pp. 443–447, 2008.

[6] K. R. Carson, A. M. Evens, E. A. Richey et al., "Progressive multifocal leukoencephalopathy after rituximab therapy in HIV-negative patients: a report of 57 cases from the Research on Adverse Drug Events and Reports project," *Blood*, vol. 113, no. 20, pp. 4834–4840, 2009.

[7] S. Bossolasco, G. Calori, F. Moretti et al., "Prognostic significance of JC virus DNA levels in cerebrospinal fluid of patients with HIV-associated progressive multifocal leukoencephalopathy," *Clinical Infectious Diseases*, vol. 40, no. 5, pp. 738–744, 2005.

[8] R. Lanzillo, R. Liuzzi, L. Vallefuoco et al., "JC virus antibody index in natalizumab-treated patients: correlations with John Cunningham virus DNA and C-reactive protein level," *Therapeutics and Clinical Risk Management*, vol. 10, pp. 807–814, 2014.

[9] M. Brickelmaier, A. Lugovskoy, R. Kartikeyan et al., "Identification and characterization of mefloquine efficacy against JC virus in vitro," *Antimicrobial Agents and Chemotherapy*, vol. 53, no. 5, pp. 1840–1849, 2009.

[10] A. Kalisch, M. Wilhelm, F. Erbguth, and J. Birkmann, "Progressive multifocal leukoencephalopathy in patients with a hematological malignancy: review of therapeutic options," *Chemotherapy*, vol. 60, no. 1, pp. 47–53, 2014.

[11] N. Epperla, R. Medina-Flores, J. J. Mazza, and S. H. Yale, "Mirtazapine and mefloquine therapy for non-AIDS-related progressive multifocal leukoencephalopathy," *Wisconsin Medical Journal*, vol. 113, no. 6, pp. 242–245, 2014.

[12] J. Paues and M. Vrethem, "Fatal progressive multifocal leukoencephalopathy in a patient with non-Hodgkin lymphoma treated with rituximab," *Journal of Clinical Virology*, vol. 48, no. 4, pp. 291–293, 2010.

7

Secretory Carcinoma of the Breast: Report of Two Cases

Vivekanand Sharma,[1] Gajendra Anuragi,[1] Suresh Singh,[1] Pinakin Patel,[1] Arpita Jindal,[2] and Raj Govind Sharma[1]

[1]*Division of Surgical Oncology, Department of Surgery, S.M.S. Medical College and Hospital, Jaipur, Rajasthan 302004, India*
[2]*Department of Pathology, S.M.S. Medical College and Hospital, Jaipur, Rajasthan 302004, India*

Correspondence should be addressed to Vivekanand Sharma; drvivekanandsharma@gmail.com

Academic Editor: Sercan Aksoy

Secretory carcinoma of the breast is an extremely rare subtype of breast cancer characterized by intracellular or extracellular secretion and granular eosinophilic cytoplasm of the neoplastic cells. The disease which was considered to be predominant in younger age group has been recognized in adult population too and tends to show slow growth and indolent behavior. The disease occurs preferentially in females and only 27 cases have been reported amongst males. An optimal treatment for the disease subtype has been debated because of the paucity of data. We report two cases (one female and one male) of this rare disease that underwent treatment at our institution.

1. Introduction

Secretory breast carcinoma (SBC) was first described by McDivitt and Stewart [1]. It is a very rare subtype of breast cancer and comprises less than 0.15% of invasive breast cancers [2]. It is identified by its distinct histomorphology and usually is associated with a favourable prognosis. Secretory carcinoma was first reported in children and the older literature identified the disease by the name of juvenile breast carcinoma. However, after the review by Tavassoli and Norris [3], it was recognised that it may occur in adult patients as well. Recently, the tumor was found to be associated with a distinct ETV6-NTRK3 mutation which confers the tumor proliferative and survival advantage.

2. Clinical Case Report 1

A 55-year-old lady with no family history of breast cancer presented to our department in January 2014. The patient had noticed a lump in the right breast a month back which had gradually grown. She underwent a lumpectomy for the same at another center and was referred with the histopathology suggestive of secretory carcinoma.

Clinical examination showed a 5 cm long healed scar in the upper outer quadrant of the right breast. The nipple and areola appeared normal. No clinical alterations in either the ipsilateral or contralateral axillae were found. There was no evidence of metastatic disease on evaluation.

The biopsy of the lumpectomy specimen showed a 3 × 2 cm mass harbouring microscopically an intraductal neoplasm with the tumor cells showing glands and microcystic spaces showing abundant pale secretions. The cells had abundant pale staining cytoplasm with small round low grade nuclei. There was no perineural or vascular invasion. The biopsy hence suggested a secretory carcinoma of the breast (Figure 1). Immunohistochemistry of the tumor on review of paraffin embedded blocks showed neoplastic cells with triple negative results (estrogen receptor and progesterone receptor and Her-2/neu protein expression negative). The tumor also stained positive for PAS, mucicarmine, and vimentin (Figure 1).

The patient opted for a modified radical mastectomy with axillary dissection citing difficulty to routinely follow-up for radiotherapy. On subsequent histopathological examination the mastectomy specimen and all 16 lymph nodes resected were negative for the presence of the tumor.

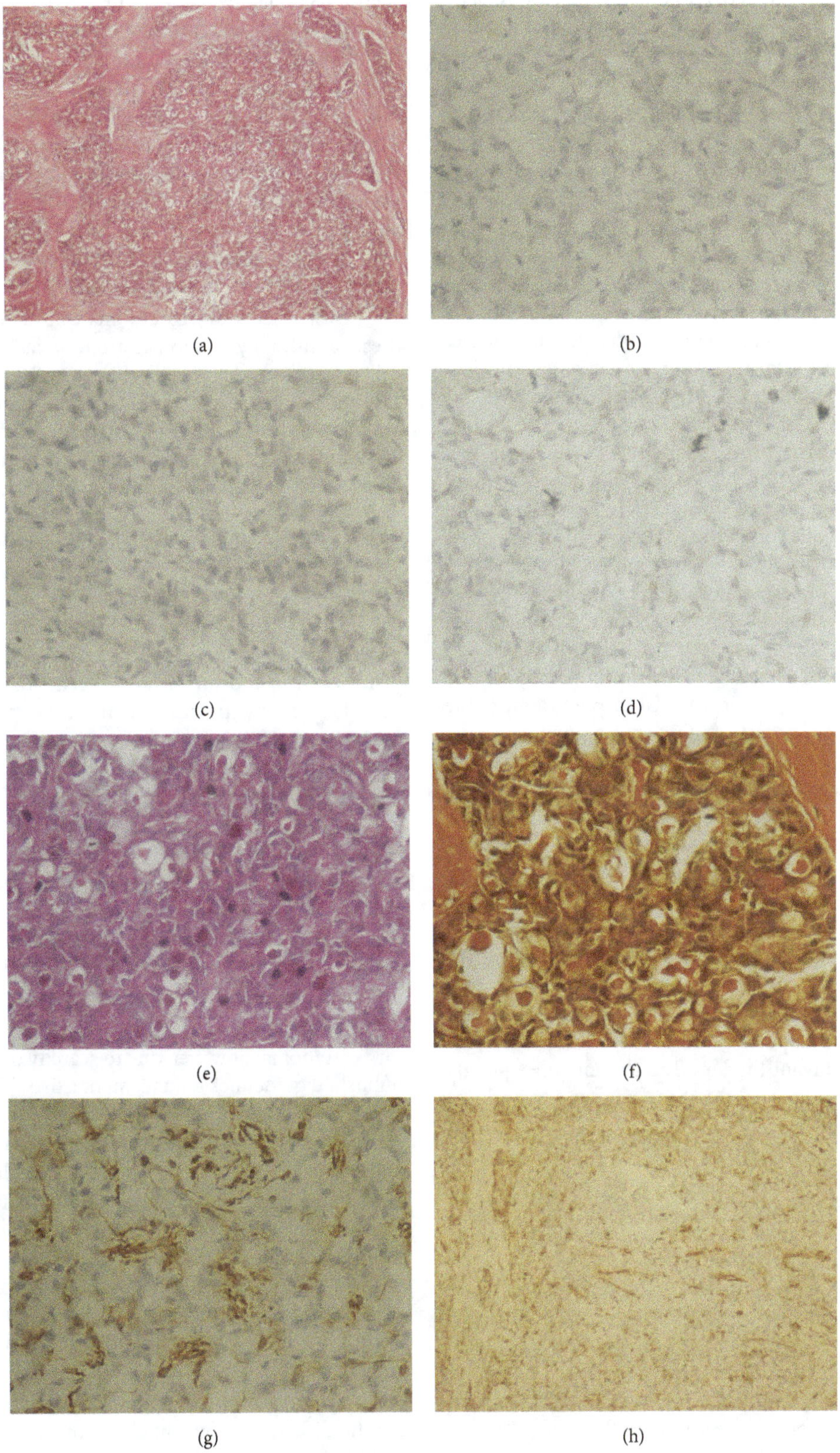

(a) (b) (c) (d) (e) (f) (g) (h)

FIGURE 1: (a) Scanner view of hematoxylin and eosin stained slide. (b), (c), (d) Immunohistochemistry for estrogen receptor (b), progesterone receptor (c), and HER 2neu (d). Special stains immunohistochemistry showing PAS staining (e), mucicarmine (f), and vimentin at 400x (g) and at 100x (h).

Postoperatively the patient made an uneventful recovery and was treated with 6 cycles of combination of Adriamycin, Cyclophosphamide, and Paclitaxel. The patient is healthy after 15 months of follow-up.

3. Case Report 2

A 12-year-old mentally subnormal boy from rural background was brought by his family with a lump in the left subareolar region which was first noticed 6 years back as a small pea sized nodule and grew painlessly to the size of presentation. The patient had no other complaints and his relatives denied any history of similar complaints in the family. The family members reported delayed milestones for the patient who performed poorly for his age and had poor speech and mental development. On examination the patient showed hypertelorism, low set ears, and left sided undescended testis. The breast examination showed a 6 × 6 cm size lump underlying the areola which was firm to hard in consistency and fixed to the overlying thinned skin. The lump was mobile over the underlying muscle. The patient had no axillary lymphadenopathy. On evaluation, otorhinolaryngoscopic evaluation of the patient was within normal limits. Core needle biopsy of the patient showed fibrocollagenous tissue with mild epithelial hyperplasia and was suggestive of gynaecomastia. Ultrasonography of the axillae and the abdomen was normal. Ultrasonography of the scrotum localised the left testis to the left inguinal region.

In view of clinical suspicion the patient was advised a wide local excision of the lump and axillary sampling which on histopathological examination revealed a 5 × 4 cm firm grey lesion harbouring secretory carcinoma with foci of stromal fibrosis and apocrine change with pathologically negative 8 lymph nodes. The margins were negative for presence of the tumor. The tumor was negative for estrogen and progesterone receptors and Her2neu. On immunohistochemistry the tumor stained positive for S-100 stain (Figure 2).

In view of the subnormal mentation of the patient and the lack of definitive supportive data in the disease subset, his relatives refused adjuvant therapy. The patient subsequently is on periodic surveillance and is healthy after 6 months of follow-up.

4. Discussion

Secretory carcinoma is a very rare type of breast carcinoma. Lamovec and Bracko reported 4 cases of SBC in their retrospective series of 7038 breast carcinoma cases [4], and Botta et al. [5] found one case of SBC among 3000 breast carcinoma cases. Li et al. reported 15 cases in their pathologic review of 10000 breast carcinoma cases [6].

The age at presentation varies from 3 to 87 years old with a mean and median age of presentation of 33 and 40 years, respectively [7]. Most of the cases occur in females with a male : female ratio of 1 : 6. In our review we found only 27 other cases of the disease in male patients [6]. Reports suggest that the disease tends to be more aggressive in males.

The patients commonly present with a slow growing, painless, well-circumscribed, mobile, palpable, subareolar mass in the breast. The mean tumor size is 3 cm. The literature mentions nodal involvement in 15% of the patients at presentation [8]. Although rare, metastatic disease at presentation has also been reported [9].

On ultrasonography a solitary, microlobulated, hypoechoic round or oval or tubular mass is seen resembling a benign lesion or well-circumscribed carcinoma. The typically slow growth and imaging make it a challenging diagnosis. The differential diagnoses include a wide range of benign conditions or malignant lesions (i.e., cystic hypersecretory hyperplasia, juvenile papillomatosis with apocrine metaplasia or mucinous carcinoma, and apocrine carcinoma).

Invasive secretory carcinoma can be differentiated from these entities by demonstration of lack of myoepithelial cell layer on a core needle biopsy. SBCs can present with several histological patterns including solid, microcystic, and ductal, with many tumors containing all three patterns [10]. The tumor cells are polygonal with granular eosinophilic cytoplasm. Atypia is minimal or absent and mitotic activity is low. The two distinctive pathological characteristics of SBC are intracellular/extracellular secretions and granular eosinophilic cytoplasm of the neoplastic cells. The intracellular and extracellular secretions can be periodic acid Schiff (diastase resistant) and mucicarmine positive. Although SBC is well circumscribed macroscopically, there may be foci of invasion in the surrounding breast tissue and associated ductal carcinoma in situ, which can be responsible for local recurrence after incomplete resection. The usefulness of FNA in pediatric patients is established but unproven in adults in whom core needle has been the preferred method.

Immunohistochemistry shows the SBC to be triple negative tumors with recently recognized balanced translocation t(12;15) ETV6-NTRK3 fusion gene. This is the first demonstration of a balanced translocation in breast cancer and was known to be associated with congenital fibrosarcoma and mesoblastic nephroma, two morphologically similar pediatric mesenchymal tumors.

Surgery is considered the mainstay of treatment of secretory carcinoma; however, due to scarcity of reported cases no published guidelines management exists. The demonstration of late local recurrence has led many to propose mastectomy for the patients with this disease [11]. Conservative surgery with delayed reconstruction is particularly lucrative in younger patients where breast development has not occurred. Considering the overall incidence of axillary lymph node infiltration is around 30% in children and adults regardless of gender an axillary lymph node dissection is advocated by some authors for tumors ≥2 cm [12]. Nevertheless, sentinel node biopsy may be useful for secretory carcinomas and recent reports suggest feasibility.

Adjuvant chemotherapy and radiation have been tried for the disease without much success. This falls contrary to the high degree of chemosensitivity shown by congenital fibrosarcomas and mesoblastic nephromas to traditional chemotherapeutic drugs. At present, they are considered mainly for the rare advanced presentation of disease. The identification of the specific gene mutation may pave way for targeted molecular therapies for this disease.

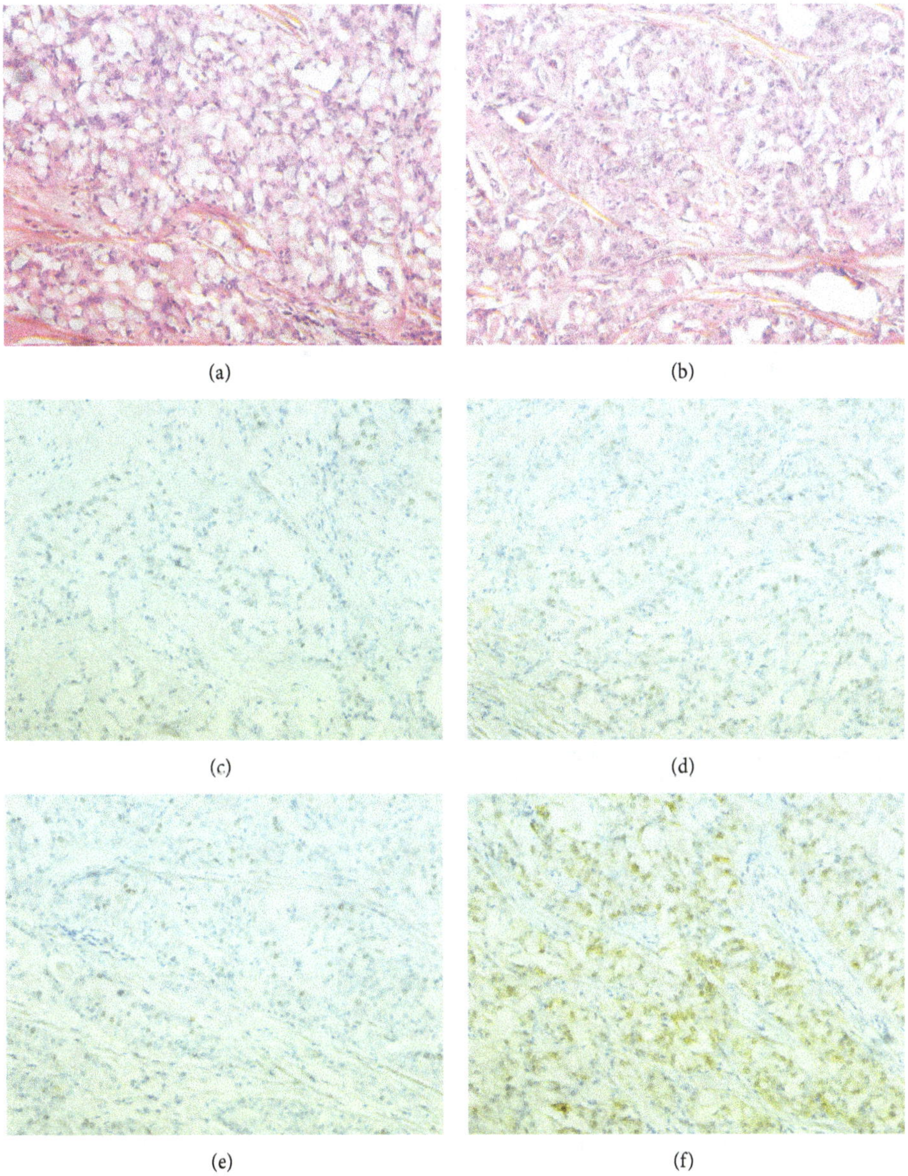

FIGURE 2: (a), (b) Hematoxylin and eosin showing sheets of glands. Immunohistochemistry for estrogen receptor (c), progesterone receptor (d), and HER 2neu (e) and S-100 positivity (f) each on 400x.

5. Conclusion

Secretory breast cancer is a rare indolent tumor that is best treated surgically. Conservative surgery owing to high rate of local recurrence has little role in adults. The role of adjuvant therapy also remains poorly defined and better understanding may allow targeted therapies in the future.

Acknowledgment

This work was done at the Division of Surgical Oncology at S.M.S. Medical College and Hospital, Jaipur, India.

References

[1] R. W. McDivitt and F. W. Stewart, "Breast carcinoma in children," *The Journal of the American Medical Association*, vol. 195, no. 5, pp. 388–390, 1966.

[2] M. Laé, P. Fréneaux, X. Sastre-Garau, O. Chouchane, B. Sigal-Zafrani, and A. Vincent-Salomon, "Secretory breast carcinomas with ETV6-NTRK3 fusion gene belong to the basal-like carcinoma spectrum," *Modern Pathology*, vol. 22, no. 2, pp. 291–298, 2009.

[3] F. A. Tavassoli and H. J. Norris, "Secretory carcinoma of the breast," *Cancer*, vol. 45, no. 9, pp. 2404–2413, 1980.

[4] J. Lamovec and M. Bracko, "Secretory carcinoma of the breast: light microscopical, immunohistochemical and flow cytometric study," *Modern Pathology*, vol. 7, no. 4, pp. 475–479, 1994.

[5] G. Botta, L. Fessia, and B. Ghiringhello, "Juvenile milk protein secreting carcinoma," *Virchows Archiv A Pathological Anatomy and Histology*, vol. 395, no. 2, pp. 145–152, 1982.

[6] D. Li, X. Xiao, W. Yang et al., "Secretory breast carcinoma: a clinicopathological and immunophenotypic study of 15 cases with a review of the literature," *Modern Pathology*, vol. 25, no. 4, pp. 567–575, 2012.

[7] K. Kawase, K. Iwase, S. Miyakawa et al., "A case of secretory carcinoma of the breast in a elderly Japanese woman," *Gan No Rinsho*, vol. 35, no. 8, pp. 943–947, 1989.

[8] S. Vieni, D. Cabibi, C. Cipolla, S. Fricano, G. Graceffa, and M. A. Latteri, "Secretory breast carcinoma with metastatic sentinel lymph node," *World Journal of Surgical Oncology*, vol. 4, article 88, 2006.

[9] F. A. Tavassoli and P. Devilee, *World Health Organization Classification of Tumors. Tumors of the Breast and Female Genital Organs*, IARC Press, Lyon, France, 2nd edition, 2003.

[10] F. Grabellus, K. Worm, A. Willruth et al., "ETV6-NTRK3 gene fusion in a secretory carcinoma of the breast of a male-to-female transsexual," *Breast*, vol. 14, no. 1, pp. 71–74, 2005.

[11] C. Arce, D. Cortes-Padilla, D. G. Huntsman et al., "Secretory carcinoma of the breast containing the ETV6-NTRK3 fusion gene in a male: case report and review of the literature," *World Journal of Surgical Oncology*, vol. 3, article 35, 2005.

[12] G. Richard, J. C. Hawk III, A. S. Baker Jr., and R. M. Austin, "Multicentric adult secretory breast carcinoma: DNA flow cytometric findings, prognostic features, and review of the world literature," *Journal of Surgical Oncology*, vol. 44, no. 4, pp. 238–244, 1990.

8

Adult Alveolar Soft Part Sarcoma of the Head and Neck

Brandon T. Mullins[1] and Trevor Hackman[2]

[1]*School of Medicine, University of North Carolina School of Medicine, 1033 Bondurant Hall, Chapel Hill, NC 27514, USA*
[2]*Division of Otolaryngology, University of North Carolina Hospitals, 101 Manning Drive, Chapel Hill, NC 27514, USA*

Correspondence should be addressed to Brandon T. Mullins; brandon_mullins@med.unc.edu

Academic Editor: Raffaele Palmirotta

Background. Alveolar soft part sarcomas (ASPS) of the head and neck are rare, aggressive soft-tissue malignancies. This study describes the clinical course and management of two patients presenting with ASPS in very rare head and neck locations, the larynx and parotid gland. *Methods.* We identified two patients presenting with ASPS of the head and neck and treated at the University of North Carolina. We compared our results to the literature from 1987 to 2013. *Results.* Patient ages at diagnosis were 27 and 39 with presenting symptoms of hoarseness and parotid swelling, respectively. Mean follow-up was 87 months. All patients received surgical resection and adjuvant radiotherapy. There were no recurrences or evidence of distant metastatic spread during the series. Disease-free survival time for the patients was 4 months and 168 months, respectively. *Conclusions.* Our study suggests that a combined-modality approach is important in the treatment of ASPS of the head and neck even in these rare locations. Continued research into new therapies is necessary to improve historically poor outcomes.

1. Introduction

Alveolar soft part sarcoma (ASPS) is a rare soft-tissue malignancy constituting less than 1% of soft-tissue sarcomas with only about 25% of those occurring in the head and neck [1–7]. In the head and neck region typical sites include the tongue and orbit, with other sites being very rare [2–4, 6–8]. It primarily affects adolescents and young adults (between the ages 15 and 35) and has a predilection for females over males [5–8]. Though they are relatively indolent in nature, due to their high rates of late-onset metastasis, they typically have a poor long-term prognosis [8, 9].

This IRB-approved retrospective case series describes two patients with ASPS of the head and neck treated at the University of North Carolina. Both patients present with very rare locations for head and neck ASPS (the larynx and parotid gland) with only a few known cases reported in the literature [2, 9–11]. They were diagnosed based on a thorough history and physical examination and pathologically confirmed through biopsy and histopathological analysis, with one case also including cytogenetic confirmation. For each case, wide-local surgical excision and adjuvant radiotherapy were the treatment of choice. Our goal is to add to the literature by reporting the clinical presentation, histopathologic and immunohistochemical findings, therapeutic considerations, and outcomes of two very rare locations for head and neck ASPS with a literature review.

2. Clinical Cases

2.1. Case 1. A 27-year-old male presented to our hospital with a 3-year history of hoarseness. He reported that the hoarseness had been worsening over the past few months and was newly associated with increased throat clearing and an occasional eating-associated cough. The past history was otherwise unremarkable.

Head and neck physical examination was unremarkable without evidence of masses, lesions, or cervical adenopathy. Endoscopy was then performed for further assessment. Flexible fiberoptic laryngoscopy revealed a left-sided submucosal mass of the false vocal cord obstructing the view of the underlying left true vocal cord. Normal mobility of the true

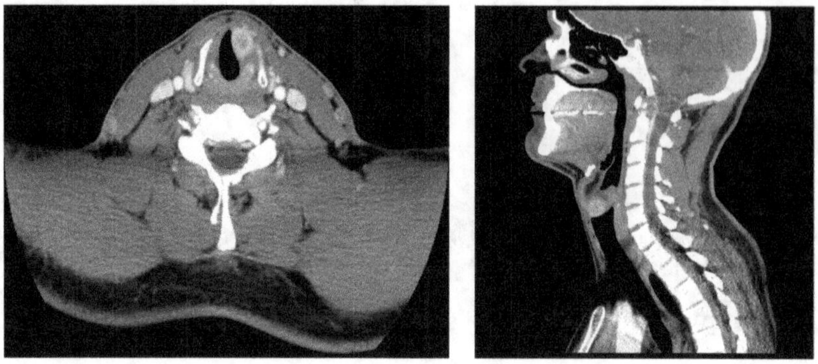

(a) (b)

Figure 1: Axial (a) and sagittal (b) CT of the avidly enhancing mass in the anterior left vocal cord.

vocal cords was noted and there was good glottis closure with pronation. The rest of the laryngeal exam was unremarkable.

Computed tomography (CT) revealed a 1.5 × 1.2 × 1.5 cm avidly enhancing mass in the anterior left vocal cord (Figure 1). The lesion involved the true left vocal cord and extended superiorly into the left laryngeal ventricle to the level of the left false vocal cord. There was no involvement of the left epiglottic fold, but there was slight infraglottic extension. A chest radiograph was obtained for staging and ruled-out pulmonary metastases and mediastinal adenopathy. Biopsy was then performed under general anesthesia revealing a firm, yellow mass somewhat alveolar and grape-like in appearance.

Microscopic examination of the biopsy specimen revealed a multilobulated spindle cell lesion. Many of the lobules were composed of nests of large polygonal cells containing finely granular eosinophilic cytoplasm and separated by delicate vessels. Based on the structure, the differential diagnosis included ASPS, perivascular epithelioid cell tumor (PEComa), or possibly metastatic carcinoma.

Immunohistochemistry then revealed negative staining results for epithelial membrane antigen (EMA), cytokeratin AE1/AE3, Cam 5.2, S-100, HMB-45, Melan-A, and smooth muscle actin, with rare cells positive for desmin. TFE-3 then showed diffuse nuclear positivity. These results narrowed the differential to ASPS or PEComa. To confirm the diagnosis, FISH analysis was then performed to evaluate for TFE-3 gene rearrangement. A characteristic feature of ASPS is the unbalanced TFE-3 translocation; however, in this case, the translocation was determined to be balanced, even on repeated analysis. Given the observed morphology and gene rearrangement results in the limited biopsy sample, PEComa was the preliminary diagnosis.

The patient was consented for excision of the mass via an endoscopic left vertical hemilaryngectomy excising the left true and false vocal cord. Intraoperatively, all frozen section margins were reported to be clear of tumor; however, on final pathologic analysis, two of the frozen section margins contained residual tumor. Also, now evaluating a larger sample, pathology concluded that the characteristic microscopic appearance and the immunohistochemical results should override the molecular results and made the final diagnosis of ASPS.

Laser reexcision was then performed to manage the initial positive margins, resulting in negative margins, and it was determined that no residual tumor was present in the reexcised specimen. Considering the initial positive margins, the narrow surgical field, and the inability to obtain wide margins while sparing the larynx, the multidisciplinary tumor board decided to include adjuvant radiotherapy in the treatment plan to reduce the risk of local recurrence. The patient received radiotherapy (59.4 Gy) at an outside hospital closer to home due to additional family support. He responded well to the therapy, had no complications, and is disease-free 4 months after the completion of treatment.

2.2. Case 2. A 37-year-old female presented to our institution with a 2-year history of left cheek swelling. The swelling was located in the region of the parotid gland and was not associated with pain. The past history was otherwise unremarkable.

Head and neck physical examination revealed a 2 × 2 cm firm, nontender mass in the left parotid area. The mass did not appear to be fixed to the underlying tissues. No adenopathy was appreciated and the remainder of the exam was unremarkable. Flexible fiberoptic nasal laryngoscopy was then performed for further evaluation, also determined to be unremarkable. CT scan was previously obtained at an outside institution and was not available to report.

Fine-needle aspiration was then performed to evaluate the mass. The initial assessment reported the presence of oncocytic cells consistent with an oncocytoma. The patient was then consented for excision of the mass via a left superficial parotidectomy, which was completed with close surgical margins.

Microscopic examination of the excised mass revealed a 2.1 cm discrete, possibly encapsulated, tumor consisting of nests and sheets of large, moderately pleomorphic, and polygonal cells bounded by broad fibrous septae with abundant small vessels. The cells showed minimal nuclear pleomorphism, prominent single central nucleoli, and abundant clear to eosinophilic granular cytoplasm. Rare mitotic figures were also noted. The differential diagnosis included oncocytoma, myoepithelioma, melanoma, adult rhabdomyoma, and ASPS.

Immunohistochemistry then revealed focal reactivity to desmin with no reactivity for actin, S100, HMB45, keratin,

Table 1: Clinical characteristics of the alveolar soft part sarcoma series.

Case	Age	Gender	Location	Tumor size	Symptoms
1	27	Male	Larynx	1.5 cm	Hoarseness
2	39	Female	Parotid gland	2.1 cm	Enlarging mass

synaptophysin, or chromogranin. This immunophenotype supported the diagnoses of adult type rhabdomyoma and alveolar soft part sarcoma and excluded the others. Periodic acid Schiff (PAS) staining was then performed revealing focal reactivity with some cells showing an intracytoplasmic crystalline material. It was then determined that the PAS positive structure combined with the desmin reactivity was most consistent with ASPS.

Since ASPS has a high metastatic rate, especially to the lung, chest CT was performed for staging and ruled out pulmonary metastases. Considering the close surgical margins, she then underwent adjuvant radiotherapy to a total dose of 63.4 Gy. There were no major complications from treatment. Since completion of radiotherapy she has had regular follow-up and has remained disease-free 168 months after the completion of her treatment.

3. Discussion

Alveolar soft part sarcomas are extremely rare soft-tissue sarcomas, typically occurring in the deep soft tissues of the lower extremities, and are especially rare in the head and neck [8, 9]. Clinically they are rather indolent in nature, with a slow clinical course, and usually present with functional impairment due to primary tumor location (i.e., hoarseness or dysphagia) or as a painless slowly enlarging mass, as seen in our cases (Table 1) [6, 8, 9]. However, due to their highly vascular nature, they also have a high rate of distant metastasis, with the lungs, brain, and bone being the most common sites [6, 8, 9]. Lung metastases are most common and are seen in 40–60% of cases [9, 12–14]. While hematogenous spread is the typical route, lymphatic metastasis is also seen in around 7–10% of cases [9, 15].

For the diagnosis of ASPS, imaging combined with analysis of the histologic, immunochemical, and molecular genetic features is beneficial. On imaging, the tumor demonstrates low attenuation on noncontrast CT and strong tumor enhancement with contrast administration. TI- and T2-weighted MRI images typically show higher signal intensity than muscle while demonstrating tubular areas of flow voids, representative of rapid blood flow within the tumor [16, 17]. Microscopically, ASPS is characterized by a pseudoalveolar appearance with clustered polygonal tumor cells, containing an abundant eosinophilic to clear granular cytoplasm, and separated by capillary-sized vascular channels and connective tissue [8, 12, 18]. On immunohistochemistry, the tumor cells are typically negative for epithelial markers (i.e., EMA and cytokeratins), chromogranin A, synaptophysin, S-100, HMB45, and Melan-A [8]. Desmin may be positive in around 50% of cases, and nonspecific markers such as neurone-specific enolase and vimentin may be positive in 30–50% of cases [8]. Most characteristically, ASPS exhibits cytoplasmic crystals containing PAS-positive and diastase-resistant material, which is seen in 80% of cases [9, 12, 15, 18]. In addition, on molecular genetic analysis, ASPS can be characterized by the der(17)t(X:17)(p11.2;p25) translocation. This unbalanced translocation between chromosomes 17q25 and Xp11.2 leads to the ASPL-TFE3 fusion gene, which activates the MET promoter and confirms the diagnosis [8, 11, 18–20]. The diagnostic features of the cases presented were mostly consistent with the literature. The tumor in case 1 demonstrated the expected enhancement on contrast imaging, microscopic examination in both cases revealed large polygonal cells with granular eosinophilic cytoplasm separated by small vessels, and immunohistochemical results in each case demonstrated either PAS-positive cytoplasmic crystalline material or TFE-3 nuclear positivity (representing the fusion gene) with most other markers staining negative. The major differing feature presented in case 1 was the balanced translocation between 17q25 and Xp11.2. However, though very rare, this balanced translocation has been reported a few times in the literature [21, 22]. The difficulty in reaching a final pathologic diagnosis in our cases, especially case 1, shows that careful and thorough diagnostic testing is essential for proper diagnosis of ASPS, especially in rarer anatomic locations.

Due to the rarity of ASPS of the head and neck, the optimal treatment plan has not been clearly elucidated. Currently, the main treatment of primary ASPS, like most soft-tissue sarcomas, is surgical removal using a wide-local excision with the goal of obtaining negative margins [6, 7, 9]. The attainment of negative margins after surgical resection has been shown to increase local control and survival rates. Due to the low rate of lymphatic spread, neck dissection is typically only utilized when palpable nodes are present rather than prophylactically [6, 9]. When metastatic lesions are present in the lung or brain, the current standard treatment is also surgical excision aiming for negative margins as it has been linked to increased median survival [18, 23, 24].

The role of radiotherapy has been controversial. Early studies reported no significant benefit with the addition of radiotherapy [24, 25]. For example, Lieberman et al., in a 102-patient review of ASPS at all sites from 1952 to 1987, reported that there was no survival advantage for patients treated with radiotherapy [24]. However, more recent studies by Sherman et al., Anderson et al., and Ogura et al., all, showed significant benefit in local control amongst their patients who received adjuvant radiotherapy after primary surgical removal [18, 26, 27]. In addition, Ogura et al. found radiotherapy benefit in treating patients with brain metastases due to ASPS [18]. Four of their patients with brain metastases were treated with gamma knife radiotherapy and all achieved satisfactory local control, with a median progression-free survival time of 12 months. They were all alive at last follow-up. Historically, the

Table 2: Treatment and outcomes of the alveolar soft part sarcoma series.

Case	Primary treatment	Margin status	Recurrence location	Time to recurrence	Disease-free survival
1	Surgery + adjuvant radiotherapy	Positive	N/A	N/A	4 months (Alive)
2	Surgery + adjuvant radiotherapy	Negative	N/A	N/A	168 months (Alive)

median survival time after brain metastases diagnosis from ASPS is 12 months [18]. There has been little study in this area, and more research should be conducted to evaluate the most efficacious treatment between gamma knife radiotherapy and surgical resection for ASPS brain metastases. The patients in our study were both treated with surgical resection and adjuvant radiotherapy which resulted in a good clinical result (Table 2). Both patients have remained recurrence-free, with progression-free survival times of 168 months and 4 months.

Conventional cytotoxic chemotherapy has been widely reported to have little benefit in the treatment of ASPS [13–15, 18, 24, 25, 27]. Many sources have cited the lack of efficacy for agents like doxorubicin, ifosfamide, dacarbazine, gemcitabine, vincristine, docetaxel, melphalan, and TNF-alpha [14, 18, 24, 25, 27–29]. Due to this, neither of the patients in our series underwent chemotherapy treatment. However, recently, more evidence has appeared for the use of antiangiogenic agents in the treatment of ASPS. Given the highly vascular nature of ASPS, antiangiogenic agents like bevacizumab, sunitinib malate, and cediranib have shown promise in small series and clinical trials for the treatment of primary and metastatic ASPS [18, 30–34]. Gardner et al. reported substantial single-agent effectiveness against ASPS in a 7-patient clinical trial [34]. Ogura et al. also noted significant tumor shrinkage with a progression-free survival period of 27 months in their patients treated with cediranib [18]. Based on early promising results such as these, continued research into the efficacy of these agents is needed to hopefully improve outcomes in ASPS. In addition, given that the ASPL-TFE3 fusion protein binds to the MET promoter and can lead to high rates of MET overexpression, molecularly targeted therapy against MET may also be a potential therapeutic target [35].

Despite current treatments, the long-term prognosis for ASPS has remained poor due to the high rate of metastatic disease. Lieberman et al. cited 2-year, 5-year, 10-year, and 20-year survival rates of 77%, 60%, 38%, and only 15%, respectively [24]. Similar 5-year and 10-year survival rates have also been reported in more recent studies [14, 18, 26]. Portera et al. reported that while the 5-year disease-free survival rate was 71% for patients presenting with localized disease, the rate dropped to 20% for patients presenting with metastases [14]. It has also been cited that median survival time decreased from a median of 11 years to 3 years when metastasis was present on presentation [9]. In recent studies, metastases on presentation have been reported in 48–65% of patients [14, 18, 20, 29], with posttreatment metastatic rates ranging from 19 to 24% [14, 18, 20]. The local recurrence rate has been similar, ranging from about 10 to 25% [14, 20, 24, 28, 36]. The rarity of ASPS in the head and neck region makes it difficult to determine prognostic factors for survival, as most studies are smaller clinical series. Though, when viewing studies based on ASPS of all sites, tumor size and AJCC stage have most readily been correlated with survival [14, 18, 24, 25, 29]. It is difficult to evaluate prognostic factor correlations in our small sample. Both patients had small tumors (less than 5 cm in size), presented at a low stage without metastasis, and received adjuvant radiotherapy despite margin status, and both patients are alive and have had good clinical outcomes.

In conclusion, our study reports two cases of head and neck ASPS in extremely rare locations, the larynx and parotid gland. When presenting in rare locations such as these, diagnosis can be difficult and analyses of the histopathologic, immunohistochemical, and molecular genetic features are beneficial for confirmation. Due to its rarity in the literature, the optimal treatment for ASPS has yet to be clearly elucidated. The most evidence seems to conclude that wide-local excision with adjuvant radiotherapy is the best current therapy, though long-term survival remains poor. Hopefully, continued research into new therapies such as antiangiogenic agents, as well as stringent follow-up for late-metastatic detection, will improve the poor outcomes of ASPS.

References

[1] K. Anbarasi, S. Sathasivasubramanian, and S. Kuruvilla, "Alveolar soft-part sarcoma of tongue," *Indian Journal of Pathology and Microbiology*, vol. 54, no. 3, pp. 581–583, 2011.

[2] T. Altuğ, E. Inci, M. G. Güvenç, D. T. Edizer, and S. Dervişoğlu, "Alveolar soft part sarcoma of the larynx," *European Archives of Oto-Rhino-Laryngology*, vol. 264, no. 4, pp. 445–449, 2007.

[3] J. G. Batsakis, "Alveolar soft-part sarcoma," *Annals of Otology, Rhinology & Laryngology*, vol. 97, no. 3, part 1, pp. 328–329, 1988.

[4] R. P. Bentley, M. J. C. Wake, and F. Raafat, "Alveolar soft part sarcoma of the tongue," *British Journal of Oral and Maxillofacial Surgery*, vol. 37, no. 6, pp. 451–454, 1999.

[5] P. P. Argyris, R. C. Reed, J. C. Manivel et al., "Oral alveolar soft part sarcoma in childhood and adolescence: report of two cases and review of literature," *Head and Neck Pathology*, vol. 7, no. 1, pp. 40–49, 2013.

[6] T. Baglam, M. E. Kalender, C. Durucu et al., "Alveolar soft part sarcoma of the tongue," *The Journal of Craniofacial Surgery*, vol. 20, no. 6, pp. 2160–2162, 2009.

[7] N. Ordonez and M. Ladanyi, "Alveolar Soft Part Sarcoma," in *World Health Organization Classification of Tumours, Pathology and Genetics, Tumours of Soft Tissue and Bone*, C. Fletcher, K. Unni, and F. Mertens, Eds., IARC Press, Lyon, France, 2002.

[8] A. L. Folpe and A. T. Deyrup, "Alveolar soft-part sarcoma: a review and update," *Journal of Clinical Pathology*, vol. 59, no. 11, pp. 1127–1132, 2006.

[9] H. S. Kim, H. K. Lee, Y.-C. Weon, and H.-J. Kim, "Alveolar soft-part sarcoma of the head and neck: clinical and imaging features in five cases," *American Journal of Neuroradiology*, vol. 26, no. 6, pp. 1331–1335, 2005.

[10] M. de Sautel, R. Gandour-Edwards, P. Donald, R. Munn, L. Barnes, and P. Vogt, "Alveolar soft part sarcoma: report of a case occurring in the larynx," *Otolaryngology—Head and Neck Surgery*, vol. 117, no. 6, pp. S95–S97, 1997.

[11] K. Kusafuka, K. Muramatsu, T. Yabuzaki et al., "Alveolar soft part sarcoma of the larynx: a case report of an unusual location with immunohistochemical and ultrastructural analyses," *Head & Neck*, vol. 30, no. 9, pp. 1257–1263, 2008.

[12] H.-W. Wang, W. Dai, X.-J. Qin, and C.-P. Zhang, "A new clinical manifestation for cheek alveolar soft-part sarcoma: a case report and review of the literature," *Journal of Oral and Maxillofacial Surgery*, vol. 72, no. 4, pp. 817–822, 2014.

[13] M. L. Kayton, P. Meyers, L. H. Wexler, W. L. Gerald, and M. P. LaQuaglia, "Clinical presentation, treatment, and outcome of alveolar soft part sarcoma in children, adolescents, and young adults," *Journal of Pediatric Surgery*, vol. 41, no. 1, pp. 187–193, 2006.

[14] C. A. Portera Jr., V. Ho, S. R. Patel et al., "Alveolar soft part sarcoma: clinical course and patterns of metastasis in 70 patients treated at a single institution," *Cancer*, vol. 91, no. 3, pp. 585–591, 2001.

[15] K. A. Eley, T. Afzal, K. A. Shah, and S. R. Watt-Smith, "Alveolar soft-part sarcoma of the tongue: report of a case and review of the literature," *International Journal of Oral and Maxillofacial Surgery*, vol. 39, no. 8, pp. 824–826, 2010.

[16] Y. Iwamoto, N. Morimoto, H. Chuman, N. Shinohara, and Y. Sugioka, "The role of MR imaging in the diagnosis of alveolar soft part sarcoma: a report of 10 cases," *Skeletal Radiology*, vol. 24, no. 4, pp. 267–270, 1995.

[17] R. Silbergleit, R. Agrawal, A. T. Savera, and S. C. Patel, "Alveolar soft-part sarcoma of the neck," *Neuroradiology*, vol. 44, no. 10, pp. 861–863, 2002.

[18] K. Ogura, Y. Beppu, H. Chuman et al., "Alveolar soft part sarcoma: a single-center 26-patient case series and review of the literature," *Sarcoma*, vol. 2012, Article ID 907179, 6 pages, 2012.

[19] A. M. Rose, J. Kabiru, and G. E. Rose, "Alveolar soft-part sarcoma of the orbit," *African Journal of Paediatric Surgery*, vol. 8, no. 1, pp. 82–84, 2011.

[20] B. Rekhi, R. Kumar, S. Menon, S. Medhi, and S. B. Desai, "Calvarial metastasis of a renal cell carcinoma, mimicking a primary alveolar soft part sarcoma, in a young girl-a rare case report," *Pathology and Oncology Research*, vol. 15, no. 1, pp. 137–141, 2009.

[21] M. Ladanyi, M. Y. Lui, C. R. Antonescu et al., "The der(17)t(X;17)(p11;q25) of human alveolar soft part sarcoma fuses the TFE3 transcription factor gene to ASPL, a novel gene at 17q25," *Oncogene*, vol. 20, no. 1, pp. 48–57, 2001.

[22] S. Uppal, H. Aviv, F. Patterson et al., "Alveolar soft part sarcoma-reciprocal translocation between chromosome 17q25 and Xp11 report of a case with metastases at presentation and review of the literature," *Acta Orthopaedica Belgica*, vol. 69, no. 2, pp. 182–187, 2003.

[23] A. Yavuz, C. Göya, A. Bora, and M. Beyazal, "Primary alveolar soft part sarcoma of the scapula," *Case Reports in Oncology*, vol. 6, no. 2, pp. 356–361, 2013.

[24] P. H. Lieberman, M. F. Brennan, M. Kimmel, R. A. Erlandson, P. Garin-Chesa, and B. Y. Flehinger, "Alveolar soft-part sarcoma. A clinico-pathologic study of half a century," *Cancer*, vol. 63, no. 1, pp. 1–13, 1989.

[25] M. Casanova, A. Ferrari, G. Bisogno et al., "Alveolar soft part sarcoma in children and adolescents: a report from the soft-tissue sarcoma italian cooperative group," *Annals of Oncology*, vol. 11, no. 11, pp. 1445–1449, 2000.

[26] N. Sherman, M. Vavilala, R. Pollock, M. Romsdahl, and N. Jaffe, "Radiation therapy for alveolar soft-part sarcoma," *Medical and Pediatric Oncology*, vol. 22, no. 6, pp. 380–383, 1994.

[27] M. E. Anderson, F. J. Hornicek, M. C. Gebhardt, K. A. Raskin, and H. J. Mankin, "Alveolar soft part sarcoma: a rare and enigmatic entity," *Clinical Orthopaedics & Related Research*, vol. 438, pp. 144–148, 2005.

[28] H. E. Auerbach and J. J. Brooks, "Alveolar soft part sarcoma: a clinicopathologic and immunohistochemical study," *Cancer*, vol. 60, no. 1, pp. 66–73, 1987.

[29] A. Ogose, Y. Yazawa, T. Ueda et al., "Alveolar soft part sarcoma in Japan: multi-institutional study of 57 patients from the Japanese Musculoskeletal Oncology Group," *Oncology*, vol. 65, no. 1, pp. 7–13, 2003.

[30] A. A. Azizi, C. Haberler, T. Czech et al., "Vascular-endothelial-growth-factor (VEGF) expression and possible response to angiogenesis inhibitor bevacizumab in metastatic alveolar soft part sarcoma," *Lancet Oncology*, vol. 7, no. 6, pp. 521–523, 2006.

[31] S. Stacchiotti, E. Tamborini, A. Marrari et al., "Response to sunitinib malate in advanced alveolar soft part sarcoma," *Clinical Cancer Research*, vol. 15, no. 3, pp. 1096–1104, 2009.

[32] S. Kummar, D. Allen, A. Monks et al., "Cediranib for metastatic alveolar soft part sarcoma," *Journal of Clinical Oncology*, vol. 31, no. 18, pp. 2296–2302, 2013.

[33] I. R. Judson, M. Scurr, K. Gardner et al., "Phase II study of cediranib in patients with advanced gastrointestinal stromal tumors or soft-tissue sarcoma," *Clinical Cancer Research*, vol. 20, no. 13, pp. 3603–3612, 2014.

[34] K. Gardner, I. Judson, M. Leahy et al., "Activity of cediranib, a highly potent and selective VEGF signaling inhibitor, in alveolar soft part sarcoma," *Journal of Clinical Oncology*, vol. 27, supplement 15, abstract 10523, 2009.

[35] H. J. Jun, J. Lee, D. H. Lim et al., "Expression of MET in alveolar soft part sarcoma," *Medical Oncology*, vol. 27, no. 2, pp. 459–465, 2010.

[36] S. Van Ruth, F. Van Coevorden, J. L. Peterse, and B. B. R. Kroon, "Alveolar soft part sarcoma: a report of 15 cases," *European Journal of Cancer*, vol. 38, no. 10, pp. 1324–1328, 2002.

9

Scalp Melanoma Diagnosed by Fine Needle Aspiration Cytology in a Tertiary Health Center

A. B. Zarami,[1] N. A. Satumari,[2] and M. Ahmed[2]

[1] *Department of Histopathology, University of Maiduguri Teaching Hospital, PMB 1414, Maiduguri, Borno State, Nigeria*
[2] *Department of Medical Laboratory Science, University of Maiduguri, PMB 1069, Maiduguri, Borno State, Nigeria*

Correspondence should be addressed to A. B. Zarami; abbabukarzarami51@yahoo.com, N. A. Satumari; nas0265@yahoo.com, and M. Ahmed; ahmedmodu21@gmail.com

Academic Editor: Jaime De la Garza

Melanoma is one of the most aggressive malignant skin neoplasms worldwide with more than 20% of world melanoma seen in black Africa and Asia. Late presentation due to ignorance, poverty, and lack of adequate health facility in Nigeria is always the norms. We present this case report because of precision in diagnosis, using fine needle aspiration cytology (FNAC) to reemphasize that the technique is cheap, cost effective, and quick that can reduce the burden of incisional biopsy before definitive surgery and improve early detection of the disease especially in developing countries.

1. Introduction

Melanoma of skin accounts for 160,000 new cases annually; worldwide there were an estimated 41,000 deaths in 2002 alone [1], and it kills about 8000 Americans each year [2]. The mortality is more in men than in women [3], probably because the site distribution permits earlier diagnosis in females [3]. The neoplasm is generally common in women than in men and particularly common in White populations living in sunny climates [3]; this is thought to be due to ultraviolet radiation; in sub-Saharan Africa trauma is being implicated [4]. Most of the lesion is found in the head and neck area [5] and on the lower extremities, the latter location being particularly common in females. Other locations of cutaneous melanomas are the subungual region ("melanotic whitlow") and the palms, soles, and nail bed [5].

The risk factors of the disease are being white, particularly those of fair complexion, red hair, and a tendency to burn or develop freckles after exposure to sunlight [5, 6]. The presence of a large number of melanocytic nevi represents a risk factor even if these nevi are not of the dysplastic type. The genetically determined disease xeroderma pigmentosum also predisposes to the development of melanoma. Cases of melanoma have been reported in association with type I Recklinghausen disease and in renal transplantation recipients [5].

Melanomas are divided into the following types: lentigo maligna, superficial spreading, acral lentiginous, mucosal, nodular, polypoid, desmoplastic, amelanotic, soft-tissue, melanoma with small nevus-like cells, melanoma with features of a spitz nevus, and uveal melanoma [7]. The superficial spreading type is the commonest and affects head and neck region; the commonest subtype of melanoma in Africa is the nodular variant that affects the feet [4]. The late presentation as always the custom in our environment and the accurate diagnosis using fine needle aspiration cytology in this index case prompted that case report.

2. Case Report

A 30-year-old man presented to our fine needle aspiration cytology (FNAC) clinic at University of Maiduguri Teaching Hospital (UMTH) from outpatient department. He presented with one-year history of scalp swelling and six-month history of cervical swelling; on examination we found scalp mass with variegated colour and ulcer measuring 14×12 cm, the floor is necrotic, and the edge is everted (Figures 1, 2, and 3).

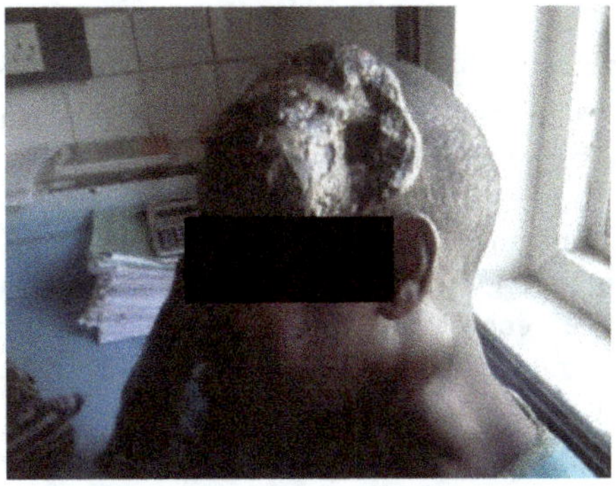

FIGURE 1

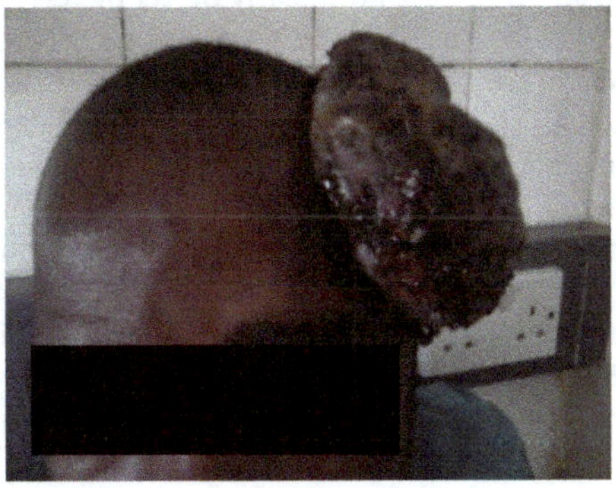

FIGURE 2

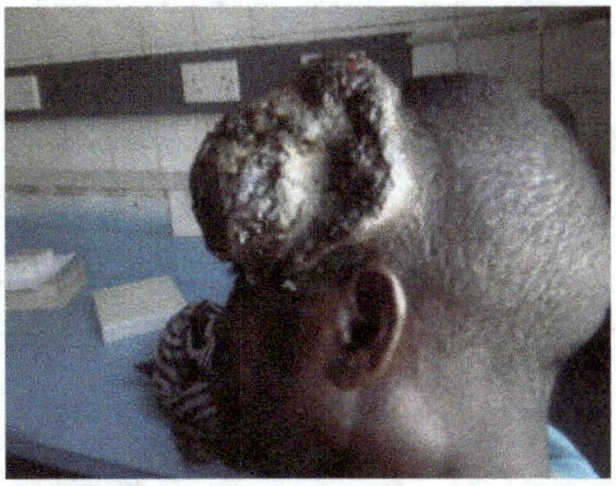

FIGURE 3

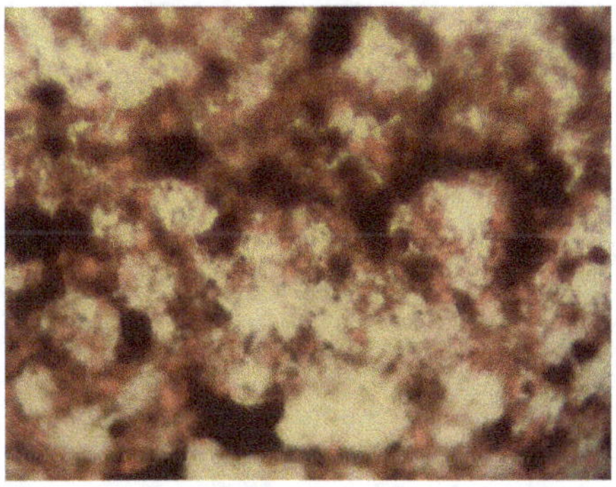

FIGURE 4: Photomicrograph of smear stained with H and E ×100.

There are multiple cervical lymphadenopathies on the ipsilateral side, the largest measuring 4 cm in the widest diameter (Figures 1 and 3).

2.1. Procedure. The FNAC was done using Cameco (needle holder) with 20 mL syringe and 23-gauge needles. Aseptic procedure was observed and verbal consent was obtained from the patient. All ethical consideration was trail before carrying out the procedure and taking photograph. Aided by the Cameco, 0.5 mL of haemorrhagic grey aspirates was obtained. It was then immediately smeared on to a glass slide and then fixed in 95% alcohol for 15 min and then stained by haematoxylin and eosin (H and E). One of the slides was stained with Fontana Masson to demonstrate melanin (Figure 5). We are limited from performing immunohistochemistry, HMB 45, S-100, and Melan-A.

3. Cytology Report

Smears show abundant dark brown pigments along with few pleomorphic cells having round to oval nuclei with moderate cytoplasm. Quite a few cells that have prominent eosinophilic nucleolus each are present (Figure 4). A Fontana Masson stain was positive (Figure 5).

3.1. Diagnosis. Scalp mass/cervical lymph nodes were positive for malignancy (consistent with melanoma).

4. Discussion

Melanoma is the commonest primary skin malignancy, the incidence of which is rising globally [4, 8, 9]. The incident has increased in the last twenty years at the rate of about 5% per year [8]. High rates of incidence are found in Australia/New Zealand, North America, and northern Europe [1]. Survival in developing countries is poorer (around 40%), in part due to late diagnosis and limited access to therapy but also because the tumours are generally acral located on the soles of the feet [1].

In Nigeria melanoma accounts for 34% of all skin malignancies, ranking second to squamous cell carcinoma of skin [9–11]. In a hospital base study in Maiduguri, 31% of all skin malignancies have been reported [4]. In another study in Cameroon, over nine-year period, melanomas represent 4.46% of all cancer and are the most frequent cancer [12]. The neoplasm has high cure rates when diagnosed early but poor survival when found at an advanced stage [13]. Most melanomas are visible on the skin, which allows for self-detection [13], though there is wide differential diagnosis. In a report based on a population-based survey, 53% of melanomas were detected by patients, 26% by physicians, 17% by family, and three percent by others [13]. Further, self-examination leads to decreased melanoma thickness in comparison to patients who do not perform self-examinations, with variable sensitivity data ranging from 25% to 93% but high specificity of 83% to 97% [3]. Despite the benefits of self-examination in early melanoma detection, this is often

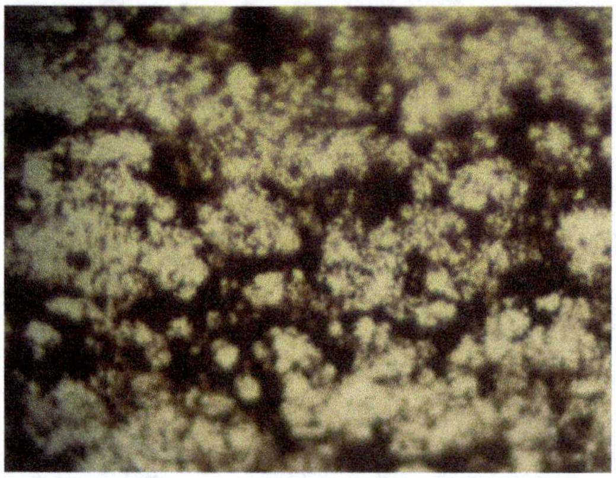

Figure 5: Photomicrograph of smear stained with Fontana Masson ×100.

very difficult on the scalp [13]; late presentations especially in Nigeria are always the norm [4].

Fine needle aspiration cytology (FNAC) is cost-effective, quick, and accurate when used appropriately and has high precision in obtaining sample [13–15], even though its sensitivity and specificity depend on the types of the lesion; however, even rare cases like intraocular and oral melanoma have been diagnosed using FNAC [14, 15]. Nggada et al. reported sensitivity of 88.9% and specificity of 96.1% of FNAC of thyroid nodules over 10-year period with concordance rate of 94.2% [16]. In metastatic melanoma, a positive predictive value of 99% has been reported [17]. FNAC offers direct sampling and identification of the minority that are definite or probable malignancies and those that are follicular neoplasms, which require surgery with full histological assessment to exclude malignancy. Fine needle aspiration is most sensitive at detecting anaplastic (almost 100%) and papillary (around 90%) carcinomas of thyroid glands [13]. Although FNAC has greater accuracy in identifying tumours than alternative imaging or biochemical methods, it misses 5–10% of cancers. Even so, its incorporation into the diagnosis of thyroid nodules reduces the requirement for excision by at least 25% and doubles the yield of cancer in those that are excised [3, 13]. Core biopsy is more traumatic and has not been shown to increase accuracy of diagnosis [13].

Generally there is suboptimal utilization of FNAC in Nigeria despite its potential in diagnosis [18, 19]. Patient with a positive aspirate of palpable regional nodes like in the index case report can proceed directly to surgery, bypassing the need for an open biopsy [20]. Therefore, FNAC is an established tool for diagnosing many tumours. Its recognized complications that have been reported are rare, with an incidence of 0.003% to 0.07%, mostly from pancreatic tumours [21].

Molecular studies unveil multiple chromosomal aberrations in melanoma; the common changes include losses of 6q, 8q, 9p, and 10q and gain of 1q, 6p 7p, 8q, 11q, and 20q [22]. This pattern of changes depends on types of melanoma and the anatomical site of the lesion. The most common gene mutation in melanoma is *BRAF* and *NRAS* which accounted for 50% and 20%, respectively; both mutations increase activity of the MAPK pathway [23]. Thymine to adenine transversion is the basic abnormality that leads to substitution within the activation segment of serine/threonine kinase gene products. However, *BRAF* mutated pathway via p13k/AKT, which promotes survival and cell cycle entry in melanoma cells, is another mechanism. *PTEN* mutation, though uncommon, inhibits AKT-p13k pathways [23]. Cytogenetics or comparative genomic hybridization is highly essential for targeted therapy. To our knowledge there is no center that is doing that in developing countries of ours.

5. Conclusion

Intensification of public health education on melanoma especially in Africa can aid in early detection, even though, to date, no prospective evidence exists to clearly demonstrate the efficacy of prevention and early detection in decreasing melanoma mortality worldwide [24]. Nevertheless, many studies suggest that both self-assessment of risk factors and clinician examination can identify a proportion of patients at highest risk for melanoma who may benefit from behavior modification and routine screening [24]. Fine needle aspiration cytology has reduced initial biopsy before definitive surgery in most centers; its utility especially in developing countries of ours is highly encouraged despite our challenges so that the disease can be diagnosed early.

References

[1] D. M. Parkin, F. Bray, J. Ferlay, and P. Pisani, "Global cancer statistics, 2002," *CA: A Cancer Journal for Clinicians*, vol. 55, no. 2, pp. 74–108, 2005.

[2] M. A. Weinstock, "Cutaneous melanoma: public health approach to early detection," *Dermatologic Therapy*, vol. 19, no. 1, pp. 26–31, 2006.

[3] B. B. L. Pillemer, M. A. Pugliano-Mauro, L. K. Ferris, and T. J. Patton, "Three cases of scalp melanomas discovered by hairdressers," *Journal of Clinical and Aesthetic Dermatology*, vol. 6, no. 8, pp. 32–34, 2013.

[4] S. Aliyu, A. G. Ibrahim, M. B. Tahir, U. D. Babayo, and A. B. Zarami, "Cutaneous melonoma in maiduguri North Eastern Nigeria," *IJOAR*, vol. 3, no. 4, 2015.

[5] J. Rosai, "Skin-tumour and tumour like condition," in *Surgical Pathology*, R. J. Ackerman's, Ed., vol. 1, pp. 160–170, Mosby Elsevier, Edinburg, UK, 10th edition, 2011.

[6] V. Beral, S. Evans, H. Shaw, and G. Milton, "Cutaneous factors related to the risk of malignant melanoma," *British Journal of Dermatology*, vol. 109, no. 2, pp. 165–172, 1983.

[7] Melanoma [Wikipedia the free encyclopedia], May 2015, https://en.wikipedia.org/wiki/Wikipedia.

[8] H. K. Koh, "Cutaneous melanoma," *The New England Journal of Medicine*, vol. 325, no. 3, pp. 171–182, 1991.

[9] M. E. Asuquo, O. Ngim, G. Ugare, J. Omotoso, and G. Ebughe, "Major dermatologic malignancies encountered in a teaching hospital surgical department in South Nigeria," *American Journal of Clinical Dermatology*, vol. 9, no. 6, pp. 383–387, 2008.

[10] A. Z. Mohammed, A. N. Manasseh, B. M. Mandong, and S. T. Edino, "Histopathological study of malignant melanoma in

highlanders," *Nigerian Journal of Surgical Research*, vol. 5, no. 1, pp. 18–22, 2003.

[11] M. O. A. Soetan Samaila and A. H. Rafindadi, "Pattern of cutaneous malignant melanoma in Zaria, Nigeria," *Annals of African Medicine*, vol. 5, no. 1, pp. 16–19, 2006.

[12] J. Mbuagbaw, C. Pisoh, C. Bengonda, B. Kegoum, and S. Takongmo, "Malignant melanoma in Cameroon," *Internet Scientific Publication*, vol. 9, no. 1, p. 5, 2013.

[13] D. E. Roskell and I. D. Buley, "Fine needle aspiration cytology in cancer diagnosis is quick, cheap, and accurate when used appropriately," *BMJ*, vol. 329, no. 7460, pp. 244–245, 2004.

[14] B. Czerniak, S. Woyke, W. Domagala, and A. Krzysztolik, "Fine needle aspiration cytology of intraocular malignant melanoma," *Acta Cytologica*, vol. 27, no. 2, pp. 157–165, 1983.

[15] S. Babburi, R. Subramanyam, V. Aparna, and P. Sowjanya, "Intraoral malignant melanoma," *Nigerian Medical Journal*, vol. 54, no. 4, pp. 278–281, 2013.

[16] H. Nggada, A. Musa, B. Gali, and M. Khalil, "Fine needle aspiration cytology of thyroid nodule(s): a Nigerian tertiary hospital experience," *Internet Journal of Pathology*, vol. 5, article 1, 2005.

[17] K. E. Lori, P. L. Stanley, L. Britt -Marie, and et al, "Fine needle anspiration in the diagnosis of metastatic melanoma," *Journal of the American Academy of Dermatology*, vol. 42, no. 5, part 1, pp. 735–740, 2000.

[18] S. A. Malami and O. Ochicha, "A review of the utilization of fine needle aspiration in clinical practice and research in Nigeria," *CytoJournal*, vol. 8, article 12, 2011.

[19] G. Schäfer, A. M. Eggermont, and C. A. Voit, "Methodology and clinical utility of ultrasound-guided fine-needle aspiration cytology of lymph nodes in melanoma patients," *Expert Review of Dermatology*, vol. 8, no. 2, pp. 145–153, 2013.

[20] H. A. Nggada, N. A. Ajayi, A. Ahidjo et al., "Fine needle aspiration cytology diagnosis of liver diseases in the University of Maiduguri Teaching Hospital, Maiduguri," *African Journal of Medicine and Medical Sciences*, vol. 33, no. 3, pp. 255–257, 2004.

[21] M. S. Metcalfe, F. H. G. Bridgewater, E. J. Mullin, and G. J. Maddern, "Useless and dangerous—fine needle aspiration of hepatic colorectal Metastases," *British Medical Journal*, vol. 328, no. 7438, pp. 507–508, 2004.

[22] B. C. Bastian, A. B. Olshen, P. E. LeBoit, and D. Pinkel, "Classifying melanocytic tumors based on DNA copy number changes," *The American Journal of Pathology*, vol. 163, no. 5, pp. 1765–1770, 2003.

[23] J. F. Solus and S. Kraft, "Ras, raf, and MAP kinase in melanoma," *Advances in Anatomic Pathology*, vol. 20, no. 4, pp. 217–226, 2013.

[24] J. A. Carlson, A. Slominski, G. P. Linette, M. C. Mihm Jr., and J. S. Ross, "Biomarkers in melanoma: predisposition, screening and diagnosis," *Expert Review of Molecular Diagnostics*, vol. 3, no. 2, pp. 163–184, 2003.

10

Clinical Outcome of Third-Line Pazopanib in a Patient with Metastatic Renal Cell Carcinoma

Michela Roberto,[1] Maria Bassanelli,[1] Elsa Iannicelli,[2] Silvana Giacinti,[1] Chiara D'Antonio,[3] Anna Maria Aschelter,[1] and Paolo Marchetti[1]

[1]*Department of Clinical and Molecular Medicine, Faculty of Medicine and Psychology "Sapienza", St. Andrea Hospital, Via di Grottarossa 1035-1030, 00189 Rome, Italy*
[2]*Department of Radiology, Faculty of Medicine and Psychology "Sapienza", St. Andrea Hospital, Via di Grottarossa 1035-1030, 00189 Rome, Italy*
[3]*Department of Medical and Surgical Sciences and Translational Medicine, Faculty of Medicine and Psychology "Sapienza", St. Andrea Hospital, Via di Grottarossa 1035-1030, 00189 Rome, Italy*

Correspondence should be addressed to Michela Roberto; mikiroberto@hotmail.it

Academic Editor: Jorg Kleeff

Background. Renal cell carcinoma accounts for about 2-3% of all malignant tumors. The prevalence of brain metastases from RCC is less than 20% of cases. Traditionally, whole brain radiotherapy as well as the latest stereotactic radiosurgery improves both survival and local tumor control. These treatments also allow stabilization of clinical symptomatology. However, validated treatment guidelines for RCC patients with brain metastases are not yet available on account of the frequent exclusion of such patients from clinical trials. Moreover, limited data about the sequential use of three therapies, changing the class of agent, have been published up to now. *Case Report.* We report the case of a patient with metastatic RCC who developed disease progression after sunitinib and everolimus as first-line and second-line therapy, respectively. Thus, he underwent a multimodality treatment with pazopanib, as third-line therapy, to control systemic disease and radiosurgery directed on the new brain metastasis. To date, the patient is still receiving pazopanib, with progression-free survival and overall survival of 43 and 103 months, respectively. *Conclusion.* In a context characterized by different emerging options, with no general consensus on the optimal treatment strategy, the use of pazopanib in pretreated patients could be a suitable choice.

1. Introduction

Renal cell carcinoma (RCC) accounts for about 2-3% of all adult, malignant tumors. Metastatic disease frequently occurs, about 50% of the cases, and a large analysis shows that the most common sites of metastases are lung, bone, lymph nodes, and liver (50, 40, 25, and 20% of cases, resp.). Adrenal and brain metastases are rarely diagnosed (about 8–10% of the patients) [1].

According to the Memorial Sloan-Kettering Cancer Center (MSKCC), three prognostic risk groups can be distinguished: favorable, intermediate, and poor [2]. Patients with advanced RCC belonging to the favorable risk group have median overall survival (OS) of 43 months; those belonging to the intermediate and poor groups have 27 and 8.8 months, respectively.

However, in the presence of brain metastases (BM), the prognosis of RCC patients worsens, with a median OS not reaching 20 months using traditional whole-brain radiotherapy (WBRT) alone [3].

Here we describe a case of long-surviving patient who experienced progression of disease after two previous lines of treatment. He underwent a multimodality treatment, consisting of stereotactic radiosurgery (SRS) of the BM and pazopanib as third-line therapy, with a good clinical outcome.

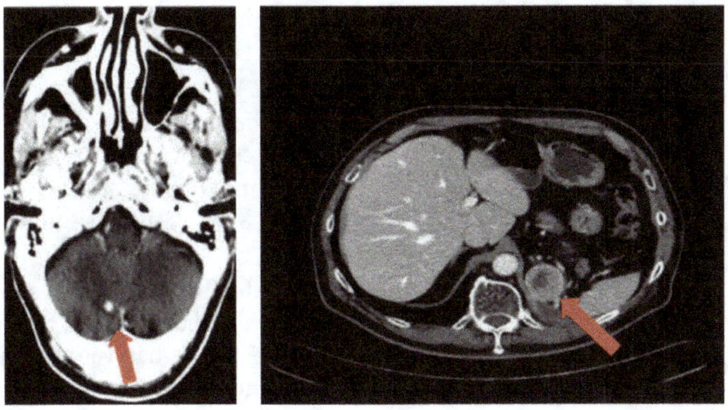

FIGURE 1: Before starting pazopanib a cerebellar lesion of 6 mm in diameter appeared and left adrenal gland solid nodule was 4 cm in size, with a little necrotic core.

2. Case Report

We report the case of a 76 year-old man who underwent a radical left nephrectomy for clear cell RCC (Fuhrman grade 1, stage II according to AJCC) in February 2007. Follow-up was negative until February 2009 when a whole-body computed tomography (CT) scan revealed lung nodule with a major diameter of 2.8 cm in the inferior left lobe. Considering the long disease-free survival time (24 months) along with the presence of single metastasis, a left lung wedge resection was performed. The histology confirmed the diagnosis of metastasis from clear cell RCC. About 5 months later, a spiral CT showed a new malignant micronodule in the right superior lung lobe and nodules ranging from 2.8 to 1.8 cm in the left and right adrenal glands, respectively. Patient's Karnofsky Performance Scale score was 90% and he was classified in the favorable risk group according to both MSKCC and Heng's score criteria. In August 2009 he started a tyrosine-kinase inhibitor (TKI), sunitinib 50 mg per day (4 weeks on and 2 weeks off). After 2 cycles of treatment, a grade 3 mucositis occurred but after 3 weeks of break it declined to grade 1. Thus, he resumed therapy at the lower dosage of 37.5 mg per day (4 weeks on and 2 weeks off). The whole-body CT scan, regularly performed every 3 months, demonstrated a stable disease (SD) as best response until June 2011 when, after 15 cycles of therapy, it revealed a progressive disease (PD) at the left adrenal gland which was confirmed by magnetic resonance imaging. Therefore, in August 2011, a second-line therapy with everolimus 10 mg per day was started. The treatment was stopped after just 4 months because of the fact that CT scan had showed a new cerebellar lesion of 6 mm in the right side and a further progression of the left adrenal nodule (4 cm) (Figure 1). The remaining malignant areas were instead stable. Patient reported grade 2 of asthenia, muscle pain, and edema of the legs during the therapy. However, on account of his good performance status and the long-lasting disease control with sunitinib, we further decided to refer him to a multimodality treatment. Thus, he received another TKI after he had undergone SRS (18 Gy, 1 fr) of the cerebellar lesion. The tolerance to SRS was good and the third-line therapy with the TKI, pazopanib (800 mg per day), was started in February 2012. The first CT evaluation showed SD in both cerebellum and adrenal glands, although the left adrenal nodule had become necrotic (Figure 2). After twelve cycles, 30% reduction of the left adrenal metastasis was observed (Figure 3) with further reduction of 10% in July 2013. The other malignant lesions appeared to be stable. Eighteen cycles were administered at full dosage. Later, dosage was firstly reduced to 600 and then to 400 mg per day for the occurrence of grade 3 hypertension and mucositis. Such a therapy is still in progress with a progression-free survival (PFS) and OS of 43 and 103 months, respectively.

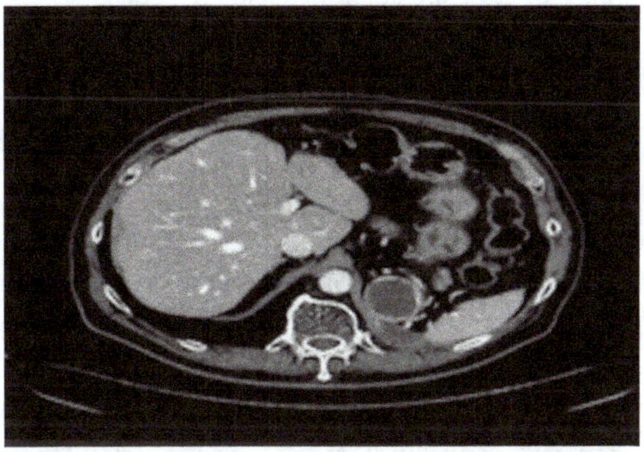

FIGURE 2: After 3 cycles of pazopanib the adrenal metastasis was stable in dimension but with more necrotic area.

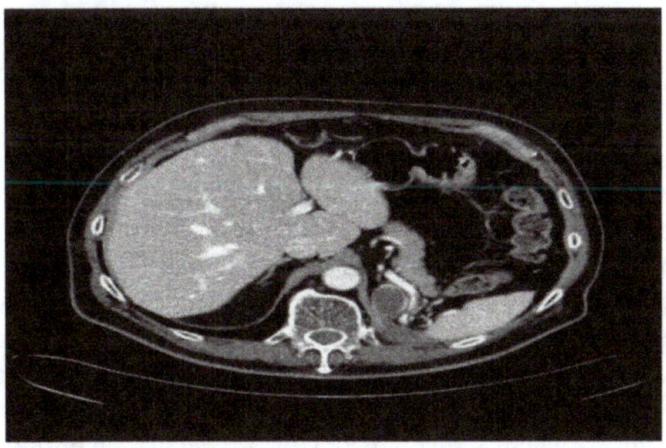

FIGURE 3: After 12 cycles of pazopanib there was a 30% reduction.

3. Discussion

Brain metastases occur in less than 20% of patients with RCC and are generally related to a very poor prognosis [3]. Shuch et al. reported that the median OS after the diagnosis of BM was 10.7 months with a 1-year, 2-year, and 5-year OS rates of 48%, 30%, and 12%, respectively [4].

The WBRT and the latest SRS are demonstrated to improve survival, local tumor control, and clinical symptomatology [5]. However, there are no validated treatment guidelines for patients with BM from RCC on account of the frequent exclusion of such patients from clinical trials [6]. Indeed, results from either expanded access or small retrospective studies are merely available [3, 7, 8]. Nevertheless, these data have showed a trend towards improved survival, mostly achieved by the application of multimodality treatment, which consists of surgery, WBRT, or SRS administration with concomitant or sequential TKI therapy.

We report a case of patient who developed BM after sunitinib as first-line therapy and everolimus as second-line therapy, with PFS of 24 and 4 months, respectively. We referred him to multimodality treatment with SRS of the cerebellar metastasis and pazopanib as third-line therapy. In our opinion, his excellent OS of more than 8 years raises particular interest. Indeed, to the best of our knowledge, none of the few previous studies about second- and third-line metastatic RCC (mRCC) reported similar outcome.

Although there are limited published data on the sequential use of three therapies in the treatment of mRCC, several studies showed an increased disease control as well as improvements in quality of life by changing the class of agent. First of all, the RECORD-1 trial showed a better outcome with everolimus (mTOR inhibitor) versus placebo (PFS was 4 and 1.9 months, resp.) in patients progressing on VEGF inhibitors (VEGFi) [9]. Another phase III study instead showed clinical benefit using sorafenib as third-line therapy [10]. In detail, a significant risk reduction of death (HR = 0.72) and progression (HR = 0.44) in the sorafenib group was reported. Moreover, data from 879 patients treated with several classes of agents as third-line therapies, such as VEGFi and mTOR inhibitors (mTORi), have been reported at recent genitourinary cancers symposium [11]. Overall, the median PFS was 5.1 months and the median OS from beginning third-line therapy was 12.0 months. Similarly, in the GOLD trial, patients previously treated with VEGFi-mTORi sequence and randomized to receive dovitinib or sorafenib as third-line therapy reached a median PFS of 3.7 versus 3.6 months, respectively [12]. Finally, Iacovelli et al. reported in third-line setting a median PFS and OS of 6.1 and 44.7 months, respectively [13]. Interestingly, when patients were stratified according to MSKCC prognostic criteria, the median OS was 59.9, 38.8, and 24.6 months in the good, intermediate, and poor prognosis groups, respectively, regardless of the treatment sequence. In this study, as a matter of fact, the VEGFi-VEGFi-mTORi sequence compared with the VEGFi-mTORi-VEGFi sequence was related to a better median total PFS (36.5 versus 29.3 months, $P = 0.059$) and OS (50.7 versus 37.8 months, $P = 0.004$). However, other retrospective studies have showed equal efficacy of these two sequences of treatments, with median OS generally not exceeding 30 months [14–16].

According to an algorithm treatment decision of changing the class of agent, having the patient received previous VEGFi-mTORi therapy, he should have been treated with another VEGFi, such as sorafenib.

Sorafenib is VEGFi-TKI approved to treat mRCC patients who have failed or cannot bear other therapies. Its main toxicity typically is hand-foot-skin (HFS) reaction that may be severe (grade 3-4) in about 15% of patients [17]. Particularly affected are hand, palm, and sole of the foot, leading in some cases to immobility.

Our patient was a musician; thus, considering the high risk of HFS occurrence, another target molecule was offered. Effectively, applying an *inverse decision-making* algorithm, as suggested by GOAL authors, we selected the best therapy by limiting toxicity and improving at the same time the treatment compliance [18].

Compared to other target therapies, such as everolimus, or axitinib, pazopanib showed clinical benefit as salvage therapy only in few studies [19, 20].

The first one included 28 patients treated with pazopanib after two previous therapies: median PFS was 16.5 months with grade 3-4 hypertension and proteinuria as the most common toxicities [19]. In the second one, pazopanib showed activity and safety also in patients with BM with up to 60% of SD and 13% of BM regression [20].

Our experience, coupled with data of literature, raises the question whether patients' clinical outcome was completely influenced by the presence of BM or rather by their exclusion from the most effective treatments such as the multimodality approach. Thus, in the evolving scenario of mRCC therapy, with no general consensus on the optimal sequence of therapies, the use of pazopanib in VEGFi-mTORi pretreated patients could represent a promising option.

References

[1] M. Bianchi, M. Sun, C. Jeldres et al., "Distribution of metastatic sites in renal cell carcinoma: a population-based analysis," *Annals of Oncology*, vol. 23, no. 4, pp. 973–980, 2012.

[2] R. J. Motzer, J. Bacik, L. H. Schwartz et al., "Prognostic factors for survival in previously treated patients with metastatic renal cell carcinoma," *Journal of Clinical Oncology*, vol. 22, no. 3, pp. 454–463, 2004.

[3] O. Bennani, S. Derrey, O. Langlois et al., "Brain metastasis from renal cell carcinoma," *Neurochirurgie*, vol. 60, no. 1-2, pp. 12–16, 2014.

[4] B. Shuch, J. C. La Rochelle, T. Klatte et al., "Brain metastasis from renal cell carcinoma: presentation, recurrence, and survival," *Cancer*, vol. 113, no. 7, pp. 1641–1648, 2008.

[5] J. P. Sheehan, M.-H. Sun, D. Kondziolka, J. Flickinger, and L. D. Lunsford, "Radiosurgery in patients with renal cell carcinoma metastasis to the brain: long-term outcomes and prognostic

factors influencing survival and local tumor control," *Journal of Neurosurgery*, vol. 98, no. 2, pp. 342–349, 2003.

[6] D. Y. C. Heng, T. K. Choueiri, B. I. Rini et al., "Outcomes of patients with metastatic renal cell carcinoma that do not meet eligibility criteria for clinical trials," *Annals of Oncology*, vol. 25, no. 1, pp. 149–154, 2014.

[7] D. A. Bastos, A. M. Molina, V. Hatzoglou et al., "Safety and efficacy of targeted therapy for renal cell carcinoma with brain metastasis," *Clinical Genitourinary Cancer*, vol. 13, no. 1, pp. 59–66, 2015.

[8] J. Verma, E. Jonasch, P. K. Allen et al., "The impact of tyrosine kinase inhibitors on the multimodality treatment of brain metastases from renal cell carcinoma," *American Journal of Clinical Oncology*, vol. 36, no. 6, pp. 620–624, 2013.

[9] R. J. Motzer, B. Escudier, S. Oudard et al., "Phase 3 trial of everolimus for metastatic renal cell carcinoma: final results and analysis of prognostic factors," *Cancer*, vol. 116, no. 18, pp. 4256–4265, 2010.

[10] G. Di Lorenzo, C. Buonerba, P. Federico et al., "Third-line sorafenib after sequential therapy with sunitinib and mTOR inhibitors in metastatic renal cell carcinoma," *European Urology*, vol. 58, no. 6, pp. 906–911, 2010.

[11] D. Y. C. Heng, C. Wells, F. Donskov et al., "Third-line therapy in metastatic renal cell carcinoma: results from the International mRCC Database Consortium," *Journal of Clinical Oncology*, vol. 33, supplement 7, abstract 430, 2015.

[12] R. J. Motzer, C. Porta, N. J. Vogelzang et al., "Dovitinib versus sorafenib for third-line targeted treatment of patients with metastatic renal cell carcinoma: an open-label, randomized phase 3 trial," *The Lancet Oncology*, vol. 15, no. 3, pp. 286–296, 2014.

[13] R. Iacovelli, G. Carteni, C. N. Sternberg et al., "Clinical outcomes in patients receiving three lines of targeted therapy for metastatic renal cell carcinoma: results from a large patient cohort," *European Journal of Cancer*, vol. 49, no. 9, pp. 2134–2142, 2013.

[14] A. Blesius, B. Beuselinck, C. Chevreau et al., "Are tyrosine kinase inhibitors still active in patients with metastatic renal cell carcinoma previously treated with a tyrosine kinase inhibitor and everolimus? Experience of 36 patients treated in France in the RECORD-1 trial," *Clinical Genitourinary Cancer*, vol. 11, no. 2, pp. 128–133, 2013.

[15] J. Busch, C. Seidel, B. Erber et al., "Retrospective comparison of triple-sequence therapies in metastatic renal cell carcinoma," *European Urology*, vol. 64, no. 1, pp. 62–70, 2013.

[16] V. Grünwald, C. Seidel, M. Fenner, A. Ganser, J. Busch, and S. Weikert, "Treatment of everolimus-resistant metastatic renal cell carcinoma with VEGF-targeted therapies," *British Journal of Cancer*, vol. 105, no. 11, pp. 1635–1639, 2011.

[17] B. Escudier, T. Eisen, W. M. Stadler et al., "Sorafenib in advanced clear-cell renal-cell carcinoma," *The New England Journal of Medicine*, vol. 356, no. 2, pp. 125–134, 2007.

[18] S. Bracarda, M. Sisani, F. Marrocolo, A. Hamzaj, S. del Buono, and V. De Simone, "GOAL: an inverse toxicity-related algorithm for daily clinical practice decision making in advanced kidney cancer," *Critical Reviews in Oncology/Hematology*, vol. 89, no. 3, pp. 386–393, 2014.

[19] S. K. Pal, D. M. S. Hossain, Q. Zhang et al., "Pazopanib as third line therapy for metastatic renal cell carcinoma: clinical efficacy and temporal analysis of cytokine profile," *The Journal of Urology*, vol. 193, no. 4, pp. 1114–1121, 2015.

[20] M. R. Matrana, C. Duran, A. Shetty et al., "Outcomes of patients with metastatic clear-cell renal cell carcinoma treated with pazopanib after disease progression with other targeted therapies," *European Journal of Cancer*, vol. 49, no. 15, pp. 3169–3175, 2013.

11

Chemoradiotherapy in a Case of Malignant Syringocystadenocarcinoma Papilliferum of Vulva with Locoregional Failure

Pamidimukkala Bramhananda Rao,[1] Saptarshi Ghosh,[1] Manisha Mohapatra,[2] N. Pramod Philip,[3] P. Ravindra Kumar,[1] Surendra Manam,[1] Pradeep Karra,[1] and Vijay Krishna Jasti[1]

[1]*Department of Radiotherapy, GSL Cancer Hospital, GSL Medical College, Rajahmundry, Andhra Pradesh 533105, India*
[2]*Department of Pathology, GSL Medical College, Rajahmundry, Andhra Pradesh 533296, India*
[3]*Department of Radiology, GSL Medical College, Rajahmundry, Andhra Pradesh 533296, India*

Correspondence should be addressed to Saptarshi Ghosh; drsaptarshi10@gmail.com

Academic Editor: Ming-Hsui Tsai

Introduction. Syringocystadenocarcinoma papilliferum (SCACP) is an extremely rare malignant adnexal tumor, which arises from syringocystadenoma papilliferum. To date, less than 30 cases of malignant SCACP have been reported, of which locoregional metastases were found in only four cases. *Case Report.* A 57-year-old female patient who presented to our Oncology Department with a recurrent malignant SCACP of the left labia along with right inguinal lymphadenopathy. Pathological examination confirmed the diagnosis of malignant SCACP with right inguinal lymph node metastases. Due to the fixity of the right inguinal nodes, neoadjuvant chemotherapy was administered with Cisplatin and 5-Fluorouracil for four cycles, following which the primary tumor and the contralateral inguinal nodes regressed completely. Then definitive chemoradiation was delivered with five cycles of weekly Cisplatin and external beam pelvic irradiation up to a dose of 59.4 Gy. Patient is disease-free 11 months after treatment. *Discussion.* We here report the fifth case of malignant SCACP with locoregional metastases. This is the first case of malignant SCACP which has been treated with neoadjuvant chemotherapy followed by concurrent chemoradiation. Although surgery has been used most commonly, chemoradiation may also have a role in the treatment of malignant SCACP, especially in cases of locoregional metastases.

1. Introduction

Syringocystadenocarcinoma papilliferum (SCACP) is a very rare entity of cutaneous adnexal tumor, which is listed in the WHO classification of skin tumors as the malignant counterpart of syringocystadenoma papilliferum (SCAP) [1, 2]. SCAP is a benign slow-growing adnexal skin tumor that mostly occurs in the scalp or face [3] and originates from apocrine or eccrine sweat glands [4]. Malignant transformation of preexisting long-standing SCAP into SCACP has been well documented now [5]. Since its first depiction in 1980 by Dissanayake and Salm [6], a total of less than 30 cases of SCACP have been reported till date, of which only four had locoregional metastases [1, 7, 8]. SCACP commonly occurs in the head and neck region, with few of them occurring in other sites [9, 10].

2. Case Report

A 57-year-old woman presented to a private practitioner with a swelling in the left labial region in last three years, which was now associated with bleeding, foul smelling discharge, and pruritus since last one month. There were no enlarged inguinal nodes at the time of presentation. She underwent wide local excision alone and was diagnosed with SCACP. Postoperative margin status was negative. Three months postoperatively, she presented to our institutional Oncology

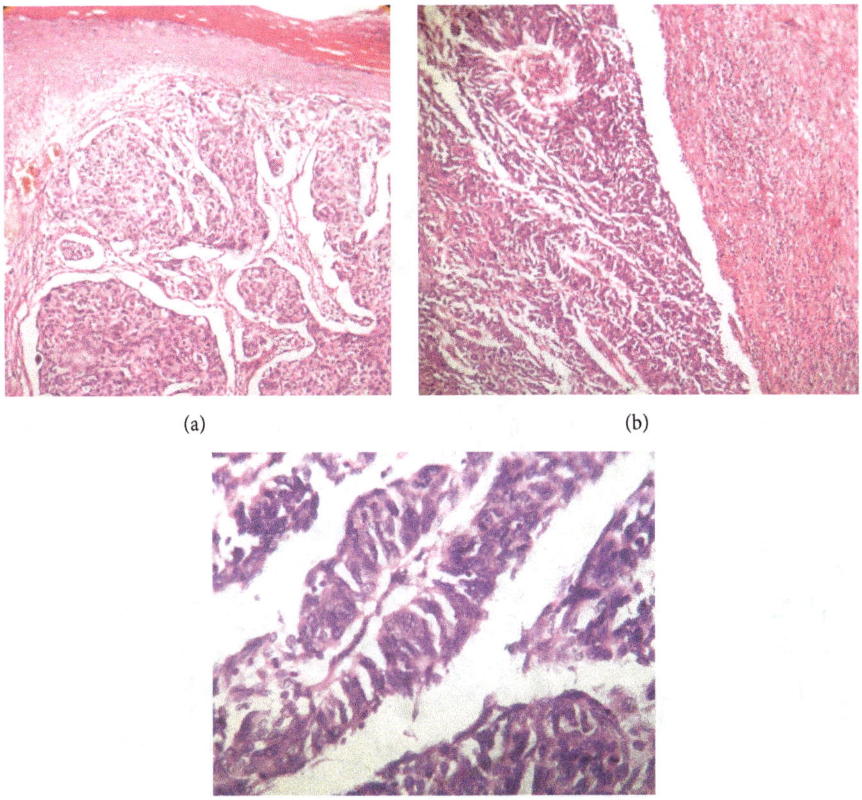

(a) (b) (c)

Figure 1: (a) Photomicrograph of the tumor showing epidermis and dermis along with a tumor arranged in tubules, nests, and islands invading into the deeper tissue (H&E, ×100). (b) Photomicrograph showing the tumor arranged in complex papillary fronds having central fibrovascular core; surrounding stroma shows dense lymphocytic infiltration (H&E, ×100). (c) Photomicrograph showing papillae lined by multilayered round to columnar cells showing mild to moderate nuclear atypia, with vesicular chromatin and some showed prominent nucleoli (H&E, ×400).

OPD with an ulcerative lesion in the left labial region along with right inguinal lymphadenopathy.

Histopathological examination of the ulcerative lesion in the left labia showed epidermis comprising of keratinized squamous epithelium and dermis showing a tumor extending from lower epidermis into deep dermis. The tumor was made up of multiple nodules comprising of duct-like structures, some appearing to be cystically dilated, papillary structures having central fibrovascular cores, solid nests, and islands (Figure 1(a)). Dense infiltrate of lymphocytes was seen inside the ducts and papillae and in the surrounding stroma (Figure 1(b)). These ductal and papillary structures were made up of multilayered round to oval to columnar cells having scanty eosinophilic cytoplasm exhibiting moderate nuclear atypia with vesicular chromatin and some showed prominent nucleoli (Figure 1(c)). Histopathological findings favoured the diagnosis of SCACP, residual disease. Fine needle aspiration (FNA) was done from the enlarged firm right inguinal lymph node. The aspirate cytosmears showed abundant cellularity comprising of clusters, nests, papillary structures, and discretely scattered malignant epithelial cells characterized by round to oval cells having scanty eosinophilic cytoplasm exhibiting hyperchromatic or vesicular nuclei with high nuclear-cytoplasmic ratio and some showed prominent nucleoli. Background showed numerous mature and transformed lymphocytes and eosinophilic proteinaceous material (Figure 2). Based on the cytomorphology, a diagnosis of metastatic papillary adenocarcinomatous deposit in right inguinal node possibly from syringocystadenocarcinoma papilliferum of vulva was offered.

Magnetic resonance imaging of the pelvis demonstrated an irregular, intermediate signal intensity lesion in the left side of the labia of size of 10 mm × 10 mm along with multiple oval to round lymph nodal masses in the right superficial inguinal region measuring 5.3 cm × 7.5 cm in size (Figures 3(a) and 3(b)). Owing to the fixity of the contralateral inguinal nodes and the large size, neoadjuvant chemotherapy with Cisplatin of 100 mg/m^2 and 5-Fluorouracil of 1000 mg/m^2 was given for four cycles. Following this, the primary tumor and the contralateral inguinal nodes regressed completely (Figures 4(a) and 4(b)). After this, definitive chemoradiation was delivered with five cycles of weekly Cisplatin of 40 mg/m^2 and external beam pelvic irradiation up to a dose of 59.4 Gy in 33 fractions. After a dose of 50.4 Gy to the whole pelvis, a boost dose of 9 Gy to the primary tumor site and the inguinal lymph nodal site along with a 2 cm margin was delivered. Patient has been followed up regularly and is disease-free 11 months after treatment.

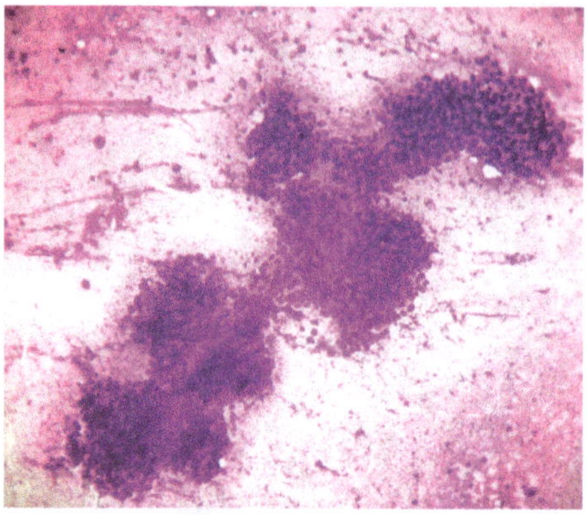

FIGURE 2: FNA cytosmears from inguinal lymph node showing round to oval tumor cells arranged in papillary structures; background shows many lymphocytes and eosinophilic proteinaceous material (Leishman, ×100).

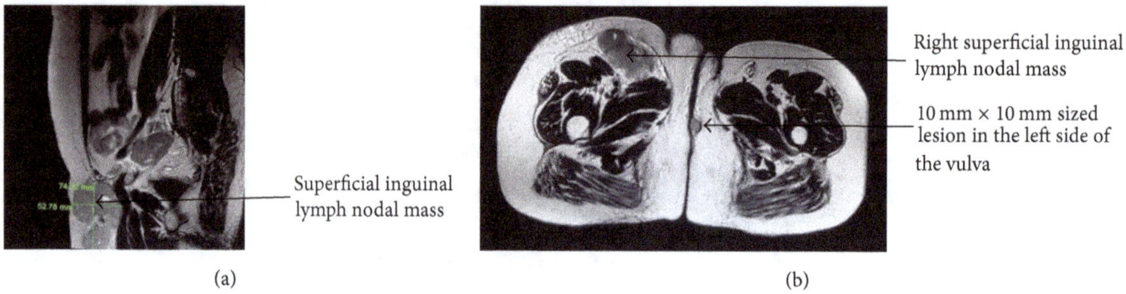

FIGURE 3: (a) Pretreatment sagittal magnetic resonance (MR) image depicting the superficial inguinal lymph nodal mass measuring 5.3 cm × 7.5 cm in size. (b) Pretreatment axial MR image showing the primary vulvar lesion and the right superficial inguinal lymph nodal mass.

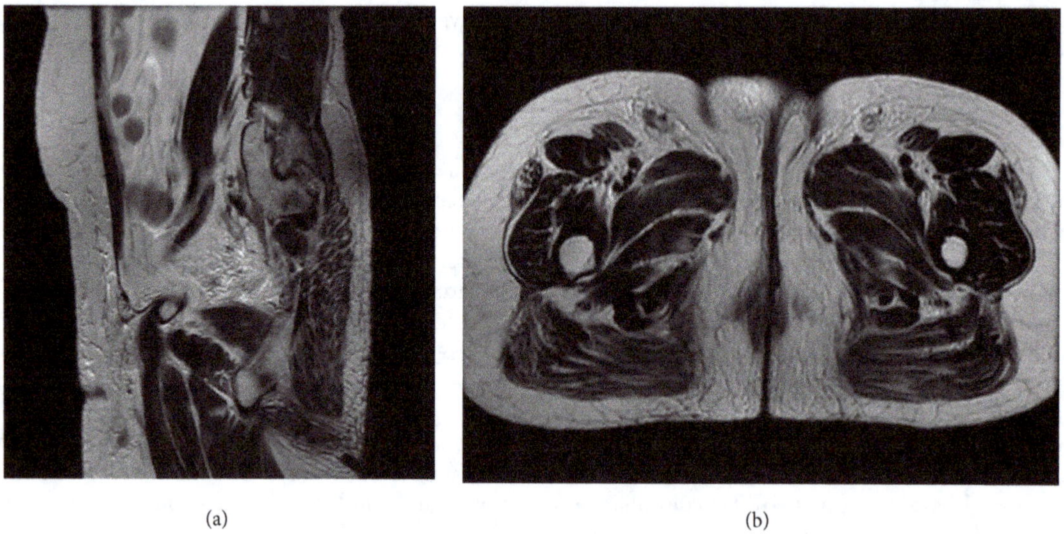

FIGURE 4: ((a) and (b)) Posttreatment MR images in sagittal and axial section show complete resolution of the inguinal lymph nodes.

3. Discussion

We describe a rare case of SCACP in vulva with locoregional metastases. A total of less than 30 cases of SCACP have been described in literature till date [7, 8]. The average age of diagnosis is 66 years [11]. Although, it most commonly occurs in the head and neck region, it may occur in other sites like perianal region, suprapubic region, calf, and arms [9]. Clinically, the lesion is long-standing, skin-coloured or yellowish, and papular in nature, which suddenly increases in size along with bleeding or ulceration [12].

The histopathological diagnosis of SCACP is sometimes difficult and may resemble hidradenocarcinoma papilliferum, apocrine ductal adenocarcinoma, and cutaneous metastases of malignancies microscopically [13]. While hidradenocarcinoma papilliferum and apocrine ductal adenocarcinoma are dermal tumors and do not show any epidermal changes, SCACP often expresses p63, which confirms its sweat gland origin, rather than a cutaneous metastasis [14, 15].

SCACP is generally a low-grade malignancy, with only two cases of recurrence being reported [7, 9]. Locoregional lymphatic metastases have been reported in only four patients to date [1, 7, 8], with none of them having any distant metastases [13, 14].

Due to the infrequent occurrence of the tumor, no standard treatment protocol has been advocated [8, 14]. Wide local excision has been advocated most commonly [8]. Sentinel lymph node biopsy has been performed along with excision in some cases [8, 14]. Mohs micrographic surgery has also been performed by Chi et al. [16] in a SCACP of the right auricle, with good disease control 6 years postoperatively. The role of chemotherapy or/and radiotherapy to SCACP is not clear. Adjuvant radiation therapy was delivered in one patient described by Arslan et al. [7], which then developed locoregional metastases.

In the current report, the patient had SCACP with locoregional failure postoperatively, which responded to chemotherapy followed by chemoradiation and is without any recurrence or distant metastases for 11 months after treatment.

4. Conclusion

SCACP is an extremely rare adnexal tumor which may occur in unusual sites like vulva. Locoregional lymphatic metastases, though infrequent, should always be investigated for. Though, as of now, wide local excision is the standard treatment, chemotherapy and radiation therapy can also achieve a good tumor control in cases of inoperable SCACP or in patients declining surgery. The role of chemoradiation has to be further investigated, especially in cases of locoregional disease spread. Regular follow-up is utterly important to detect any locoregional failure or recurrence early, as aggressive treatment may achieve good tumor control.

References

[1] M. Numata, S. Hosoe, N. Itoh, Y. Munakata, S. Hayashi, and Y. Maruyama, "Syringadenocarcinoma papilliferum," *Journal of Cutaneous Pathology*, vol. 12, no. 1, pp. 3–7, 1985.

[2] H. Woestenborghs, P. Van Eyken, and A. Dans, "Syringocystadenocarcinoma papilliferum in situ with pagetoid spread: a case report," *Histopathology*, vol. 48, no. 7, pp. 869–870, 2006.

[3] E. B. Helwig and V. C. Hackney, "Syringocystadenoma papilliferum: lesions with and without naevus sebaceous and basal cell carcinoma," *Archives of Dermatology*, vol. 71, pp. 361–372, 1955.

[4] K. Niizuma, "Syringocystadenoma papilliferum: light and electron microscopic studies," *Acta Dermato-Venereologica*, vol. 56, no. 5, pp. 327–336, 1976.

[5] R. Hoekzema, M. F. E. Leenarts, and E. W. P. Nijhuis, "Syringocystadenocarcinoma papilliferum in a linear nevus verrucosus," *Journal of Cutaneous Pathology*, vol. 38, no. 2, pp. 246–250, 2011.

[6] R. V. P. Dissanayake and R. Salm, "Sweat-gland carcinomas: prognosis related to histological type," *Histopathology*, vol. 4, no. 4, pp. 445–466, 1980.

[7] H. Arslan, M. Diyarbakrl, Ş. Batur, and C. Demirkesen, "Syringocystadenocarcinoma papilliferum with squamous cell carcinoma differentiation and with locoregional metastasis," *Journal of Craniofacial Surgery*, vol. 24, no. 1, pp. e38–e40, 2013.

[8] E. Satter, D. Grady, and C. T. Schlocker, "Syringocystadenocarcinoma papilliferum with locoregional metastases," *Dermatology Online Journal*, vol. 20, no. 4, Article ID 22335, 2014.

[9] N. Leeborg, M. Thompson, S. Rossmiller, N. Gross, C. White, and K. Gatter, "Diagnostic pitfalls in syringocystadenocarcinoma papilliferum: case report and review of the literature," *Archives of Pathology and Laboratory Medicine*, vol. 134, no. 8, pp. 1205–1209, 2010.

[10] A. Abrari and U. Mukherjee, "Syringocystadenocarcinoma papilliferum at unusual site: inherent lesional histologic polymorphism is the pathognomon," *BMJ Case Reports*, 2011.

[11] J. Peterson, K. Tefft, J. Blackmon, A. Rajpara, and G. Fraga, "Syringocystadenocarcinoma papilliferum: a rare tumor with a favorable prognosis," *Dermatology Online Journal*, vol. 19, no. 9, Article ID 19620, 2013.

[12] S. H. Park, Y. M. Shin, D. H. Shin, J. S. Choi, and K. H. Kim, "Syringocystadenocarcinoma papilliferum: a case report," *Journal of Korean Medical Science*, vol. 22, no. 4, pp. 762–765, 2007.

[13] L. Requena, H. Kiryu, and A. B. Ackerman, "Ackerman's histologic diagnosis of neoplastic skin disease: a method by pattern analysis," in *Neoplasms with Apocrine Differentiation*, pp. 665–675, Lippincott-Raven Publishers, Philadelphia, Pa, USA, 1998.

[14] O. E. Aydin, B. Sahin, H. S. Ozkan, and O. Gore, "A rare tumor: syringocystadenocarcinoma papilliferum," *Dermatologic Surgery*, vol. 37, no. 2, pp. 271–274, 2011.

[15] B. Paradiso, E. Bianchini, P. Cifelli, L. Cavazzini, and G. Lanza, "A new case of syringocystadenocarcinoma papilliferum: a rare pathology for a wide-ranging comprehension," *Case Reports in Medicine*, vol. 2014, Article ID 453874, 8 pages, 2014.

[16] C.-C. Chi, R.-Y. Tsai, and S.-H. Wang, "Syringocystadenocarcinoma papilliferum: successfully treated with Mohs micrographic surgery," *Dermatologic Surgery*, vol. 30, no. 3, pp. 468–471, 2004.

12

Mucoepidermoid Carcinoma of the Palatine Tonsil

Lucas Novaes Teixeira, Victor Angelo Martins Montalli, Luiz Carlos Santana Teixeira, Fabrício Passador-Santos, Andresa Borges Soares, and Vera Cavalcanti de Araújo

Department of Oral Pathology, São Leopoldo Mandic Institute and Research Center, Rua José Rocha Junqueira 13, Ponte Preta, 13045-755 Campinas, SP, Brazil

Correspondence should be addressed to Lucas Novaes Teixeira; novaesrp@yahoo.com.br

Academic Editor: Ossama W. Tawfik

Mucoepidermoid carcinoma (MEC) is the most common primary salivary gland malignancy in both adults and children. It has a slight female predilection and usually presents as a painless, rubber-like or soft mass, which may be fixed or mobile. Histologically, MEC is comprised of a mixture of cell types including mucous, epidermoid, and intermediate cells that can be arranged in solid nests or cystic structures. In the oral cavity, it most frequently occurs at the palate or buccal mucosa. The present paper aimed to describe an unusual case of MEC arising in the palatine tonsil.

1. Introduction

Many different malignant neoplasms may arise from the palatine tonsils, with the most common histological type being the squamous cell carcinoma (SCC), which accounts for up to 85% of all cases [1–3]. Malignant lymphoproliferative diseases are the second most frequent malignancy of the palatine tonsil, with the diffuse large B-cell lymphoma (DLBCL) comprising approximately 30% of all lymphomas [4]. Metastatic deposits of lung [5] and gastric carcinomas [6], as well as melanoma [7], renal carcinoma [8], and adenocarcinoma of the colon [9], have also been described in the palatine tonsils.

Minor salivary gland tumors exhibit diverse histopathological features as well as a varied clinical behavior [10]. They may be derived from any of the minor salivary glands distributed throughout the oral cavity [11]. Interestingly, despite the presence of minor salivary glands in the palatine tonsils, the development of malignant salivary tumors here is unusual. Indeed, a scarce number of case reports have been documented in the scientific literature [12–14]. The present paper, therefore, aimed to report a case of MEC arising in the palatine tonsil.

2. Case History

A 47-year-old man reported experiencing dysphagia and a sore throat for 4 months. The patient was both a heavy smoker (40 cigarettes daily) and an alcoholic. His medical history was significant for Type 2 Diabetes Mellitus. The patient presented with a swelling on the right side of the neck (Figure 1(a)). Intraoral examination revealed an ulcerated mass on the right palatine tonsil (Figure 1(b)). Axial computed tomography (CT) revealed a solid lesion with lobulated and ill-defined margins (Figure 1(c)). An incisional biopsy was performed and the specimen was fixed in 10% buffered formalin.

Paraffin sections were prepared for light microscopy using routine procedures. The sections were stained with hematoxylin and eosin (H&E). Microscopic examination revealed a fragment of oral mucosa covered with a nonkeratinized stratified squamous epithelium. A neoplasm of glandular epithelial origin was identified in the lamina propria (Figure 2(a)). The tumor cells were arranged in sheets, exhibiting a uniform morphology with few cells showing atypia and mitotic figures (Figure 2(b)). Clear cells were observed in some areas of the tumor (Figure 2(c)).

TABLE 1: Specifications of the primary antibodies.

Primary antibody	Source	Dilution	Retrieval	Incubation time
CK-7	Dako	1:100	Water bath 95°C (citric acid): 30 min	60 min
CK-13	Dako	1:100	Water bath 95°C (citric acid): 30 min	60 min
CK-14	NeoMarkers	1:1200	Water bath 95°C (citric acid): 30 min	60 min
Vimentin	Dako	1:300	Water bath 95°C (citric acid): 30 min	60 min
Smooth muscle actin	Dako	1:100	Water bath 95°C (citric acid): 30 min	60 min
Chromogranin	Abcam	1:500	Water bath 95°C (citric acid): 30 min	60 min
p16	CINtec Histology	1:250	Water bath 95°C (citric acid): 30 min	60 min

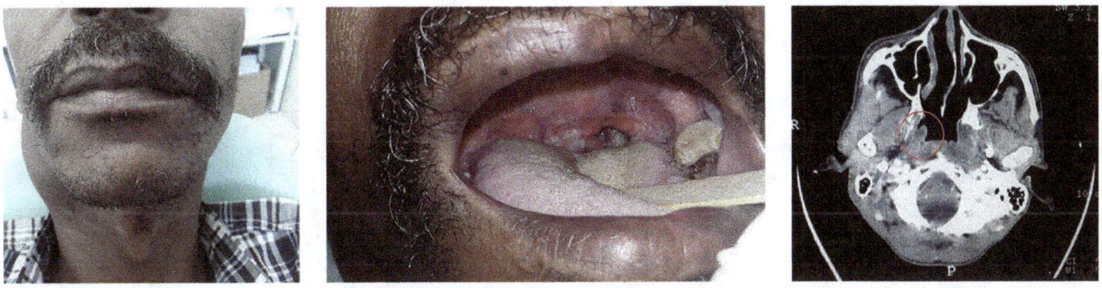

(a) (b) (c)

FIGURE 1: (a) The swelling on the right side of the neck, (b) ulcerated mass on the right palatine tonsil, and (c) CT image exhibiting a lobulated and ill-defined lesion (red circle).

TABLE 2: Immunohistochemistry results.

Primary antibody	Result
CK-7	+
CK-13	+
CK-14	+
Vimentin	−
Smooth muscle actin	−
Chromogranin	−
p16	−

The samples were subsequently submitted to immunohistochemistry for a subset of cytokeratins (CK), vimentin, smooth muscle actin, chromogranin, and p16, the latter indicating the presence of HPV. The source, clone, concentration, and incubation time of the primary antibodies are described in Table 1. PAS with diastase digestion (PAS + DD) and mucicarmine staining were also performed. CK-7 was positive in the neoplastic cells, while the superficial oral epithelium was negative (Figure 2(d)). CK-13 and CK-14 positivity was also observed in the neoplastic cells (Figures 2(e) and 2(f)), while vimentin, smooth muscle actin, and p16 were negative (Figure 2(g)). Some areas containing mucous were identified within the tumor, as demonstrated by positivity to PAS + DD and mucicarmine (Figures 2(h) and 2(i)). These results in combination support the diagnosis of MEC (Table 2). The patient was referred to the Hospital of the State University of Campinas (UNICAMP), where the tumor was considered inoperable. The patient underwent chemotherapy and radiotherapy but unfortunately died 6 months after diagnosis.

3. Discussion

MEC is one of the most common malignancies of the minor salivary glands [15–17] and is currently described as "a malignant glandular epithelial neoplasm characterized by mucous, intermediate, and epidermoid cells, with columnar, clear cell and oncocytoid features" [18]. According to histopathologic features and the relationship among its cellular components, MEC is classified as low-grade, intermediate-grade, or high-grade [19]. MEC of the minor salivary glands most frequently occurs at the palate and buccal mucosa followed by tongue, gingiva, floor of the mouth, and nasal cavity [20].

This case report describes a case of MEC affecting the right palatine tonsil. The palatine tonsils are considered part of Waldeyer's ring, whose main role is antibody synthesis [21]. Due to its position at the entrance of the oropharynx, the tonsils are the first soft tissue to encounter inhaled and ingested microorganisms. Thus, they are considered the first line of defense against exogenous aggressors [22]. A large number of tumors occur in the palatine tonsils, including SCC, the most common neoplasm of this region [3]. Histologically, SCC is characterized by marked cellular pleomorphism, abnormally large nuclei, increased nuclear to cytoplasmic ratio, and numerous typical and atypical mitotic figures, with or without necrosis [23]. In the present case, neoplastic cells exhibited a homogenous morphology, with mitoses being detected rarely.

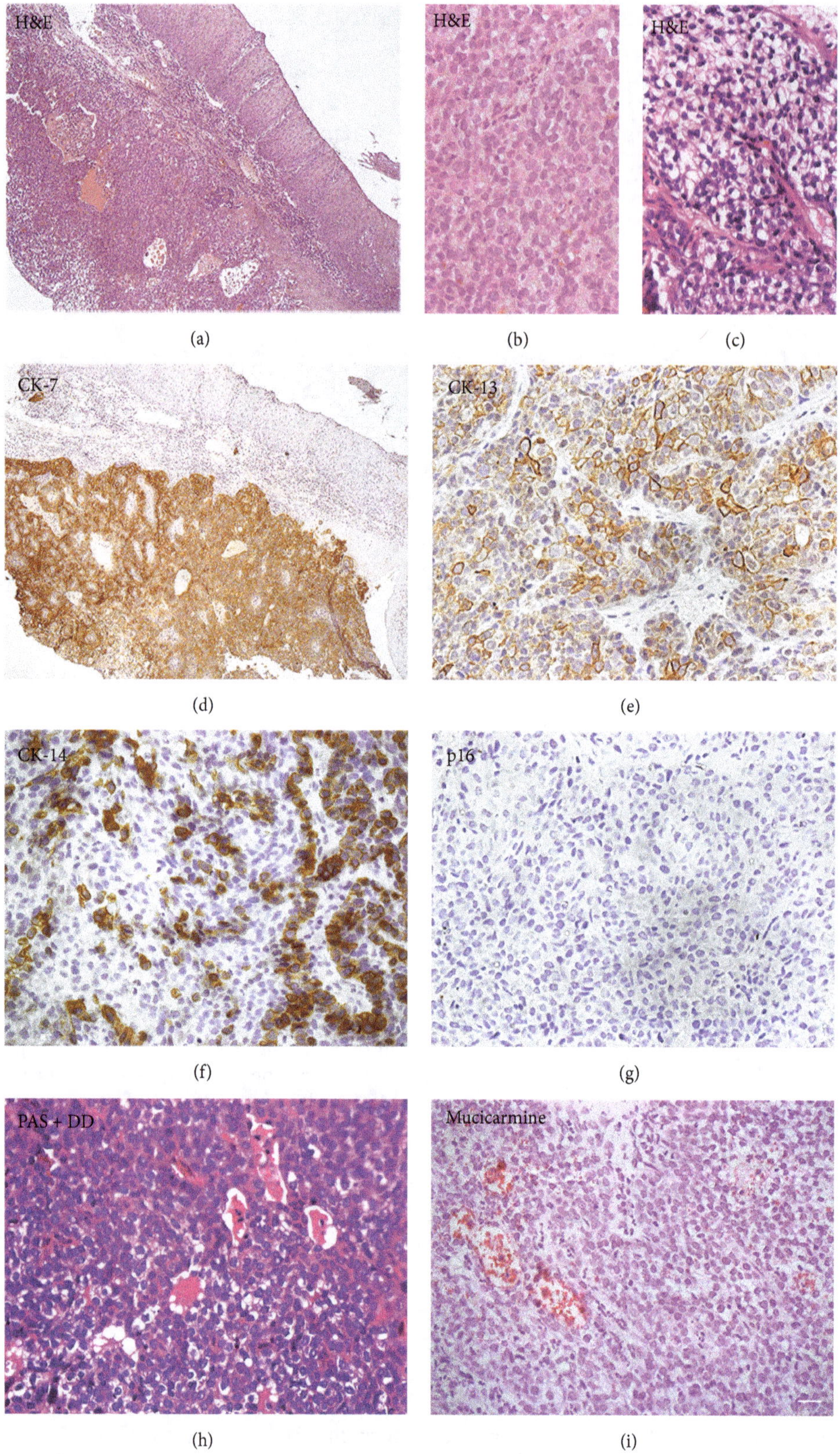

FIGURE 2: (a) H&E revealing a neoplasm of glandular epithelial origin within the lamina propria. (b) The cells showed a homogenous morphology with few cells showing atypia and mitotic figures. (c) Clear cells were observed in some areas. The neoplastic cells were positive for (d) CK-7, (e) CK-13, and (f) CK-14 and negative for (g) p16. (h) PAS with diastase digestion (i) and mucicarmine were also detected within the tumor. Scale bar: (a, c) = 80 μm; (b, d, e, f, g, h) = 20 μm.

The primary risk factors traditionally associated with the development of oral SCC development are smoking and alcohol consumption [24–26]. However, cases of SCC arising from the tonsil area may also be associated with HPV infection [27]. Indeed, approximately 51% of these carcinomas contain HPV DNA [28], with the most prevalent HPV subtype identified being HPV-16, detected in 84% HPV DNA positive tumors [28]. The chance of HPV infection associated with the development of the carcinoma described in the present case report should be discarded, since immunostaining for p16, which is indicative of the presence of HPV, was negative.

Adenocarcinomas account for less than 1% of all malignancies of the palatine tonsils [3], with only a few studies having described the presence of such tumors at this site. The most frequent histological subtypes are represented by adenoid cystic carcinoma [13, 14] and polymorphous low-grade adenocarcinoma [12]. Regarding MEC, only two cases arising in the palatine tonsils have been described in the literature [29, 30].

Approximately 70% of all cases of MEC are comprised by low-grade and intermediate-grade tumors [31, 32]. Thus, routine diagnosis of MEC is generally based on conventional H&E staining looking to identify the presence of cystic structures and mucous cells [20]. High-grade MEC, however, can resemble SCC, as observed in the present case report. In this context, immunohistochemical analysis represents a useful diagnostic tool for salivary gland tumors [33]. The use of this technique to improve understanding of salivary gland tumors was initiated in the 1980s with studies of intermediate keratin filaments, vimentin, and desmin [34–39]. Keratins are a group of intermediate filaments restricted to the epithelium, which are preserved in both malignant transformation and metastasis [40, 41]. During the development of normal human minor salivary glands, one may observe the expression of different CK subtypes [42]. CK-7 was the first CK identified in salivary glands, with its expression remaining in adult salivary glands [38, 42, 43]. In the present case report, immunohistochemistry revealed the presence of large areas showing positivity to CK-7, confirming its glandular origin. Interestingly, Regauer et al. detected a subset of CK-7 positive carcinomas in the Waldeyer's ring area [44]. They suggested that these neoplasms are better classified as basaloid SCC. Although CK-7 was reported in this case report, the morphologic characteristics of basaloid SCC were not encountered, namely, lobules of basaloid cells with central areas of comedonecrosis [45].

Immunohistochemistry for the present case indicated that, besides CK-7, the neoplastic cells were also positive for CK-13 and CK-14, as described previously [33, 46]. Some authors have suggested that positivity for CK-14 may be a distinctive marker in the diagnosis of oral SCC [47, 48]. However, one should note that this CK can also be detected in MEC [33, 46]. Indeed, the basal cells of the epithelium of the oral mucosa, as well as the basal cells of the excretory duct in normal salivary tissues, are positive for CK-14 [47–49]. Thus, positive immunostaining for CK-14 is most likely related to the excretory duct origin of MEC [50]. Moreover, the neoplastic cells exhibited CK-7 positivity, which excludes the chance of SCC. The expression of CK-13 may be detected in MEC, since luminal cells of excretory ducts are positive for this CK, which may also be used as a marker in the differential diagnosis of other salivary gland tumors [33]. In addition to the CKs, staining with PAS + DD and mucicarmine can also be useful markers to discriminate SCC from MEC [51]. Positive areas of PAS and mucicarmine detected in some areas of the tumor corroborated the diagnosis of MEC described in the present case report.

The standard approach for the treatment of MEC is total excision of the tumor [52]. However, minor salivary gland carcinomas of the oropharynx are often challenging to manage [53], with radical tonsillectomy and ipsilateral neck dissection having been used as a treatment option [30, 54]. In the present case, due to the advanced stage of the tumor at presentation, the treatment of choice was chemo- and radiotherapy. Some studies have advised the use of radiotherapy for both high-grade MEC and patients with unclear surgical margins [55–57]. On the other hand, the data regarding chemotherapy in MEC is scarce, with this treatment generally being adopted in palliative management of inoperable tumors [58]. Despite the use of these two modalities in the treatment of the present case, the patient unfortunately died.

In conclusion, this case report highlights the possibility of salivary gland tumor affecting the oropharynx. Thus, during the differential diagnosis of a tumor mass at this specific site, whether asymptomatic or not, salivary gland tumors should not be ignored, since early diagnosis and appropriate management are a determining factor in the prognosis of the patient.

Acknowledgments

The authors would like to thank Jeruza Pinheiro da Silveira Bossonaro and Nadir Freitas for their helpful technical assistance.

References

[1] M. E. Guay and P. Lavertu, "Tonsillar carcinoma," *European Archives of Oto-Rhino-Laryngology*, vol. 252, no. 5, pp. 259–264, 1995.

[2] G. S. Mizono, R. F. Diaz, K. K. Fu, and R. Boles, "Carcinoma of the tonsillar region," *Laryngoscope*, vol. 96, no. 3, pp. 240–244, 1986.

[3] S. M. Golas, "Trends in palatine tonsillar cancer incidence and mortality rates in the United States," *Community Dentistry and Oral Epidemiology*, vol. 35, no. 2, pp. 98–108, 2007.

[4] A. López-Guillermo, L. Colomo, M. Jiménez et al., "Diffuse large B-cell lymphoma: clinical and biological characterization and outcome according to the nodal or extranodal primary originc," *Journal of Clinical Oncology*, vol. 23, no. 12, pp. 2797–2804, 2005.

[5] W. Hong, X. Wang, X.-M. Yu, B. Chen, G.-J. Ding, and Y.-P. Zhang, "Palatine tonsillar metastasis of lung cancer during chemotherapy," *International Journal of Clinical and Experimental Pathology*, vol. 5, no. 5, pp. 468–471, 2012.

[6] E. Yamaguchi, M. Uchida, Y. Makino et al., "Tonsillar metastasis of gastric cancer," *Clinical Journal of Gastroenterology*, vol. 3, no. 6, pp. 289–295, 2010.

[7] R. Cecchi, M. Pavesi, P. Calamandrei, V. Rapicano, and C. De Gaudio, "Tonsil metastasis from cutaneous melanoma: first clinical sign of recurrence after complete lymph node dissection," *Journal of Cutaneous Medicine and Surgery*, vol. 14, no. 1, pp. 43–45, 2010.

[8] M. Massaccesi, A. G. Morganti, G. Serafini et al., "Late tonsil metastases from renal cell cancer: a case report," *Tumori*, vol. 95, no. 4, pp. 521–524, 2009.

[9] L.-M. Sheng, L.-Z. Zhang, H.-M. Xu, and Y. Zhu, "Ascending colon adenocarcinoma with tonsillar metastasis: a case report and review of the literature," *World Journal of Gastroenterology*, vol. 14, no. 46, pp. 7138–7140, 2008.

[10] A. Dalgic, O. Karakoc, U. Aydin et al., "Minor salivary gland neoplasms," *Journal of Craniofacial Surgery*, vol. 25, no. 3, pp. e289–e291, 2014.

[11] K. Balogh and L. Pantanowitz, "Mouth, nose, and paranasal sinuses," in *Histology for Pathologists*, S. E. Mills, Ed., pp. 403–430, Lippincott Williams & Wilkins, Philadelphia, Pa, USA, 2007.

[12] C. B. Pittman and R. P. Zitsch III, "Polymorphous low-grade adenocarcinoma of the tonsil: report of a case and review of the literature," *American Journal of Otolaryngology: Head and Neck Medicine and Surgery*, vol. 23, no. 5, pp. 297–299, 2002.

[13] N. Azarpira, M. J. Ashraf, and M. Shishegar, "Fine-needle aspiration biopsy of adenoid cystic carcinoma of the palatine tonsil," *Indian Journal of Pathology and Microbiology*, vol. 54, no. 2, pp. 424–425, 2011.

[14] E. Azizli, M. Akpinar, F. Gunver, and O. Yigit, "Bilateral tonsillar adenoid cystic carcinoma," *Journal of Craniofacial Surgery*, vol. 22, no. 6, pp. 2408–2409, 2011.

[15] F. A. de Oliveira, E. C. B. Duarte, C. T. Taveira et al., "Salivary gland tumor: a review of 599 cases in a Brazilian population," *Head and Neck Pathology*, vol. 3, no. 4, pp. 271–275, 2009.

[16] X.-D. Wang, L.-J. Meng, T.-T. Hou, and S.-H. Huang, "Tumours of the salivary glands in northeastern China: a retrospective study of 2508 patients," *British Journal of Oral and Maxillofacial Surgery*, vol. 53, no. 2, pp. 132–137, 2015.

[17] R. H. Spiro, "Management of malignant tumors of the salivary glands," *Oncology*, vol. 12, no. 5, pp. 671–680, 1998.

[18] R. K. Goode and A. K. El-Naggar, "Mucoepidermoid carcinoma," in *World Health Organization Classification of Tumours. Pathology and Genetics of Head and Neck Tumours*, L. Barnes, J. W. Eveson, P. Reichart, and D. Sidransky, Eds., pp. 219–220, IARC Press, Lyon, France, 2005.

[19] A. Coca-Pelaz, J. P. Rodrigo, A. Triantafyllou et al., "Salivary mucoepidermoid carcinoma revisited," *European Archives of Oto-Rhino-Laryngology*, vol. 272, no. 4, pp. 799–819, 2015.

[20] M. A. Luna, "Salivary mucoepidermoid carcinoma: revisited," *Advances in Anatomic Pathology*, vol. 13, no. 6, pp. 293–307, 2006.

[21] S. Masieri, D. Trabattoni, C. Incorvaia et al., "A role for Waldeyer's ring in immunological response to allergens," *Current Medical Research and Opinion*, vol. 30, no. 2, pp. 203–205, 2014.

[22] P. Hellings, M. Jorissen, and J. L. Ceuppens, "The Waldeyer's ring," *Acta Oto-Rhino-Laryngologica Belgica*, vol. 54, no. 3, pp. 237–241, 2000.

[23] A. Cardesa, N. Gale, A. Nadal, and N. Zidal, "Squamous cell carcinoma," in *World Health Organization Classification of Tumours. Pathology and Genetics of Head and Neck Tumours*, L. Barnes, J. W. Eveson, P. Reichart, and D. Sidransky, Eds., pp. 118–121, IARC Press, Lyon, France, 2005.

[24] C. Scully and J. V. Bagan, "Oral squamous cell carcinoma: overview of current understanding of aetiopathogenesis and clinical implications," *Oral Diseases*, vol. 15, no. 6, pp. 388–399, 2009.

[25] A. G. Zygogianni, G. Kyrgias, P. Karakitsos et al., "Oral squamous cell cancer: early detection and the role of alcohol and smoking," *Head & Neck Oncology*, vol. 6, no. 3, pp. 1–12, 2011.

[26] A. H. Madani, M. Dikshit, D. Bhaduri, T. Aghamolaei, S. H. Moosavy, and A. Azarpaykan, "Interaction of alcohol use and specific types of smoking on the development of oral cancer," *International Journal of High Risk Behaviors and Addiction*, vol. 3, no. 1, pp. 1–4, 2014.

[27] T. Ramqvist, N. Grün, and T. Dalianis, "Human papillomavirus and tonsillar and base of tongue cancer," *Viruses*, vol. 7, no. 3, pp. 1332–1343, 2015.

[28] S. Syrjänen, "HPV infections and tonsillar carcinoma," *Journal of Clinical Pathology*, vol. 57, no. 5, pp. 449–455, 2004.

[29] L. Jing-Xian, "Clinico-pathologic studies on 143 cases of tonsillar malignancies with special reference to lymphomas," *Zhonghua Zhong Liu Za Zhi*, vol. 14, no. 6, pp. 433–436, 1992.

[30] S. J. Jarvis, V. Giangrande, and P. A. Brennan, "Mucoepidermoid carcinoma of the tonsil: a very rare presentation," *Acta Otorhinolaryngologica Italica*, vol. 33, no. 4, pp. 286–288, 2013.

[31] S. A. Miguens Jr., A. C. Uchoa Vasconcelos, M. A. Figueiredo, L. Soares Yurgel, F. Salum, and K. Cherubini, "Mucoepidermoid carcinoma: a retrospective study," *Minerva Stomatologica*, vol. 59, no. 6, pp. 325–332, 2010.

[32] K. Yamazaki, H. Ohta, R. Shodo, H. Matsuyama, and S. Takahashi, "Clinicopathological features of mucoepidermoid carcinoma," *The Journal of Laryngology and Otology*, vol. 128, no. 1, pp. 91–95, 2014.

[33] V. C. de Araújo, S. O. M. de Sousa, Y. R. Carvalho, and N. S. de Araújo, "Application of immunohistochemistry to the diagnosis of salivary gland tumors," *Applied Immunohistochemistry & Molecular Morphology*, vol. 8, no. 3, pp. 195–202, 2000.

[34] J. Caselitz and T. Löning, "Specific demonstration of actin and keratin filaments in pleomorphic adenomas by means of immunoelectron microscopy," *Virchows Archiv A Pathological Anatomy and Histology*, vol. 393, no. 2, pp. 153–158, 1981.

[35] J. Caselitz, M. Osborn, G. Seifert, and K. Weber, "Intermediate-sized filament proteins (prekeratin, vimentin, desmin) in the normal parotid gland and parotid gland tumours," *Virchows Archiv A*, vol. 393, no. 3, pp. 273–286, 1981.

[36] J. Caselitz, M. Osborn, J. Wustrow, G. Seifert, and K. Weber, "The expression of different intermediate-sized filaments in human salivary glands and their tumours," *Pathology Research and Practice*, vol. 175, no. 2-3, pp. 266–278, 1982.

[37] R. M. Palmer, "The identification of myoepithelial cells in human salivary glands. A review and comparison of light microscopical methods," *Journal of Oral Pathology & Medicine*, vol. 15, no. 4, pp. 221–229, 1986.

[38] H. Gustafsson, U. Kjorell, A. Eriksson, I. Virtanen, and L.-E. Thornell, "Distribution of intermediate filament proteins in

developing and adult salivary glands in man," *Anatomy and Embryology*, vol. 178, no. 3, pp. 243–257, 1988.

[39] H. Gustafsson, I. Virtanen, and L.-E. Thornell, "Glial fibrillary acidic protein and desmin in salivary neoplasms," *Virchows Archiv B*, vol. 57, no. 1, pp. 303–313, 1989.

[40] P. Chu, E. Wu, and L. M. Weiss, "Cytokeratin 7 and cytokeratin 20 expression in epithelial neoplasms: a survey of 435 cases," *Modern Pathology*, vol. 13, no. 9, pp. 962–972, 2000.

[41] G. A. Stopyra, M. J. Warhol, and H. A. B. Multhaupt, "Cytokeratin 20 immunoreactivity in renal oncocytomas," *Journal of Histochemistry & Cytochemistry*, vol. 49, no. 7, pp. 919–920, 2001.

[42] M. D. Martins, V. Cavalcanti de Araujo, R. Raitz, and N. Soares de Araújo, "Expression of cytoskeletal proteins in developing human minor salivary glands," *European Journal of Oral Sciences*, vol. 110, no. 4, pp. 316–321, 2002.

[43] P. G. Chu and L. M. Weiss, "Keratin expression in human tissues and neoplasms," *Histopathology*, vol. 40, no. 5, pp. 403–439, 2002.

[44] S. Regauer, A. Beham, and S. Mannweiler, "CK7 expression in carcinomas of the Waldeyer's ring area," *Human Pathology*, vol. 31, no. 9, pp. 1096–1101, 2000.

[45] A. Cardesa, N. Zidar, and C. Ereño, "Basaloid squamous cell carcinoma," in *World Health Organization Classification of Tumours. Pathology and Genetics of Head and Neck Tumours*, L. Barnes, J. W. Eveson, P. Reichart, and D. Sidransky, Eds., pp. 124–125, IARC Press, Lyon, France, 2005.

[46] E. J. D. da Silveira, S. S. L. Veras Barros, R. F. B. de Amorim, L. M. G. Queiroz, R. D. A. Freitas, and L. B. de Souza, "Cytokeratin profile in mucoepidermoid carcinoma is not related to its histological grading of malignancy," *Experimental and Molecular Pathology*, vol. 81, no. 1, pp. 72–76, 2006.

[47] V. C. de Araüjo and S. O. M. de Sousa, "Expression of different keratins in salivary gland tumours," *European Journal of Cancer Part B: Oral Oncology*, vol. 32, no. 1, pp. 14–18, 1996.

[48] A. P. V. Sobral, S. V. L. Loducca, L. P. Kowalski et al., "Immunohistochemical distinction of high-grade mucoepidermoid carcinoma and epidermoid carcinoma of the parotid region," *Oral Oncology*, vol. 38, no. 5, pp. 437–440, 2002.

[49] R. B. Presland and B. A. Dale, "Epithelial structural proteins of the skin and oral cavity: function in health and disease," *Critical Reviews in Oral Biology & Medicine*, vol. 11, no. 4, pp. 383–408, 2000.

[50] R. S. Azevedo, O. P. de Almeida, L. P. Kowalski, and F. R. Pires, "Comparative cytokeratin expression in the different cell types of salivary gland mucoepidermoid carcinoma," *Head and Neck Pathology*, vol. 2, no. 4, pp. 257–264, 2008.

[51] G. L. Ellis and P. L. Auclair, *Atlas of Tumor Pathology: Tumors of the Salivary Glands*, Armed Forces Institute of Pathology, Washington, DC, USA, 1996.

[52] H. Ozawa, T. Tomita, K. Sakamoto et al., "Mucoepidermoid carcinoma of the head and neck: clinical analysis of 43 patients," *Japanese Journal of Clinical Oncology*, vol. 38, no. 6, pp. 414–418, 2008.

[53] N. G. Iyer, L. Kim, I. J. Nixon et al., "Factors predicting outcome in malignant minor salivary gland tumors of the oropharynx," *Archives of Otolaryngology - Head and Neck Surgery*, vol. 136, no. 12, pp. 1240–1247, 2010.

[54] V. Vander Poorten, J. Hunt, P. J. Bradley et al., "Recent trends in the management of minor salivary gland carcinoma," *Head and Neck*, vol. 36, no. 3, pp. 444–455, 2014.

[55] Y. Hosokawa, H. Shirato, K. Kagei et al., "Role of radiotherapy for mucoepidermoid carcinoma of salivary gland," *Oral Oncology*, vol. 35, no. 1, pp. 105–111, 1999.

[56] M. S. Brandwein, K. Ivanov, D. I. Wallace et al., "Mucoepidermoid carcinoma: a clinicopathologic study of 80 patients with special reference to histological grading," *The American Journal of Surgical Pathology*, vol. 25, no. 7, pp. 835–845, 2001.

[57] K. Triantafillidou, J. Dimitrakopoulos, F. Iordanidis, and D. Koufogiannis, "Mucoepidermoid carcinoma of minor salivary glands: a clinical study of 16 cases and review of the literature," *Oral Diseases*, vol. 12, no. 4, pp. 364–370, 2006.

[58] S. A. Laurie and L. Licitra, "Systemic therapy in the palliative management of advanced salivary gland cancers," *Journal of Clinical Oncology*, vol. 24, no. 17, pp. 2673–2678, 2006.

13

Innovative Approaches to Radiation Treatment for Mycosis Fungoides in the Setting of Collagen Vascular Disease

Stephanie A. Terezakis,[1,2] George C. Bohle III,[3,4] Ying-Chun Lo,[5,6] Sean L. Berry,[2] and Joachim Yahalom[2]

[1] *Department of Radiation Oncology and Molecular Radiation Sciences, Johns Hopkins Hospital, Baltimore, MD 21287, USA*
[2] *Department of Radiation Oncology, Memorial Sloan-Kettering Cancer Center, New York, NY 10065, USA*
[3] *Dental Service, Department of Surgery, Memorial Sloan-Kettering Cancer Center, New York, NY 10065, USA*
[4] *College of Dentistry, University of Oklahoma, Oklahoma City, OK 73117, USA*
[5] *Department of Oncology, Johns Hopkins School of Medicine, Baltimore, MD 21287, USA*
[6] *Department of Pathology, Yale-New Haven Hospital, New Haven, CT 06510, USA*

Correspondence should be addressed to Stephanie A. Terezakis; stereza1@jhmi.edu

Academic Editor: Marcel W. Bekkenk

Patients with connective tissue disorders are clinically challenging for radiation oncologists as these patients may be at increased risk for radiation-related skin toxicity. A clinical dilemma presents itself in a patient with lupus who presents with confluent skin lesions from mycosis fungoides requiring radiotherapy. In this report, we discuss an innovative technique used to develop an immobilization device that also effectively functioned as a uniform bolus with distinct dosimetric advantages to the use of a facial moulage.

1. Introduction

Patients with connective tissue disorders present a formidable clinical challenge to the treating radiation oncologist as numerous reports have suggested that these patients may be at an increased risk of toxicity secondary to radiation treatment (RT) [1–6]. It has been hypothesized that patients with connective tissue disorder have increased radiosensitivity and possibly increased risk of pathological damage to the microvasculature from radiation therapy [7, 8]. Due to prior published case reports describing enhanced radiation-induced toxicity in these patients, it is likely that radiation is not offered to all those who may benefit even though the extent of these risks is still largely unknown [9]. Therefore, in current clinical practice, lupus is a relative but not an absolute contraindication of radiation therapy and radiation is only delivered when absolutely necessary [10]. Rather than avoiding radiation as a therapeutic modality, these patients may benefit from treatment techniques that minimize the risk of toxicity and maximize therapeutic benefit. We were presented with a difficult case of a patient with erythematous lupus and mycosis fungoides (MF) of the bilateral face. The patient had already progressed through known topical therapies and there were no additional treatment options that would address her facial skin lesions except radiation therapy. Current widely available techniques for treatment include combining the use of a normal thermoplastic mask for immobilization with supplemental bolus material (e.g., SuperFlab or PlayDoh). However, during the course of daily treatments that could extend over several weeks, it becomes challenging to guarantee the reproducibility of the bolus position, the daily adherence of the bolus to the patient's surface over the entire treatment area, and the integrity of the bolus material itself. The face contains many topographical variations and poorly fit bolus materials will degrade the delivered dose distribution, particularly at the patient's skin surface [11]. We describe and evaluate the clinical feasibility of a novel approach to creating an immobilization device that

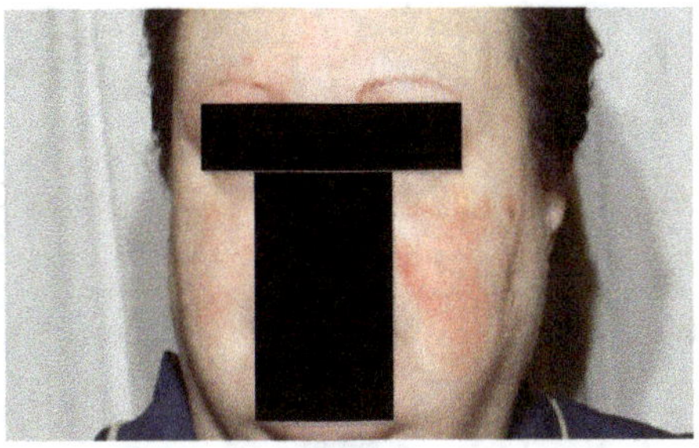

FIGURE 1: Pretreatment extent of clinically apparent disease.

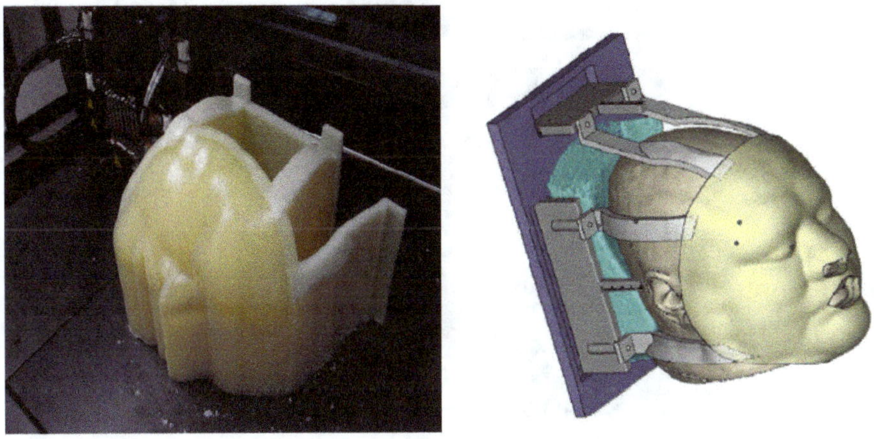

FIGURE 2: Fabrication of immobilization mold using customized bolus.

also functions as a bolus material. This device is customized and form-fitted using a digital model of the patient.

2. Case Report

This 60-year-old patient with history of erythematous lupus presented with a confluent facial eruption of classical (epidermotropic) MF and was referred to radiation oncology after several courses of topical therapies failed (Figure 1). Before being referred to radiation oncology, the patient received ultraviolet radiation therapy with no improvement. There were multiple lesions on the face beyond the very obvious lesion on the left cheek. There were multiple pathologic skin biopsies throughout the face performed which confirmed mycosis fungoides. Her treatment plan needed to target the disease sites on the surface of the face including the bilateral eyebrows, eyelids, cheeks, and temples. Given this patient's history of erythematous lupus and the eloquent location of her radiation field, it was decided that a low dose of 1800 cGy in 200 cGy fractions would be delivered to the face to a depth of 5 mm. An electron energy of 6 MeV was chosen with a desired bolus thickness of 1 cm in order to deliver the prescribed dose both at depth and to the skin surface. Immobilization was also an important component of treatment setup to minimize the margins required in the design of the planning target volume. To adequately cover the involved sites, the bolus would necessarily be placed over nearly the entire face, under the mask, which would be intolerable for the patient due to difficulty with breathing and claustrophobia. Therefore, an alternative technique was explored to create an immobilization device that would effectively function as a uniform bolus that would be tolerable to the patient on a daily basis.

The patient presented for simulation for radiation planning and to acquire mask measurements. A computed tomography (CT) scan of the patient's head and neck was obtained from crown to the hyoid bone for the fabrication of a custom face mask. The CT scan was reconstructed into 0.625 mm slices to provide a high resolution image. The Orfit (Orfit Industries, Antwerp, Belgium) head and neck immobilization device baseboard was measured with calipers to the nearest 0.01 mm and a virtual model was made using engineering software (SolidWorks 2008, Dassault Systèmes SolidWorks Corp., Concord, MA, USA). Lastly the neck pillow used was scanned using cone beam CT (ILUMA, IMTEC/3M) and a high resolution image was saved in.STL format.

The separate virtual images of the patient, neck pillow, and immobilization device baseboard were combined into one model. The mask was designed using medical software (Mimics, Materialise, Ann Arbor, MI, USA) and coupled with the attachment apparatus designed on the virtual model (Figure 2). Using PolyJet printing technology (Connex500, Objet Geometries), the soft, pliable mask and rigid connecting apparatus were fabricated (Figure 3). The mask material was a proprietary "rubber-like" material (TangoPlus, Objet Geometries, Billerica, MA, USA) with a density of

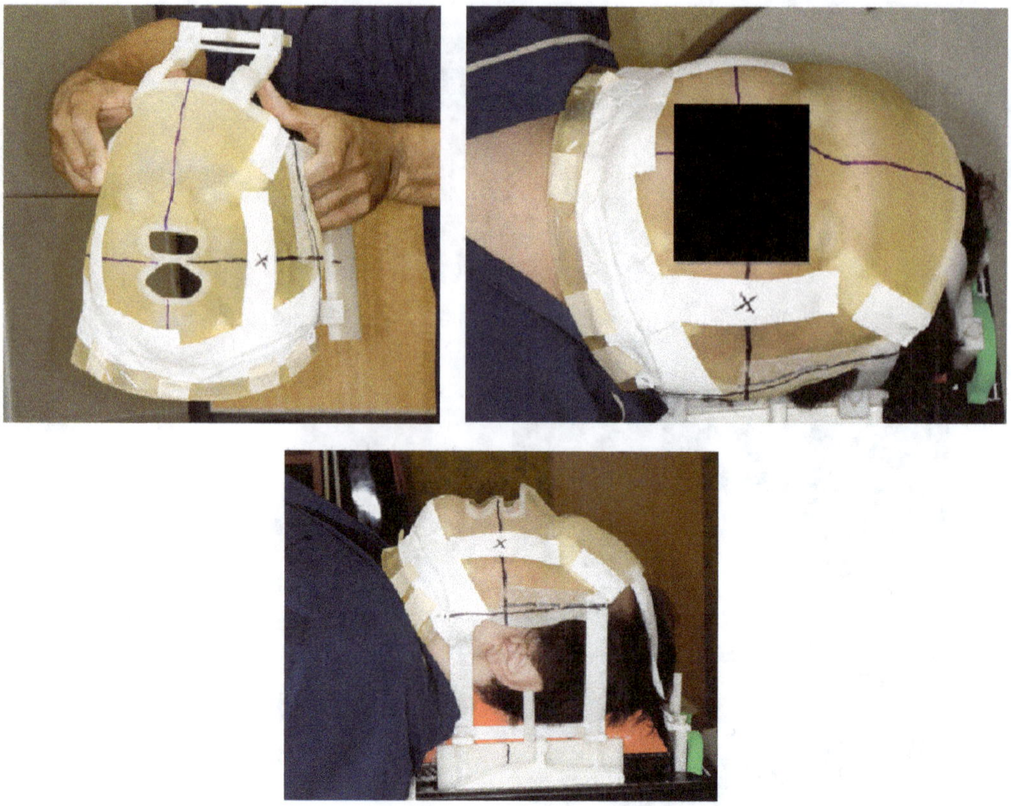

Figure 3: Final immobilization mold using customized bolus.

1.141 gr/cm^3. The patient returned for a second simulation appointment, at which time the mask and stabilization apparatus were fit to the patient.

The water equivalent thickness of the rubber material was studied using phantom measurements. A depth ionization distribution in polystyrene was measured for a 6 MeV electron beam using the Memorial Pipe chamber, a thin-window (0.05 mm) parallel-plate ionization chamber. Then, the measurement was repeated with a flat, 1.29 cm thick, sample of the material placed on top of the polystyrene. The offset between the two resulting depth ionization distributions represents the radiological equivalent thickness of the bolus material.

3. Results

Figure 4 is a representative slice of the resulting treatment plan (Figure 4). A beam arrangement of two en face electron beams was chosen. One beam was directed towards each cheek using a source to surface distance of 105 cm. An in-house treatment planning system (TPS) was employed with dose calculations conducted via pencil beam convolution with a calculation grid size of 2 mm. A gap between the field edges was used at the skin surface along the midline of the face such that hot spots that were deemed intolerable were minimized and the best possible prescription dose coverage throughout the entire face was maintained.

From measurement, the radiological equivalent thickness of the bolus was equal to 1.024 times the geometric thickness. The measured HU in the TPS was 100, and calculations within

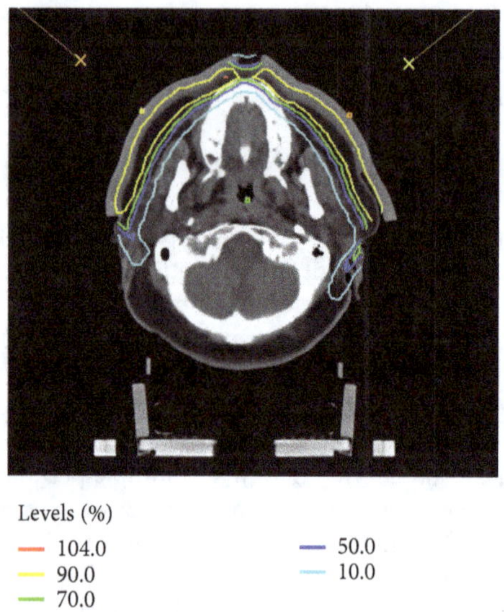

Figure 4: Dose distribution of 6 MeV electrons with customized bolus face mask in place; dose was prescribed to the 90% isodose line (yellow contour).

the TPS result in a radiological equivalent bolus thickness of 1.08 cm. This indicates that the TPS will predict the penetration depth of the electron beam within approximately 0.5 mm.

The intaglio surface of the mask was cleaned daily with mild soap and water as the material does not breathe well and

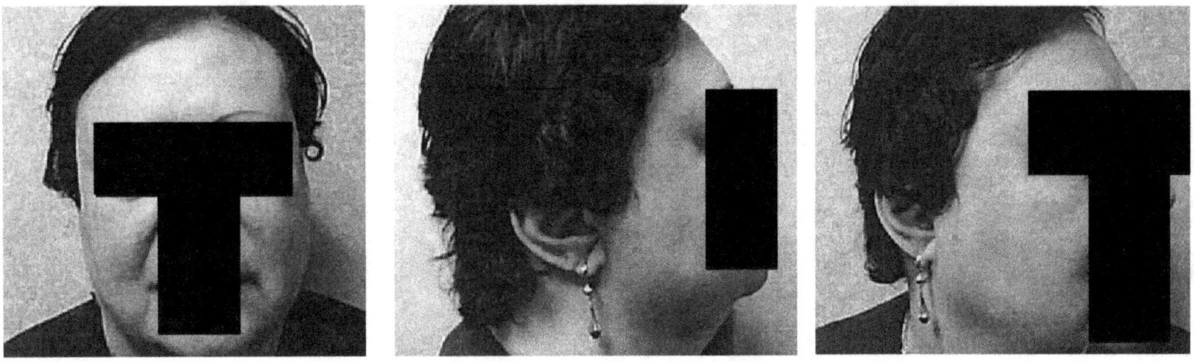

FIGURE 5: Follow-up of patient at 4 years demonstrating excellent cosmesis.

the patient perspires during treatment. The mask maintained integrity throughout daily treatment with no evidence of stretch or deformation. The patient sustained mild grade I erythema during the course of radiation which resolved within several weeks after completion of her radiation course. Her facial lesions sustained a complete response at four-year follow-up with no evidence of radiation-related sequelae (Figure 5).

4. Discussion

Traditionally and currently in clinical practice, lupus can be a relative contraindication for patients to receive radiation therapy. Here we demonstrate that radiation therapy can be performed in patients who require it using innovative approaches and should not be avoided altogether. For the patient we presented in this report, she had no other treatment options. Rather than assuming that radiotherapy could not be done safely and effectively, we used an innovative approach to utilize radiotherapy, which was effective (as evidenced by no progression of disease) and safe (as evidenced by no manifestation of skin toxicity after RT).

In this report, we describe an approach to the development of an immobilization device with integrated bolus used to develop a plan in a TPS. Widely available current techniques utilize a normal thermoplastic mask for immobilization and a commonly used bolus material. In this patient, for example, there would have been concerns with the use of a thermoplastic mask with supplemental SuperFlab. Sheets of SuperFlab cannot stay tight in all of the crevices of the face such as the eyelid and nasal ala, leading to localized air gaps and subsequent hot and cold spots. Since we are treating the "whole face," the concerns with dose homogeneity with this more commonly used technique are more exaggerated than the typical patient. The technique using a thermoplastic mask in addition to PlayDoh could also pose a problem as PlayDoh is very difficult to mold in a uniform thickness while avoiding internal air bubbles. Also, it would be difficult to avoid compressing and reshaping the mold with repeated applications and thus, reproducibility may be compromised. The technique we describe brings a level of precision unavailable in most treatment techniques. Use of a digital patient model also avoids the local deformations in the face that can occur when a thermoplastic mask is held tight while it dries or when creating a moulage.

An alternative plan would have been to produce a stone cast of the patient from a facial moulage and fabricate the mask in medical grade silicone by hand. The advantages to a moulage are cost and the shorter mask production turnaround time. However, the moulage has inherent inaccuracies due to the physical material properties of expansion or contraction and the actual weight of the impression that can distort soft tissues. After the moulage is made and the stone cast poured, the mask must be designed by hand which can lead to a nonuniform thickness of bolus leading to hot/cold spots in the treatment plan. Additionally, even if the thickness is precisely controlled, silicone manipulated by hand will contain air bubbles thus leading to a nonuniform density and again causing hot/cold spots. By utilizing CAD/CAM technology, the above factors are controlled as the imaging does not distort the soft tissues of the face. Additionally, the machines that manipulate the material and fabricate the shape are extremely accurate and control for factors such as expansion/contraction, density, and thickness.

The amount of time spent in the design, fabrication, and quality assurance of this device can be broken into two parts: device-specific and patient-specific parts. The device-specific aspects are time consuming in which detailed measurements of the immobilization device base plate and head rest need to be taken and modeled in the CAD software. Further, the water equivalent thickness of the bolus material has to be determined. However, this only has to be done during initial commissioning of the system or if there are any modifications to the materials. The patient-specific aspect requires 2 CT scans, a high resolution scan to get the model of the patient's face and a subsequent scan to verify how well the mask fits and to verify its thickness. The fabrication of the mask itself is either performed by a third-party service or, as 3D printers become more widely available, in-house.

5. Conclusions

The possibility that radiation may be withheld from patients for whom it may be curative is concerning. This report describes an innovative technique that may be used to minimize risks to a patient with a complicated clinical scenario and raises awareness to a clinical practice trend in which patients with CVD may receive suboptimal care despite limited data [12, 13]. In this report, we describe an approach to the development of an immobilization device with integrated bolus for a difficult treatment site with excellent clinical results.

References

[1] M. Abu-Shakra and P. Lee, "Exaggerated fibrosis in patients with systemic sclerosis (scleroderma) following radiation therapy," *Journal of Rheumatology*, vol. 20, no. 9, pp. 1601–1603, 1993.

[2] T. Hölscher, S. M. Bentzen, and M. Baumann, "Influence of connective tissue diseases on the expression of radiation side effects: a systematic review," *Radiotherapy and Oncology*, vol. 78, no. 2, pp. 123–130, 2006.

[3] A. Lin, E. Abu-Isa, K. A. Griffith, and E. Ben-Josef, "Toxicity of radiotherapy in patients with collagen vascular disease," *Cancer*, vol. 113, no. 3, pp. 648–653, 2008.

[4] C. Phan, M. Mindrum, C. Silverman, K. Paris, and W. Spanos, "Matched-control retrospective study of the acute and late complications in patients with collagen vascular diseases treated with radiation therapy," *Cancer Journal*, vol. 9, no. 6, pp. 461–466, 2003.

[5] M. E. Pinn, D. G. Gold, I. A. Petersen, T. G. Osborn, P. D. Brown, and R. C. Miller, "Systemic lupus erythematosus, radiotherapy, and the risk of acute and chronic toxicity: the Mayo Clinic Experience," *International Journal of Radiation Oncology Biology Physics*, vol. 71, no. 2, pp. 498–506, 2008.

[6] J. G. Ross, D. H. Hussey, N. A. Mayr, and C. S. Davis, "Acute and late reactions to radiation therapy in patients with collagen vascular diseases," *Cancer*, vol. 71, no. 11, pp. 3744–3752, 1993.

[7] I. A. Olivotto, R. N. Fairey, J. H. Gillies, and H. Stein, "Fatal outcome of pelvic radiotherapy for carcinoma of the cervix in a patient with systemic lupus erythematosis," *Clinical Radiology*, vol. 40, no. 1, pp. 83–84, 1989.

[8] R. Fleck, M. D. McNeese, N. A. Ellerbroek, T. A. Hunter, and F. A. Holmes, "Consequences of breast irradiation in patients with pre-existing collagen vascular diseases," *International Journal of Radiation Oncology, Biology, Physics*, vol. 17, no. 4, pp. 829–833, 1989.

[9] V. Benk, A. Al-Herz, D. Gladman, M. Urowitz, and P. R. Fortin, "Role of radiation therapy in patients with a diagnosis of both systemic lupus erythematosus and cancer," *Arthritis Care & Research*, vol. 53, no. 1, pp. 67–72, 2005.

[10] A. B. Patel, C. L. Hallemeier, I. A. Petersen, A. W. Jensen, T. G. Osborn, and R. C. Miller, "Acute and late toxicities of radiotherapy for patients with discoid lupus erythematosus: a retrospective case-control study," *Radiation Oncology*, vol. 7, article 22, 2012.

[11] S. C. Sharma and M. W. Johnson, "Surface dose perturbation due to air gap between patient and bolus for electron beams," *Medical Physics*, vol. 20, no. 2, part 1, pp. 377–378, 1993.

[12] Y. H. Kim, S. Chow, A. Varghese, and R. T. Hoppe, "Clinical characteristics and long-term outcome of patients with generalized patch and/or plaque (T2) mycosis fungoides," *Archives of Dermatology*, vol. 135, no. 1, pp. 26–32, 1999.

[13] J. M. Robertson, D. H. Clarke, M. M. Pevzner, and R. C. Matter, "Breast conservation therapy: severe breast fibrosis after radiation therapy in patients with collagen vascular disease," *Cancer*, vol. 68, no. 3, pp. 502–508, 1991.

14

Small Bowel Adenocarcinoma as the Cause of Gastrointestinal Bleeding in Celiac Disease: A Rare Malignancy in a Common Disease

Jaleh Fallah,[1,2] Maxwell Eyram Afari,[1,2] Alfredo C. Cordova,[2,3] Adam J. Olszewski,[1,2] and Taro Minami[2,4]

[1]*Department of Medicine, Memorial Hospital of Rhode Island, Pawtucket, RI 02860, USA*
[2]*The Warren Alpert Medical School of Brown University, Pawtucket, RI 02860, USA*
[3]*Department of Surgery, Memorial Hospital of Rhode Island, Pawtucket, RI 02860, USA*
[4]*Division of Pulmonary, Critical Care and Sleep Medicine, Memorial Hospital of Rhode Island, Pawtucket, RI 02860, USA*

Correspondence should be addressed to Jaleh Fallah; jfallah1191@gmail.com

Academic Editor: Yoshihito Yokoyama

Introduction. Celiac disease is associated with an increased risk of small bowel malignancies, particularly lymphoma. Its association with small bowel carcinoma is less known. *Case Description.* We report a case of an 89-year-old woman with celiac disease who experienced recurrent episodes of gastrointestinal bleeding and was ultimately found to have adenocarcinoma of the small intestine. *Discussion and Evaluation.* Diagnosis of small bowel adenocarcinoma is often delayed because of the need for specialized modalities, which are often deferred in the inpatient setting. Although resection is the modality of choice for small bowel tumors, a majority is either locally advanced or metastatic at diagnosis, and even localized cancers have worse prognosis than stage-matched colorectal tumors. The role of adjuvant chemotherapy is uncertain, but it is often offered extrapolating data from other gastrointestinal cancers. Small bowel carcinomas occurring in the context of celiac disease appear to be associated with higher rates of microsatellite instability than sporadic tumors, although other specific genomic abnormalities and mechanisms of carcinogenesis in celiac disease remain unknown. *Conclusion.* Recurrent episodes of gastrointestinal bleeding in a patient with celiac disease should prompt an early evaluation of the small bowel to assure timely diagnosis of carcinoma at an early curable stage.

1. Introduction

Celiac disease is a common disease, with a prevalence of approximately 1-2% in North and South America, North Africa, India, and the Middle East [1]. Iron deficiency is a common clinical feature of this disease and is related to malabsorption rather than gastrointestinal blood loss. Celiac disease is known to be associated with an increased risk of malignancy, particularly lymphoma [2, 3]. However, less is known about the risk of gastrointestinal carcinoma associated with celiac disease. We have encountered a case of adenocarcinoma of the small intestine with celiac disease, a rare malignancy in a common disease.

2. Case Presentation

An 89-year-old woman with a history of celiac disease, prior gastrointestinal bleeding, and dementia was admitted to our Intensive Care Unit for a recurrent gastrointestinal bleeding. The celiac disease had been diagnosed two years earlier by an endoscopic biopsy of the duodenum (demonstrating a subtotal villous atrophy) and with a correlative serum tissue transglutaminase IgA antibody (162 units, reference range 0–19 units). The patient had not been compliant with the recommended gluten-free diet because of early dementia and was treated with additional oral budesonide because of chronic abdominal discomfort. She was in her usual state

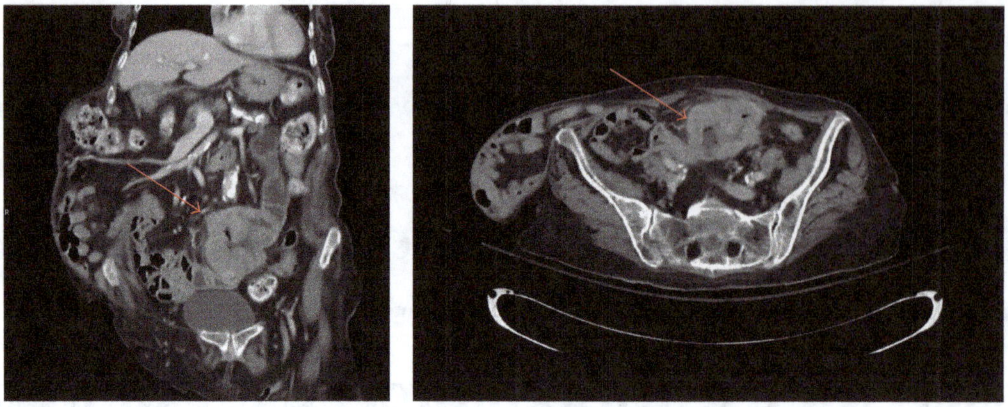

(a) (b)

Figure 1: Axial (a) and coronal (b) projections of the computerized tomography of the abdomen. Arrows point to the small bowel tumor.

of health until two days prior to this admission when she developed nausea and had multiple bouts of coffee ground emesis, with which she presented to the emergency room. She reported poor appetite and significant weight loss during the prior year, which had been ascribed to celiac disease-related malabsorption and led to therapy with oral budesonide. Her medical history was additionally significant for prior admission with similar symptoms of nausea, vomiting, and gastrointestinal bleeding with severe anemia three, six, and twelve months prior to the index presentation. Esophagogastroduodenoscopy (EGD) had been performed on all these occasions, showing gastritis and duodenitis with biopsies consistent with celiac disease. There was no history of tobacco or alcohol use and no family history of celiac disease or malignancies.

On admission, the patient was hypotensive with blood pressure of 93/49 mm Hg and heart rate of 86 beats per minute and afebrile and her respiratory rate was 18 breaths per minute. Physical examination revealed a palpable left paraumbilical mass and a 20 cm × 20 cm reducible hernia in the right abdominal wall. Laboratory work-up revealed hemoglobin of 6.9 g/dL (reference range, 12.0–16.0 g/dL). Serum chemistry, liver function tests, electrocardiogram, and chest radiograph were within normal limits. Abdominal computed tomography (CT) with intravenous contrast revealed a proximal dilatation of an abnormally thickened segment of the small bowel suspicious for a malignancy (Figure 1). The patient was resuscitated with intravenous fluids and a red cell transfusion.

On third admission day, after hemodynamic stability was established, she underwent laparotomy. A large (15 × 10 cm) small bowel tumor located approximately 20 cm from the ligament of Treitz was resected (Figure 2). There was no evidence of metastatic lesions in the peritoneum or liver during intraoperative inspection of all quadrants of the abdominal cavity. Pathologic examination revealed a poorly differentiated adenocarcinoma (final tumor size 6.5 cm) with invasion into an adjacent portion of the small intestine and to the serosal surface, with metastases to 4 out of 12 resected lymph nodes, staged as pT4b pN2 M0 or stage III according to the American Joint Commission on Cancer staging system (Figure 3). The tumor cells were positive for immunohistochemical markers of adenocarcinoma (CDX2 and CK7) and negative for CK20, vimentin, neuroendocrine markers (synaptophysin, chromogranin, and CD56), and lymphoid antigens (CD3, CD20, and CD45). After the surgery, the patient elected palliative care and did not receive any further cancer-directed therapy.

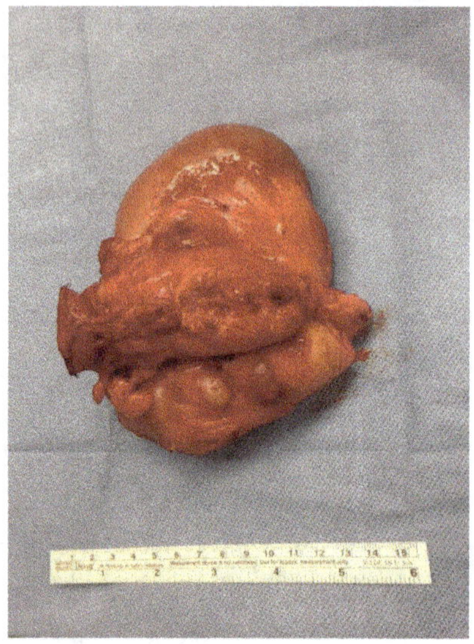

Figure 2: Photograph of the gross resection specimen of the small bowel segment containing adenocarcinoma.

3. Discussion

Small bowel carcinoma is a rare clinical entity with an annual incidence of 0.66 cases per 100,000 person-years in the United States, which is higher for men (0.80 per 100,000) than for women (0.55) [4]. Neuroendocrine tumors (39%, mostly carcinoids) are more common than carcinomas (31%), while less common histologies encompass lymphomas (18%) and

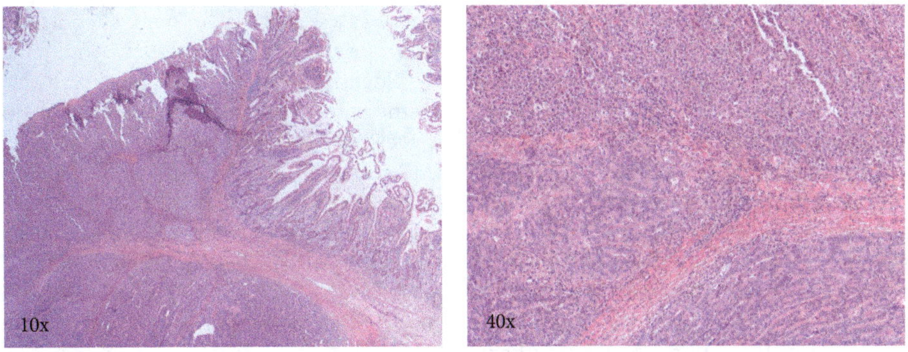

(a) (b)

FIGURE 3: Microscopic images of the tumor from the histopathologic specimen, hematoxylin and eosin stain. (a) Low-power magnification (10x) shows normal small bowel mucosa (right) and invasive adenocarcinoma (left). (b) High-power magnification (40x) shows two patterns of differentiation, with poorly differentiated carcinoma in the upper part of the panel.

sarcomas (10%). Although the small intestine is three times longer than the large intestine, it is the primary location for only 5% of all gastrointestinal malignancies [5].

Despite the fact that lower gastrointestinal bleeding is a common cause of hospitalization in the elderly, the diagnosis can be challenging and the diagnostic differential is broad. In a study of 1,112 patients admitted to an urban emergency medical center, diverticulosis (33.5%), hemorrhoids (22.5%), and carcinoma (12.7%) were the most common etiologies [6]. In general the causes of gastrointestinal bleeding can be grouped into anatomic (diverticular disease), vascular (hemorrhoid, ischemic colitis, and angiodysplasia), neoplastic, and inflammatory (infectious colitis, inflammatory bowel disease) causes.

The diagnosis of small bowel carcinoma is difficult and often delayed. Clinical presentation is typically nonspecific with symptoms that include nausea, vomiting, weight loss, abdominal pain, and anemia. In our patient, the diagnostic process was further complicated by presence of a known small bowel disease (celiac disease) commonly associated with iron deficiency anemia, negative endoscopy, and colonoscopy. Iron deficiency anemia is present in 46% of patients with celiac disease and is typically caused by malabsorption of iron in the proximal small intestine and usually resolves with strict adherence to gluten-free diet and oral iron supplementation, although it may be refractory in up to 20% [7]. In our case, the correct diagnosis for the underlying cause of recurrent anemia was only made during the fourth hospital admission.

Serum cancer markers carcinoembryonic antigen (CEA) and Ca19.9 may be elevated in cases of small bowel carcinoma but are neither sensitive nor specific and should not be used for diagnostic purposes. Even in metastatic disease CEA is elevated only in 30% and Ca19.9 in 41% of cases [8]. Extrapolating the established guidelines for colorectal carcinoma, these markers, if elevated at diagnosis, can be used for surveillance after surgery or for assessment of disease activity in patients with metastatic cancer [9]. Values of CEA or Ca19.9 were not obtained in our patient who elected palliative care only after her cancer diagnosis.

Because small bowel is not accessible during standard endoscopic procedures performed in the setting of gastrointestinal bleeding, a high index of suspicion is required to identify pathology in this segment of the gastrointestinal tract. Clinical examination has a low sensitivity for small bowel tumors until they become palpable, as it was in our case. CT may provide suggestive information about nodal, extramucosal involvement and distant metastases. However, it can miss superficial lesions and presence of overlapping bowel loops may lead to false negative diagnosis. The addition of enterography to CT circumvents these problems and increases the sensitivity [10]. Magnetic resonance imaging (MRI) is rapidly gaining clinical utility in the evaluation of small bowel disease. It advantageously avoids ionizing radiation, can assess bowel peristalsis, and provides a higher resolution, but it has its own challenges such as cost and accessibility. CT is better in the assessment of a perforation or bowel obstruction and concomitantly helps in directing interventional therapies [10].

Capsule endoscopy may identify a site of occult bleeding or malignancy but poses a risk of capsule retention when there is an impending obstruction [11]. Double balloon enteroscopy overcomes the above limitation and has the advantage of ability to obtain biopsy or providing endoscopic therapy [12]. These newer diagnostic techniques can expedite the diagnosis, but in clinical practice they are often deferred to the outpatient setting in patients presenting with acute gastrointestinal bleeding. Our case illustrates the importance of pursuing such evaluations when repeated episodes of unexplained gastrointestinal bleeding occur in order to avoid delay in the diagnosis of a potentially curable malignancy.

The pathogenesis of small bowel adenocarcinoma is not entirely known due to the rarity of the disease. Genetic syndromes like Peutz-Jeghers (relative risk, 520), hereditary nonpolyposis colon cancer (relative risk, 103 to 291 depending on specific mutation), and familial adenomatous polyposis (relative risk, 330) are risk factors for small bowel adenocarcinoma [13]. Conditions associated with chronic inflammation of the small intestine are also major risk factors for this malignancy and include Crohn's disease and celiac disease.

Thirteen percent of small bowel adenocarcinomas have been shown to be associated with celiac disease [14]. Cases of small bowel adenocarcinoma in patients with celiac disease have been previously reported [15–17].

Celiac disease is an autoimmune disorder which results from the interplay of immune, genetic, and environmental factors. The lymphocytic infiltrate could potentially induce an immunological response disrupting the epithelium and causing premalignant changes. In a series of 94 cases of small bowel adenocarcinoma from the Mayo Clinic, evidence of flat dysplasia at the tumor margin was noted in 50% of cases associated with celiac disease [18]. Although some authors suggested that carcinomas in celiac disease may arise from adenomatous polyp [19], others found no increased incidence of duodenal adenomas in celiac disease [20].

Microsatellite instability, a hallmark of the hereditary nonpolyposis colon cancer (Lynch) syndrome, is a molecular feature commonly encountered in small bowel adenocarcinoma, where it is present in about 20–40% of cases [21–23]. Several studies have demonstrated particularly high prevalence of microsatellite instability (70–80%) in tumors associated with celiac disease [24, 25]. A comparative genomic hybridization study of 15 celiac disease-related and 33 unrelated small bowel adenocarcinomas showed similar chromosomal aberrations between the two subsets, but there was a higher rate of *APC* gene promoter hypermethylation and of microsatellite instability in celiac disease-related tumors (67% versus 33%) [26].

Small bowel carcinogenesis in Crohn's disease differs from celiac disease. Cytokines, released due to the chronic inflammatory state, interact with cell surface receptors and target genes thus promoting carcinogenesis [27]. Unlike in celiac disease where proximal jejunum predominates as the location of adenocarcinomas, Crohn's disease affects mostly the distal ileum.

In the absence of randomized trials, the optimal treatment for small bowel carcinoma is still uncertain and is essentially extrapolated from the clinical experience in colorectal cancer. Surgery remains the treatment of choice in the absence of metastatic disease and is often required even in the metastatic setting due to high likelihood of obstruction or severe hemorrhage [28]. Because most patients are diagnosed with advanced disease and have high-grade histology [4], small bowel adenocarcinoma generally carries a poor prognosis with 5-year relative survival of 28% without surgery and 32% after resection [29]. Adjuvant chemotherapy using fluorouracil-based regimens approved in colorectal cancer is commonly offered for patients with stage II or III disease [30]. It may also provide benefits in selected patients with metastatic disease, where a 27% response rate, median progression-free survival of 6.6 months and median overall survival of 15 months, was reported among patients receiving palliative chemotherapy [8]. In one phase II trial of the combination of capecitabine and oxaliplatin, a response rate of 50% was observed, with median time to progression of 11.3 months and median overall survival of 20.4 months [31]. It is important however to recognize that patients with significant comorbidities or poor performance status may not derive any benefit from adjuvant or palliative chemotherapy, and, in those cases, as it was in ours, supportive care alone may be appropriate.

Identification of molecular pathways involved in the pathogenesis of small bowel cancer holds a promise of developing more efficacious therapies. A screening assay of 140 compounds suggested utility of the halichondrin B analogue eribulin in cases with *Wnt-β-catenin* pathway mutation present in 20% of cases [21]. A multiplex assay analysis of 83 cases showed frequent mutations in *KRAS* (43%), *TP53* (41%), *PIK3CA* (8%), *BRAF* (6%), and *ERBB2* (8%) genes, for which targeted agents are available or currently studied [32].

4. Conclusion

When patients with celiac disease present with gastrointestinal bleeding, small intestinal malignancy has to be included in differential diagnosis if endoscopy and colonoscopy do not reveal an obvious source of blood loss. Early evaluation for a malignancy using a high-yield technique should be considered to avoid a diagnostic delay and the poor prognosis associated with advanced cancers.

Abbreviations

CT: Computerized tomography
EGD: Esophagogastroduodenoscopy.

Consent

Written informed consent for the publication of this paper could not be obtained due to patient death. All patient identifiers have been removed to ensure patient's privacy.

Authors' Contribution

All authors were involved in the formulation and drafting of the case report. All authors have read and approved the final paper. Alfredo C. Cordova was the surgeon operating on the patient.

Acknowledgment

The authors extend their sincere gratitude to Dr. Stanley Schwartz for the preparation and review of pathology.

References

[1] N. E. Castillo, T. G. Theethira, and D. A. Leffler, "The present and the future in the diagnosis and management of celiac disease," *Gastroenterology Report*, vol. 3, no. 1, pp. 3–11, 2015.

[2] C. Catassi, E. Fabiani, G. Corrao et al., "Risk of non-Hodgkin lymphoma in celiac disease," *Journal of the American Medical Association*, vol. 287, no. 11, pp. 1413–1419, 2002.

[3] J. F. Ludvigsson, S. M. Montgomery, A. Ekbom, L. Brandt, and F. Granath, "Small-intestinal histopathology and mortality risk

in celiac disease," *Journal of the American Medical Association*, vol. 302, no. 11, pp. 1171–1178, 2009.

[4] O. Qubaiah, S. S. Devesa, C. E. Platz, M. M. Huycke, and G. M. Dores, "Small intestinal cancer: a population-based study of incidence and survival patterns in the United States, 1992 to 2006," *Cancer Epidemiology Biomarkers and Prevention*, vol. 19, no. 8, pp. 1908–1918, 2010.

[5] A. I. Neugut, J. S. Jacobson, S. Suh, R. Mukherjee, and N. Arber, "The epidemiology of cancer of the small bowel," *Cancer Epidemiology, Biomarkers & Prevention*, vol. 7, no. 3, pp. 243–251, 1998.

[6] C. Gayer, A. Chino, C. Lucas et al., "Acute lower gastrointestinal bleeding in 1,112 patients admitted to an urban emergency medical center," *Surgery*, vol. 146, no. 4, pp. 600–607, 2009.

[7] T. R. Halfdanarson, M. R. Litzow, and J. A. Murray, "Hematologic manifestations of celiac disease," *Blood*, vol. 109, no. 2, pp. 412–421, 2007.

[8] A. Zaanan, L. Costes, M. Gauthier et al., "Chemotherapy of advanced small-bowel adenocarcinoma: a multicenter AGEO study," *Annals of Oncology*, vol. 21, no. 9, pp. 1786–1793, 2010.

[9] G. Y. Locker, S. Hamilton, J. Harris et al., "ASCO 2006 update of recommendations for the use of tumor markers in gastrointestinal cancer," *Journal of Clinical Oncology*, vol. 24, no. 33, pp. 5313–5327, 2006.

[10] G. Masselli and G. Gualdi, "CT and MR enterography in evaluating small bowel diseases: when to use which modality?" *Abdominal Imaging*, vol. 38, no. 2, pp. 249–259, 2013.

[11] R. Srai, L. Tullie, A. Wadoodi, and M. Saunders, "Capsule endoscopy: a dangerous but diagnostic tool," *BMJ Case Reports*, 2013.

[12] H. Suzuki, A. Yamada, H. Watabe et al., "Successful treatment of early-stage jejunum adenocarcinoma by endoscopic mucosal resection using double-balloon endoscopy: a case report," *Diagnostic and Therapeutic Endoscopy*, vol. 2012, Article ID 521960, 4 pages, 2012.

[13] T. Aparicio, A. Zaanan, M. Svrcek et al., "Small bowel adenocarcinoma: epidemiology, risk factors, diagnosis and treatment," *Digestive and Liver Disease*, vol. 46, no. 2, pp. 97–104, 2014.

[14] P. D. Howdle, P. K. Jalal, G. K. T. Holmes, and R. S. Houlston, "Primary small-bowel malignancy in the UK and its association with coeliac disease," *QJM*, vol. 96, no. 5, pp. 345–353, 2003.

[15] H. Benhammane, F. Z. El M'rabet, K. Idrissi Serhouchni et al., "Small bowel adenocarcinoma complicating coeliac disease: a report of three cases and the literature review," *Case Reports in Oncological Medicine*, vol. 2012, Article ID 935183, 4 pages, 2012.

[16] M. Gwiggner and P. Patel, "An unusual case of obscure gastrointestinal bleeding in a patient with coeliac disease," *Case Reports in Gastrointestinal Medicine*, vol. 2011, Article ID 634684, 3 pages, 2011.

[17] S. D. Rampertab, K. A. Forde, and P. H. R. Green, "Small bowel neoplasia in coeliac disease," *Gut*, vol. 52, no. 8, pp. 1211–1214, 2003.

[18] C. J. Bruno, K. P. Batts, and D. A. Ahlquist, "Evidence against flat dysplasia as a regional field defect in small bowel adenocarcinoma associated with celiac sprue," *Mayo Clinic Proceedings*, vol. 72, no. 4, pp. 320–322, 1997.

[19] C. Catassi, I. Bearzi, and G. K. T. Holmes, "Association of celiac disease and intestinal lymphomas and other cancers," *Gastroenterology*, vol. 128, no. 4, pp. S79–S86, 2005.

[20] S. D. Rampertab, A. Fleischauer, A. I. Neugut, and P. H. R. Green, "Risk of duodenal adenoma in celiac disease," *Scandinavian Journal of Gastroenterology*, vol. 38, no. 8, pp. 831–833, 2003.

[21] H. Suzuki, Y. Hirata, N. Suzuki et al., "Characterization of a new small bowel adenocarcinoma cell line and screening of anti-cancer drug against small bowel adenocarcinoma," *The American Journal of Pathology*, vol. 185, no. 2, pp. 550–562, 2015.

[22] M. Planck, K. Ericson, Z. Piotrowska, B. Halvarsson, E. Rambech, and M. Nilbert, "Microsatellite instability and expression of MLH1 and MSH2 in carcinomas of the small intestine," *Cancer*, vol. 97, no. 6, pp. 1551–1557, 2003.

[23] T. Aparicio, M. Svrcek, A. Zaanan et al., "Small bowel adenocarcinoma phenotyping, a clinicobiological prognostic study," *British Journal of Cancer*, vol. 109, no. 12, pp. 3057–3066, 2013.

[24] D. D. Potter, J. A. Murray, J. H. Donohue et al., "The role of defective mismatch repair in small bowel adenocarcinoma in celiac disease," *Cancer Research*, vol. 64, no. 19, pp. 7073–7077, 2004.

[25] F. Bergmann, S. Singh, S. Michel et al., "Small bowel adenocarcinomas in celiac disease follow the CIM-MSI pathway," *Oncology Reports*, vol. 24, no. 6, pp. 1535–1539, 2010.

[26] B. Diosdado, T. E. Buffart, R. Watkins et al., "High-resolution array comparative genomic hybridization in sporadic and celiac disease-related small bowel adenocarcinomas," *Clinical Cancer Research*, vol. 16, no. 5, pp. 1391–1401, 2010.

[27] V. Palascak-Juif, A. M. Bouvier, J. Cosnes et al., "Small bowel adenocarcinoma in patients with Crohn's disease compared with small bowel adenocarcinoma de novo," *Inflammatory Bowel Diseases*, vol. 11, no. 9, pp. 828–832, 2005.

[28] M. S. Talamonti, L. H. Goetz, S. Rao, and R. J. Joehl, "Primary cancers of the small bowel: analysis of prognostic factors and results of surgical management," *Archives of Surgery*, vol. 137, no. 5, pp. 564–571, 2002.

[29] S. Y. Pan and H. Morrison, "Epidemiology of cancer of the small intestine," *World Journal of Gastrointestinal Oncology*, vol. 3, no. 3, pp. 33–42, 2011.

[30] M. J. Overman, S. Kopetz, E. Lin, J. L. Abbruzzese, and R. A. Wolff, "Is there a role for adjuvant therapy in resected adenocarcinoma of the small intestine," *Acta Oncologica*, vol. 49, no. 4, pp. 474–479, 2010.

[31] M. J. Overman, G. R. Varadhachary, S. Kopetz et al., "Phase II study of capecitabine and oxaliplatin for advanced adenocarcinoma of the small bowel and ampulla of vater," *Journal of Clinical Oncology*, vol. 27, no. 16, pp. 2598–2603, 2009.

[32] A. Laforest, T. Aparicio, A. Zaanan et al., "ERBB2 gene as a potential therapeutic target in small bowel adenocarcinoma," *European Journal of Cancer*, vol. 50, no. 10, pp. 1740–1746, 2014.

15

Migrating Polyarthritis as a Feature of Occult Malignancy

Geoffrey Alan Watson,[1] Lorraine O'Neill,[1] Ruth Law,[1] Geraldine McCarthy,[2] and Douglas Veale[1]

[1] *St. Vincent's University Hospital, Dublin, Ireland*
[2] *Mater Misericordiae University Hospital, Dublin, Ireland*

Correspondence should be addressed to Geoffrey Alan Watson; geoff_watson7@hotmail.com

Academic Editor: Annekathryn Goodman

Malignant disease may be associated with a wide variety of musculoskeletal syndromes. Rarely the musculoskeletal system can be indirectly affected by paraneoplastic phenomena, such as carcinomatous polyarthritis (CP). The differential diagnosis for CP is broad and is often a diagnosis of exclusion. CP often presents similarly to other forms of inflammatory arthritis, and a detailed history and physical examination can often distinguish CP from other more common causes of polyarticular arthritis. However serological tests such as rheumatoid factor (RF) and anti-citrullinated peptide (anti-CCP) antibody positivity, while rare, can be misleading. Clinical awareness and suspicion are paramount in achieving an accurate diagnosis and early detection of an occult neoplasm is critical for prompt management and therapy. We report two cases presenting with this unique clinical phenotype associated with paraneoplastic polyarthropathy and review the literature.

1. Introduction

Malignant disease may be associated with a wide variety of musculoskeletal syndromes [1–3]. Mechanisms include direct local invasion of the primary tumor, metastasis, and synovial response to juxta-articular masses. Rarely the musculoskeletal system can in addition be indirectly affected by paraneoplastic phenomena, such as carcinomatous polyarthritis (CP). CP is a poorly understood clinical entity and may present similarly to other forms of inflammatory arthritis. Distinguishing features have been proposed and include late age and abrupt onset, asymmetric joint involvement, negative family history, and resolution of symptoms after diagnosis and treatment of the underlying malignancy [2]. However CP remains a diagnosis of exclusion and positive serological tests such as rheumatoid factor (RF) may be misleading. It has previously been postulated that the absence of anti-citrullinated peptide (anti-CCP) antibodies may distinguish CP from other more common rheumatic conditions such as rheumatoid arthritis (RA) [2]. However, while rare, isolated case reports are emerging linking CP with anti-CCP positivity, suggesting that serology may not be wholly reliable in providing this distinction. Here we report two cases presenting with a polyarthropathy including one case where anti-CCP antibodies were detectable.

2. Case Reports

Our first case involves 80-year-old female who presented with a three-day history of right-sided shoulder pain and associated fever. On further questioning the patient described asymmetric migratory joint pain over the preceding three-week period, affecting her left wrist, knees, and right shoulder. She had been taking nonsteroidal anti-inflammatory drugs (NSAIDs) without relief and was also receiving a two-week course of ciprofloxacin for a urinary tract infection. Physical examination revealed tenderness and painful restriction of motion of the right shoulder. There was also a right-sided knee effusion. The remainder of the physical examination was unremarkable.

Her medical history was significant for type 2 diabetes, ischaemic heart disease, and congestive heart failure. She

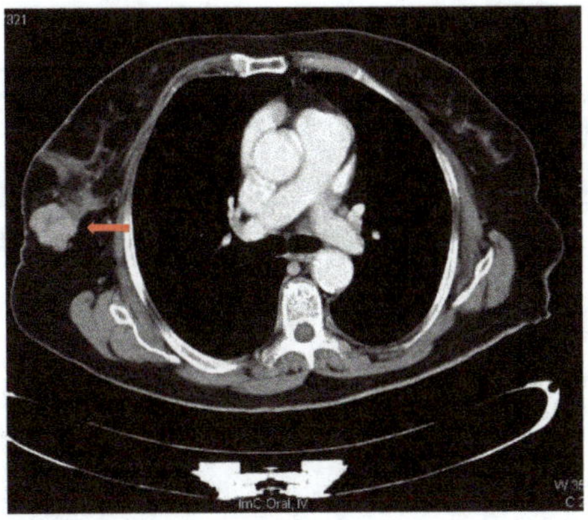

FIGURE 1: CT of abdomen. The red arrow illustrates a well circumscribed, multilobulated 3.3 cm lesion in the inferior outer quadrant of the right breast.

was a lifelong nonsmoker and did not consume any alcohol. Review of systems was otherwise unremarkable.

Initial laboratory results revealed a white cell count of 11.9×10^9/L, hemoglobin 11.2 g/dL, and platelets 384×10^9/L. A metabolic panel was significant for mild hyponatremia (131 mmol/L) (normal levels 135–145 mmol/L) and a slightly raised urea (7.7 mmol/L) and creatinine (93 μmol/L). Her erythrocyte sedimentation rate (ESR) was 21 mm/h and C-reactive protein (CRP) was elevated at 111.8 mg/L. Uric acid was 0.29 mmol/L. Rheumatoid factor was marginally elevated at 42 IU/mL. Anti-CCP was also elevated at 36 IU/mL. An X-ray of her right shoulder showed moderate degenerative changes at the acromioclavicular joint. Imaging of the knees and pelvis showed mild degenerative changes. Urine dipstick was positive for leukocytes but negative for nitrites. She was initially suspected of having polyarticular gout based on her slightly elevated uric acid levels and was subsequently treated with colchicine.

During her admission she developed nonspecific abdominal pain and tenderness in the right iliac fossa. A CT of abdomen was requested and reported no intra-abdominal pathology. However there was an incidental finding of a 3.3 cm multilobulated lesion in the inferior outer quadrant of the right breast (Figure 1). Subsequent mammogram revealed a 3.5 cm irregular hypoechoic mass highly suggestive of malignancy. This was confirmed after tissue biopsy, with microscopy revealing a papillary carcinoma (Figure 2).

During that time her right shoulder pain spontaneously resolved. However she then developed new onset right wrist pain, swelling, and erythema. X-ray revealed moderate degenerative changes. Joint aspiration revealed markedly increased inflammatory cells but no crystals. Colchicine and NSAIDs were stopped and she was given IM methylprednisolone to which she responded well, and her CRP decreased to 70. She was seen in clinic one week later and had no appreciable synovitis on examination.

Six weeks later she underwent chemotherapy and radiotherapy for her breast cancer. She was seen again in clinic ten weeks later and she did not report any recurrence of her joint symptoms.

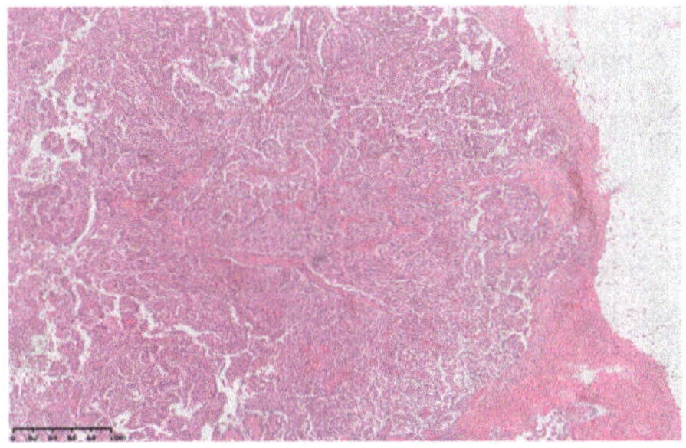

FIGURE 2: Encapsulated papillary carcinoma showing classical papillary architecture with surrounding fibrous capsule.

Our second patient, 71-year-old female, was referred by her general practitioner for evaluation of a six-month history of pain and swelling of her hands and feet. This was associated with early morning stiffness lasting greater than two hours daily. NSAIDs and a short course of prednisolone had failed to improve her symptoms.

Her past medical history was significant for ischaemic heart disease, hypertension, hyperlipidaemia, and peptic ulcer disease. She had a thirty-pack year history of smoking. Three of her four siblings had been treated for colorectal or breast neoplasms.

On examination she had thirteen tender and ten swollen joints including metacarpophalangeal (MCP), proximal interphalangeal (PIP), wrist, shoulder, ankle, and knee joints. Grade 2 clubbing was evident as was a multinodular goitre. Other than a raised CRP at 12 mg/L and serum calcium at 2.68 mmol/L, baseline laboratory investigations were normal. Rheumatoid factor and anti-CCP antibodies were both negative. Chest radiograph revealed a left upper lobe lesion, which was confirmed on CT. Subsequent biopsy identified a non-small cell adenocarcinoma. She underwent a lobectomy with a rapid resolution of her joint symptoms.

3. Discussion

Migratory polyarthritis is a common presentation with a broad differential diagnosis [1–4]. Common causes include inflammatory arthritis including crystal arthropathy and other forms of systemic rheumatic disease such as connective tissue disorders and occasionally infectious agents [4]. Less commonly, joint symptoms may be attributed to neoplastic disease.

CP is associated with a wide variety of solid tumours and haematologic malignancies, particularly cancers of the lung and ovaries (Table 1). Cancer polyarthritis was first described by Lansbury in 1953 [5] and by MacKenzie and Scherbel in 1963 [6]. The topic has since been reviewed by Naschitz et al. [7] and most recently by Larson et al. [8]. Hypertrophic osteoarthropathy, dermatomyositis, paraneoplastic vasculitis, and most recently palmar fasciitis have all been described as paraneoplastic disorders [1, 9]. However, carcinomatous polyarthritis remains a rare and poorly understood clinical entity [2, 3]. CP is historically defined by the following criteria [1, 2]:

TABLE 1: Malignancies associated with carcinomatous polyarthritis. Four cases, highlighted in bold, have shown anti-CCP positivity. Rheumatoid factor (RF), anti-citrullinated protein antibody (anti-CCP), positive (+), negative (−), not included (NI), Non-Small Cell Lung Cancer (NSCLC), Squamous Cell Cancer (SCC), Small Cell Lung Cancer (SCLC), Acute Lymphoblastic Leukemia (ALL), Chronic Myeloid Leukemia (CML), and Chronic Lymphoid Leukemia (CLL).

Case report and reference	Type of malignancy	RF	Anti-CCP
Present case	**Breast**	+	+
Present case	NSCLC	−	−
Zupancic et al. [2]	SCC lung	+	NI
Stummvoll et al. [3]	Adenocarcinoma colon	−	NI
Stummvoll et al. [3]	SCC Lung	−	NI
Larson et al. [8]	**NSCLC (adenocarcinoma)**	+	+
Nadal et al. [10]	Prostate cancer	NI	−
Bradley and Pinals [11]	Spindle cell cancer	+	NI
Pines et al. [12]	Breast	−	NI
Pines et al. [12]	Unknown primary	−	NI
Pines et al. [12]	SCLC	−	NI
Acosta Madiedo et al. [13]	NSCLC	−	NI
Chuan et al. [9]	Tubular adenocarcinoma stomach	−	NI
Eggelmeijer and Macfarlane [14]	Supraglottic SCC	−	NI
Bennett et al. [15]	Ovarian adenocarcinoma	+	NI
Simon and Ford [16]	Adenocarcinoma colon	−	NI
Mok and Kwan [17]	Unknown primary	+	NI
Handy et al. [18]	**T cell ALL**	+	+
Kumar et al. [19]	**Pancreas**	+	+
Sheehy et al. [20]	NSCLC (adenocarcinoma)	+	NI
Bivalacqua et al. [21]	NSCLC (adenocarcinoma)	NI	NI
Docquier et al. [22]	Uterine adenocarcinoma	−	NI
Haroon and Phelan [23]	Pancreatic cancer	−	NI
Ardalan and Shoja [24]	Multiple myeloma	−	NI
Leslie [25]	Cervical cancer	NI	NI
Baijens and Manni [26]	cT4N2cM0 hypopharynx carcinoma	NI	NI
Martorell et al. [27]	Serocystadenocarcinoma ovary	−	NI
Martorell et al. [27]	Serocystadenocarcinoma ovary	+	NI
Martorell et al. [27]	Ovarian carcinoma	−	NI
Martorell et al. [27]	Serocystadenocarcinoma ovary	−	NI
Medsger et al. [28]	Ovarian adenocarcinoma	NI	NI
Medsger et al. [28]	Ovarian adenocarcinoma	NI	NI
Medsger et al. [28]	Ovarian adenocarcinoma	NI	NI
Medsger et al. [28]	Ovarian adenocarcinoma	NI	NI
Medsger et al. [28]	Ovarian adenocarcinoma	NI	NI
Medsger et al. [28]	Ovarian adenocarcinoma	NI	NI
Baron [29]	SCLC	−	NI
Baer and Phillips [30]	Pancreatic adenocarcinoma	NI	NI
Taggart et al. [31]	Adenocarcinoma Fallopian tube	−	NI
Taggart et al. [31]	Ovarian adenocarcinoma	NI	NI
Michaels and Sorber [32]	Pancreatic adenocarcinoma	−	NI
Shiel et al. [33]	SCLC	NI	NI
Shiel et al. [33]	Ovarian adenocarcinoma	NI	NI
Pfinsgraff et al. [34]	CML	−	NI
Pfinsgraff et al. [34]	Pancreatic adenocarcinoma, parathyroid adenoma	NI	NI
Pfinsgraff et al. [34]	Squamous cell carcinoma unknown primary	−	NI
Pfinsgraff et al. [34]	Adenocarcinoma unknown primary	NI	NI

Table 1: Continued.

Case report and reference	Type of malignancy	RF	Anti-CCP
Pfinsgraff et al. [34]	Hodgkin disease	NI	NI
Valverde-Garcia et al. [35]	Breast cancer	NI	NI
Cammilleri et al. [36]	Follicular B cell lymphoma	–	NI
Willemse et al. [37]	Adenocarcinoma of the coelomic epithelium	–	NI
Van den Bergh et al. [38]	Adenocarcinoma of prostate prolactinoma	–	NI
Mathieu et al. [39]	CLL	NI	NI
Vinker et al. [40]	Ovarian adenocarcinoma	NI	NI
Saxman and Seitz [41]	Breast carcinoma	–	NI
Grados et al. [42]	Transitional cell carcinoma of the renal pelvis	–	NI
Grados et al. [42]	Adenocarcinoma of the uterus	–	NI
Enomoto et al. [43]	Early-stage gastric carcinoma	+	NI
Denschlag et al. [44]	Fallopian tube carcinoma	–	NI
Giannakopoulos et al. [45]	Ovarian adenocarcinoma	–	NI
Yogarajah et al. [46]	Ovarian adenocarcinoma	NI	NI
Bolibar et al. [47]	Ovarian adenocarcinoma	–	NI
Preda et al. [48]	Ovarian adenocarcinoma	NI	NI
Krishna et al. [49]	Breast cancer	–	NI
Qureshi and Saavedra [50]	Ovarian adenocarcinoma	–	NI
Clarke et al. [51]	Transitional cell carcinoma of the bladder	–	NI
Nahar and Al-Rajhi [52]	Ovarian adenocarcinoma	–	NI
Sandhya and Danda [53]	Breast carcinoma	NI	NI
Mcgivern and Mcaleese [54]	NSCLC	NI	NI
Salmon et al. [55]	Ovarian adenocarcinoma	–	NI
Salmon et al. [55]	Ovarian adenocarcinoma	–	NI
Salmon et al. [55]	Uterine cancer	NI	NI
Shetty et al. [56]	Neuroendocrine tumour of adrenal gland	–	NI

(i) Close temporal relationship (12 months) between onset of arthritis and malignancy
(ii) Late age at onset
(iii) Asymmetric joint involvement
(iv) Explosive onset
(v) Predominance of lower extremity involvement with sparing of wrists and small joints of hands
(vi) Absence of Rheumatoid Factor (RF)
(vii) Absence of rheumatoid nodules
(viii) No family history of rheumatic disease
(ix) Non-specific histopathologic appearance of synovial lining
(x) Absence of characterisitic radiologic lesions

Box 1: Features of cancer polyarthritis (Stummvoll et al. [3], Larson et al. [8], Caldwell and McCallum [57], and Pfitzenmeyer et al. [58]).

(i) It must occur during the course of an identified malignant disease or precede clinical evidence of a malignancy.

(ii) Symptoms cannot be the result of direct tumor invasion or compression.

(iii) Symptoms improve with treatment of the underlining neoplasm.

In 1985, Caldwell and McCallum published the key features of cancer polyarthritis and suggested distinguishing features to aid in narrowing the differential [57]. Pfitzenmeyer et al. [58] later added the absence of characteristic radiologic lesions to the list of typical features (Box 1). These features have been supported by recent case reviews [2, 3, 8, 10]. It is now well recognised that rheumatic syndromes often precede the diagnosis of malignant disease [1–3, 8, 57]. Racanelli et al. found that, in patients with solid tumours, only 11.5% had a malignancy diagnosed at the time of their rheumatic presentation, while 88.5% were diagnosed after their initial presentation [59]. Thus new presentations of polyarthropathy may represent an important clue in the detection of an occult malignancy.

CP however remains a diagnosis of exclusion and must be distinguished from other more common causes of polyarthritis. Infectious causes due to bacteria or Lyme disease may be associated with fever, acute symptom onset, and monoarthritis. A thorough clinical history is useful in detecting seronegative spondyloarthropathies. Reactive arthritis is usually preceded by an infection such as campylobacter-induced diarrhea, while enteric arthritis may be seen in patients with a history of inflammatory bowel disease. Finally the crystal arthropathies can be easily distinguished by joint aspiration and visualisation of crystals under the microscope.

Distinguishing CP from a late onset form of RA, however, is challenging. Previous studies have shown that the incidence of both increases with age. Both may present over the course of weeks to months with similar signs and symptoms, namely, soft tissue swelling, limited range of motion of affected joints, and morning stiffness [3, 9, 11–16]. Features suggestive of chronic disease and inflammation (anaemia, elevated ESR/CRP) are also seen [2, 3, 11–13, 16, 20, 22, 28, 29, 42, 49, 55]. The joint fluid generally shows nonspecific inflammatory changes [1, 2, 11, 16, 17]. Imaging studies are largely unremarkable [1–3, 14, 16, 60]. In addition symptoms often fail to resolve with the use of conventional therapy such as NSAIDs and steroids [2, 27–32, 41, 42, 44, 48, 50].

Several case reports included in Box 1 have emerged documenting findings that challenge the traditional distinguishing features of CP. Several noted symmetric joint involvement involving the wrists, knees, and small joints of the hands as the predominant rheumatic manifestation [2, 3, 8–16, 23, 27, 28, 31, 34, 35, 38–40, 42, 43, 48, 49].

Our first case had a positive rheumatoid factor, which can be partially explained by the underlying malignancy, which is associated with a positive rheumatoid factor in 10–20 percent of patients [58]. Morel et al. documented symptom relief for 9 out of 20 patients who were treated with NSAIDs, while most responded to steroid therapy [60].

An additional means to differentiate these two disorders was postulated by measuring anti-cyclic citrullinated peptide (anti CCP) antibodies. Anti-CCP has a similar sensitivity to RF (50–75%) with a higher specificity (90–95%) [61]. Due to this high specificity, however, a positive Anti-CCP may result in an inaccurate diagnosis of rheumatoid arthritis, thus resulting in delayed diagnosis and treatment of the underlying malignancy. To our knowledge, only four case reports, including the present case, have reported an association between CP and elevated anti-CCP levels [8, 18, 19] (Box 1). Thus, many features that have been proposed to distinguish between CP and RA are not always reliable.

One prevailing theme however is resolution of rheumatic symptoms after treatment of the underlying malignancy [2, 3, 9, 11–16, 22, 27, 28, 33–35, 39–41, 43–48, 50, 52, 55]. Resolution of symptoms after chemotherapy or surgery may vary, and while our first patient's symptoms may have been masked by steroids, our second patient showed a rapid improvement just days after undergoing surgery. The return of arthritic symptoms in these patients should provoke further investigation to rule out any evidence of tumour recurrence [2].

To date, the pathogenesis of this disorder remains unclear. Bradley and Pinals suggested that circulating immune complexes (CIC), which have been observed in over 60 percent of some types of cancers, may play a pivotal role [11]. Theories suggesting that elevated levels of platelet activating factors may be deposited in the synovium and trigger an inflammatory response have also been postulated [2, 15]. Additional mechanisms have been proposed including autoimmune phenomena involving lymphocytes originating in hyperplastic lymph nodes draining tumour sites [1, 9, 11, 14]; however these theories all remain speculative.

4. Summary

Carcinomatous polyarthritis is a rare disorder associated with a wide variety of malignancies. The differential diagnosis for CP is broad and is often a diagnosis of exclusion. Several of the classical features initially proposed to distinguish CP may be unreliable, and positive serological tests such as rheumatoid factor and anti-CCP antibody positivity can be misleading. A comprehensive history and physical examination is paramount in distinguishing CP from other more common causes of polyarticular arthritis, with careful attention to social and family history to detect any possible risk factors for cancer. Clinical awareness and suspicion remain the most important factors in achieving an accurate diagnosis. Early diagnosis of an occult neoplasm is critical for prompt management and therapy and can ultimately be lifesaving.

References

[1] G. Fam Adel, "Paraneoplastic rheumatic syndromes," *Baillière's Best Practice & Research. Clinical Rheumatology*, vol. 14, no. 3, pp. 515–533, 2000.

[2] M. Zupancic, A. Annamalai, J. Brenneman, and S. Ranatunga, "Migratory polyarthritis as a paraneoplastic syndrome," *Journal of General Internal Medicine*, vol. 23, no. 12, pp. 2136–2139, 2008.

[3] G. H. Stummvoll, M. Aringer, K. P. Machold, J. S. Smolen, and M. Raderer, "Cancer polyarthritis resembling rheumatoid arthritis as a first sign of hidden neoplasms," *Scandinavian Journal of Rheumatology*, vol. 30, no. 1, pp. 40–44, 2001.

[4] A. M. Richie and M. L. Francis, "Diagnostic approach to polyarticular joint pain," *American Family Physician*, vol. 68, no. 6, pp. 1151–1160, 2003.

[5] J. Lansbury, "Collagen disease complicating malignancy," *Annals of the Rheumatic Diseases*, vol. 12, no. 4, pp. 301–305, 1953.

[6] A. H. MacKenzie and A. L. Scherbel, "Connective tissue syndromes associated with carcinoma," *Geriatrics*, vol. 18, article 753, 1963.

[7] J. E. Naschitz, I. Rosner, M. Rozenbaum, E. Zuckerman, and D. Yeshurun, "Rheumatic syndromes: clues to occult neoplasia," *Seminars in Arthritis and Rheumatism*, vol. 29, no. 1, pp. 43–55, 1999.

[8] E. Larson, D. Etwaru, C. Siva, and K. Lawlor, "Report of anti-CCP antibody positive paraneoplastic polyarthritis and review of the literature," *Rheumatology International*, vol. 31, no. 12, pp. 1635–1638, 2011.

[9] H. Chuan, C. E. Robinson, W. H. Sutherland, and W. L. Dunn, "Polyarthritis associated with gastric carcinoma," *Canadian Medical Association Journal*, vol. 131, no. 8, pp. 909–911, 1984.

[10] R. Nadal, Z. H. McMahan, and E. S. Antonarakis, "Paraneoplastic palmar fasciitis and polyarthritis syndrome in a patient with advanced prostate cancer," *Clinical Genitourinary Cancer*, vol. 11, no. 4, pp. e15–e23, 2013.

[11] J. D. Bradley and R. S. Pinals, "Carcinoma polyarthritis: role of immune complexes in pathogenesis," *Journal of Rheumatology*, vol. 10, no. 5, pp. 826–828, 1983.

[12] A. Pines, N. Kaplinsky, D. Olchovsky, and O. Frankl, "Rheumatoid arthritis-like syndrome: a presenting symptom of malignancy. Report of 3 cases and review of the literature," *European Journal of Rheumatology and Inflammation*, vol. 7, no. 2, pp. 51–55, 1984.

[13] J. M. Acosta Madiedo, A. Murthy, D. A. Cortese, and M. D. Cohen, "An unusual case of carcinoma polyarthritis with associated vasculitis," *Arthritis and Rheumatism*, vol. 40, no. 4, pp. 779–782, 1997.

[14] F. Eggelmeijer and J. D. Macfarlane, "Polyarthritis as the presenting symptom of the occurrence and recurrence of a laryngeal carcinoma," *Annals of the Rheumatic Diseases*, vol. 51, no. 4, pp. 556–557, 1992.

[15] R. M. Bennett, M. H. Ginsberg, and S. Thomsen, "Carcinomatous polyarthritis: the presenting symptom of an ovarian tumor and association with a platelet activating factor," *Arthritis & Rheumatism*, vol. 19, no. 5, pp. 953–958, 1976.

[16] R. D. Simon Jr. and L. E. Ford, "Rheumatoid-like arthritis associated with a colonic carcinoma," *Archives of Internal Medicine*, vol. 140, no. 5, pp. 698–700, 1980.

[17] C. C. Mok and Y. K. Kwan, "Rheumatoid-like polyarthritis as a presenting feature of metastatic carcinoma: a case presentation and review of the literature," *Clinical Rheumatology*, vol. 22, no. 4-5, pp. 353–354, 2003.

[18] C. E. Handy, G. Robles, U. Haque, and B. Houston, "T cell ALL presenting as seropositive rheumatoid arthritis: case report and review of the literature on seropositive paraneoplastic arthritis," *Clinical Rheumatology*, vol. 34, no. 9, pp. 1647–1650, 2015.

[19] S. Kumar, S. Sethi, F. Irani, and B. Y. Bode, "Anticyclic citrullinated peptide antibody-positive paraneoplastic polyarthritis in a patient with metastatic pancreatic cancer," *The American Journal of the Medical Sciences*, vol. 338, no. 6, pp. 511–512, 2009.

[20] C. Sheehy, J. G. Ryan, M. Kelly, and M. Barry, "Palmar fasciitis and polyarthritis syndrome associated with non-small-cell lung carcinoma," *Clinical Rheumatology*, vol. 26, no. 11, pp. 1951–1953, 2007.

[21] T. J. Bivalacqua, H. Alphs, I. Aksentijevich, E. M. Schaeffer, and M. P. Schoenberg, "Paraneoplastic polyarthritis from non-small-cell lung cancer metastatic to the bladder," *Journal of Clinical Oncology*, vol. 25, no. 18, pp. 2621–2623, 2007.

[22] C. Docquier, F. Majois, and C. Mitine, "Palmar fasciitis and arthritis: association with endometrial adenocarcinoma," *Clinical Rheumatology*, vol. 21, no. 1, pp. 63–65, 2002.

[23] M. Haroon and M. Phelan, "A paraneoplastic case of palmar fasciitis and polyarthritis syndrome," *Nature Clinical Practice Rheumatology*, vol. 4, no. 5, pp. 274–277, 2008.

[24] M. R. Ardalan and M. M. Shoja, "Multiple myeloma presented as acute interstitial nephritis and rheumatoid arthritis-like polyarthritis," *American Journal of Hematology*, vol. 82, no. 4, pp. 309–313, 2007.

[25] B. M. Leslie, "Palmar fasciitis and polyarthritis associated with a malignant neoplasm: a paraneoplastic syndrome," *Orthopedics*, vol. 15, no. 12, pp. 1436–1439, 1992.

[26] L. W. J. Baijens and J. J. Manni, "Paraneoplastic syndromes in patients with primary malignancies of the head and neck. Four cases and a review of the literature," *European Archives of Oto-Rhino-Laryngology*, vol. 263, no. 1, pp. 32–36, 2006.

[27] E. A. Martorell, P. M. Murray, J. J. Peterson, D. M. Menke, and K. T. Calamia, "Palmar fasciitis and arthritis syndrome associated with metastatic ovarian carcinoma: a report of four cases," *Journal of Hand Surgery*, vol. 29, no. 4, pp. 654–660, 2004.

[28] T. A. Medsger Jr., J. A. Dixon, and V. F. Garwood, "Palmar fasciitis and polyarthritis associated with ovarian carcinoma," *Annals of Internal Medicine*, vol. 96, no. 4, pp. 424–431, 1982.

[29] M. Baron, "Palmar fasciitis, polyarthritis, and carcinoma," *Annals of Internal Medicine*, vol. 97, article 616, 1982.

[30] A. N. Baer and R. M. Phillips Jr., "Pancreatic carcinoma and palmar fasciitis," *Annals of Internal Medicine*, vol. 99, no. 3, pp. 411–412, 1983.

[31] A. J. Taggart, J. M. I. Iveson, and V. Wright, "Shoulder-hand syndrome and symmetrical arthralgia in patients with tubo-ovarian carcinoma," *Annals of the Rheumatic Diseases*, vol. 43, no. 3, pp. 391–393, 1984.

[32] R. M. Michaels and J. A. Sorber, "Reflex sympathetic dystrophy as a probable paraneoplastic syndrome: case report and literature review," *Arthritis and Rheumatism*, vol. 27, no. 10, pp. 1183–1185, 1984.

[33] W. C. Shiel Jr., P. E. Prete, M. Jason, and B. S. Andrews, "Palmar fasciitis and arthritis with ovarian and non-ovarian carcinomas. New syndrome," *The American Journal of Medicine*, vol. 79, no. 5, pp. 640–644, 1985.

[34] J. Pfinsgraff, R. B. Buckingham, P. J. Killian et al., "Palmar fasciitis and arthritis with malignant neoplasms: a paraneoplastic syndrome," *Seminars in Arthritis and Rheumatism*, vol. 16, no. 2, pp. 118–125, 1986.

[35] J. Valverde-Garcia, X. Juanola-Roura, J. M. Ruiz-Martin, J. M. Nolla-Sole, J. Rodriguez-Moreno, and D. Roig-Escofet, "Paraneoplastic palmar fasciitis-polyarthritis syndrome associated with breast cancer," *Journal of Rheumatology*, vol. 14, no. 6, pp. 1207–1209, 1987.

[36] S. Cammilleri, M. C. Guzian, J. Mattei, O. Mundler, and S. Guis, "Whole-body ^{18}FDG-PET in an arthritis paraneoplastic syndrome revealed an underlying hematological neoplasm," *Case Reports in Medicine*, vol. 2013, Article ID 594704, 3 pages, 2013.

[37] P. H. B. Willemse, N. H. Mulder, H. J. van de Tempel, J. G. Aalders, and D. T. Sleijfer, "Palmar fasciitis and arthritis in a patient with an extraovarian adenocarcinoma of the coelomic epithelium," *Annals of the Rheumatic Diseases*, vol. 50, no. 1, pp. 53–54, 1991.

[38] L. Van den Bergh, S. B. Vanneste, and D. C. Knockaert, "Palmar fasciitis and arthritis associated with cancer of the prostate.," *Acta Clinica Belgica*, vol. 46, no. 2, pp. 106–110, 1991.

[39] E. Mathieu, A. C. Koeger, A. Coutellier, S. Rozenberg, B. De La Tour, and P. Bourgeois, "Palmar fasciitis arthritis syndrome revealing relapse of chronic lymphoid leukemia," *Presse Medicale*, vol. 20, no. 11, article 521, 1991.

[40] S. Vinker, R. Dgani, B. Lifschitz-Mercer, Z. M. Sthoeger, and L. Green, "Palmar fasciitis and polyarthritis associated with ovarian carcinoma in a young patient: a case report and review of the literature," *Clinical Rheumatology*, vol. 15, no. 5, pp. 495–497, 1996.

[41] S. B. Saxman and D. Seitz, "Breast cancer associated with palmar fasciitis and arthritis," *Journal of Clinical Oncology*, vol. 15, no. 12, pp. 3515–3516, 1997.

[42] F. Grados, E. Houvenagel, G. Cayrolle, R. Bellony, P. Fardellone, and L. Sebert J.-, "Two new cancer locations accompanied with palmar fasciitis and polyarthritis," *Revue du Rhumatisme (English Edition)*, vol. 65, no. 3, pp. 212–214, 1998.

[43] M. Enomoto, H. Takemura, M. Suzuki et al., "Palmar fasciitis and polyarthritis associated with gastric carcinoma: complete resolution after total gastrectomy," *Internal Medicine*, vol. 39, no. 9, pp. 754–757, 2000.

[44] D. Denschlag, E. Riener, P. Vaith, C. Tempfer, and C. Keck, "Palmar fasciitis and polyarthritis as a paraneoplastic syndrome associated with tubal carcinoma: a case report," *Annals of the Rheumatic Diseases*, vol. 63, no. 9, pp. 1177–1178, 2004.

[45] C. K. Giannakopoulos, G. K. Kyriakidou, and G. E. Toufexi, "Palmar fasciitis and polyarthritis associated with secondary ovarian carcinoma. Case report," *European Journal of Gynaecological Oncology*, vol. 26, no. 3, pp. 339–341, 2005.

[46] M. Yogarajah, J. Soh, B. Lord, N. Goddard, and R. Stratton, "Palmar fasciitis and polyarthritis syndrome: a sign of ovarian malignancy," *Journal of the Royal Society of Medicine*, vol. 101, no. 9, pp. 473–475, 2008.

[47] E. P. Bolibar, J. S. Raya, C. P. Simeon, L. Montesinos, N. Jou, and A. Cuxart, "Palmar fascitis and polyarthritis as a paraneoplastic syndrome associated with ovarian carcinoma: a case report," *BMJ Case Reports*, vol. 2009, 2009.

[48] V. A. Preda, P. Frederiksen, and S. Kossard, "Indurated reticulate palmar erythema as a sign of paraneoplastic palmar fasciitis and polyarthritis syndrome," *Australasian Journal of Dermatology*, vol. 50, no. 3, pp. 198–201, 2009.

[49] K. Krishna, A. Yacoub, L. F. Hutchins, and P. M. Kortebein, "Palmar fasciitis with polyarthritis syndrome in a patient with breast cancer," *Clinical Rheumatology*, vol. 30, no. 4, pp. 569–572, 2011.

[50] A. A. Qureshi and A. Saavedra, "Palmar fasciitis and polyarthritis syndrome in patients with ovarian cancer-a case report and review of the literature," *Hand*, vol. 6, no. 2, pp. 220–223, 2011.

[51] L. L. Clarke, C. T. C. Kennedy, and P. Hollingworth, "Palmar fasciitis and polyarthritis syndrome associated with transitional cell carcinoma of the bladder," *Journal of the American Academy of Dermatology*, vol. 64, no. 6, pp. 1159–1163, 2011.

[52] I. K. Nahar and M. S. Al-Rajhi, "Palmar fasciitis and arthritis syndrome associated with metastatic ovarian cancer: a paraneoplastic syndrome," *The Gulf Journal of Oncology*, no. 12, pp. 59–61, 2012.

[53] P. Sandhya and D. Danda, "Paraneoplastic palmar fasciitis in carcinoma breast," *Journal of Clinical Rheumatology*, vol. 18, no. 2, article 112, 2012.

[54] U. Mcgivern and J. Mcaleese, "Palmar fasciitis: a para-neoplastic phenomenon indicating recurrence of non small cell lung cancer—case report and review of the literature," *International Journal of Rheumatic Diseases*, vol. 15, no. 1, pp. 8–9, 2012.

[55] C. Salmon, G. Gill, D. Loeuille, and I. Chary-Valckenaere, "Three new cases of palmar fasciitis with polyarthritis including a patient with atypical mutilating osteolysis," *Joint Bone Spine*, vol. 80, no. 2, pp. 217–220, 2013.

[56] S. Shetty, J. Hephzibah, B. Borah et al., "Paraneoplastic polyarthritis in association with metastatic neuroendocrince tumour of the adrenal gland," *The Australasian Medical Journal*, vol. 7, no. 8, pp. 345–349, 2014.

[57] D. S. Caldwell and R. M. McCallum, "Rheumatologic manifestations of cancer," *Medical Clinics of North America*, vol. 70, no. 2, pp. 385–417, 1986.

[58] P. Pfitzenmeyer, P. Bielefeld, C. Tavernier, J. F. Besancenot, and M. Gaudet, "Current aspects of paraneoplastic acute polyarthritis," *La Revue de Medecine Interne*, vol. 13, no. 3, pp. 195–199, 1992.

[59] V. Racanelli, M. Prete, C. Minoia, E. Favoino, and F. Perosa, "Rheumatic disorders as paraneoplastic syndromes," *Autoimmunity Reviews*, vol. 7, no. 5, pp. 352–358, 2008.

[60] J. Morel, V. Deschamps, E. Toussirot et al., "Characteristics and survival of 26 patients with paraneoplastic arthritis," *Annals of the Rheumatic Diseases*, vol. 67, no. 2, pp. 244–247, 2008.

[61] A. Wilk and W. van Venrooij, *The Use of Anti-Cyclic Citrullinated Peptide (anti-CCP) Antibodies in RA*, American College of Rheumatology, 2003.

16

Bilateral Bronchiectasis as a Presentation Form of Pulmonary Marginal Zone B-Cell Lymphoma of Bronchus Associated Lymphoid Tissue

Glenda Ernst,[1] Carla Torres,[2] Eduardo Borsini,[1] Félix Vigovich,[1] Daniel Downey,[3] Alajandro Salvado,[1] and Martín Bosio[1]

[1]*Hospital Británico de Buenos Aires, C1280AEB Buenos Aires, Argentina*
[2]*Hospital San Juan de Dios, Buenos Aires, Argentina*
[3]*Hospital Español, Buenos Aires, Argentina*

Correspondence should be addressed to Martín Bosio; marbosio@hotmail.com

Academic Editor: Josep M. Ribera

The pulmonary marginal zone B-cell lymphoma of bronchus associated lymphoid tissue of the lung (BALT) is a rare illness that can remain without symptoms. Radiological findings of pulmonary lymphoma are heterogeneous. In literature, bronchiectasis is only described in one patient who also had besides adenomegalies. We reported on a 48-year-old female patient. She showed symptoms consistent with dyspnea with productive cough; there were crepitant sounds in the auscultation. Pulmonary functional test has shown a severe restrictive pattern with a low FVC and DLCO. CT scan showed bronchiectasis in the medium lobule without adenomegalies. Echocardiogram was normal, and the laboratory findings only showed leukocytosis. There were no findings in the bronchoscopy, but the lung biopsy showed a B-cell pulmonary lymphoma (positive to CD20 and CD79a in immunostaining). A wide variety of radiological manifestations has been previously described; however, we have presented this rare case, with bronchiectasis, as unique radiological finding.

1. Introduction

Pulmonary marginal zone B-cell lymphoma of bronchus associated lymphoid tissue of the lung (BALT) lymphoma is characterized by an abnormal infiltration of lymphoid cells in the lung parenchyma. These pulmonary primary neoplasms are commonly localized in the extranodal marginal zone tissue without extrathoracic involvement at the beginning of the illness [1]. BALT constitutes an infrequent entity representing only the 0.5% of pulmonary primary neoplasm; however, it is the major type of lung lymphoma (between 72 and 90%) [2].

Radiological manifestation of BALT lymphomas has included multiple pulmonary nodules, pulmonary tumors, and consolidative areas [3]. Although cavitation and pleural involvement are rare, these findings have been described in a reduced number of patients [4].

We present a particular patient, who showed bilateral bronchiectasis in the CT scan and was diagnosed with pulmonary BALT lymphoma.

2. Case Presentation

A 48-year-old female patient with BMI of 23.3 is without illnesses history, is nonalcoholic, and is not smoker or exposed to other toxic expositions. She went to consulting room with dyspnea (mMRC: 3) that had begun to affect her daily activities. She also presented with productive cough, which has lasted the last two months.

Despite this, the patient presented a good health state and was without fever at the time of the consulting. The auscultation in the pulmonary examination showed crepitated sounds, with a good oxygen saturation (95% on room air). No other evidences were found.

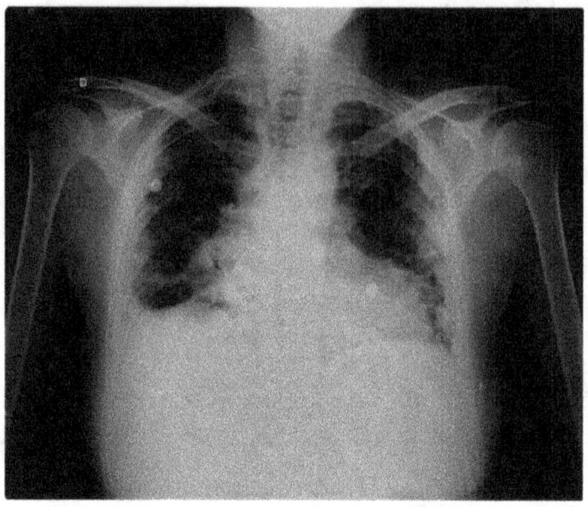

Figure 1: Loss of volume observed with peripheral infiltrates and pleural bilateral involvement.

Table 1: Pulmonary function test.

	Pulmonary function test After bronchoscopy
FVC (L)	1.61
FVC (%)	42
FEV1 (L)	1.52
FEV1 (%)	50
FEV1/FVC (%)	95
TLC (L)	2.8
DLCO unc (mL/min/mmHg)	13.88
DLCO unc (%)	50

The laboratory findings showed leukocytosis. The acute face reactants were normal (VSG and PCR). AISD and Koch bacillus culture were negative. Immunological panel: FR, antibodies for DNA, FAN, C3, C4, C-ANCA, and P-ANCA were also negative. Values of α1-antitrypsin and β2-microglobulin were normal.

Pulmonary functional test had shown a severe restrictive pattern with a diminished vital capacity (FVC) and diffusion capacity (DLCO) (Table 1). A six-minute walking test was performed in which the patient walked 500 meters with an initial saturation of 93% (BORG 0) and finishing with 86% (BORG 3).

Chest X-ray revealed images with bilateral opacities with right pleural effusion (Figure 1). CT scan showed bronchiectasis in the medium and lower lobule and pleural bilateral thickening (Figure 2(a)), without adenomegalies (Figure 2(b)). PET-scan showed SUV of 10.4 with involvement of parenchyma in the medium lobule and supradiaphragmatic nodules.

Echocardiogram was normal, systolic functions in both ventricles (FSVI and FSVD) were conserved, TAPSE was 22 mm, and PSAP was 25 mmHg. The filled pattern was normal.

Fibrobronchoscopy was performed without evidencing abnormal findings in the trachea or bronchi. The cytology of bronchoalveolar lavage was negative for tumoral cells and cellular count was normal. The bacteriological cultures were also negative.

Pulmonary and mediastinum lymph node biopsies were carried out. Histopathology findings revealed a lymphoid proliferative process in the lung parenchyma; the lymphocytes were immune-histochemically positive for CD20 and CD79a, PAX5, and BCL2 and negative for CD3, CD5, CD23, CD10, and cyclin-D1. These findings have contributed to demonstrate a B-cell lymphoma consistent with marginal zone lymphoma of the lung. Pulmonary and mediastinal lymph nodes showed follicular lymphoid hyperplasia without lymphomatous changes. Bone marrow biopsy did not show an involvement of the disease (Figure 3).

Patient started the treatment with rituximab for 12 months, showing an improvement of clinical symptoms. Currently (18 months after), she is being continuously examined as out-patient, showing PET-scans control with SUV 2.5.

3. Discussion

Primary lung lymphoma is a rare illness that presents different pathological variants and degrees of malignancy: most B-cell lymphomas are low grade malignancy and they are usually associated with the bronchial mucosa (BALT lymphomas/MALT) and represent about 90% of all primary lung lymphomas; large B-cell lymphomas show an intermediate to high grade malignancy; and finally peripheral T cell lymphomas occur as part of a systemic process with lymphoid granulomatosis or peripheral T cell lymphomas [3].

Most of the patients remain without symptoms until diagnosis (between 37.5 and 50%). Usually, the symptoms are nonspecific like cough, dyspnea, thoracic pain, and hemoptysis. Extrapulmonary manifestations are unusual but include fever, weight loss, and nocturnal sweating. Acute reactants as PCR, ERS, or LDH could be increased; however, these findings are nonspecific [5].

To diagnose pulmonary primary lymphoma criteria established by Saltzstein that show unilateral or bilateral pulmonary involvement should be kept, having mediastinal or hilar lymphadenopathy or not, and it must not have evidence of extrathoracic disease within 3 months of diagnosis [6].

The pathogenesis of this illness remains unclear; however, chronic antigenic stimulation, as in autoimmune disease, infection, and/or smoking, has been suggested as a trigger, which supports the fact that deregulation of lymphoid cell function may be involved [7, 8].

In 30–40% of patients autoimmune diseases (Sjögren's syndrome, rheumatoid arthritis, systemic lupus erythematosus, pernicious anemia, and Hashimoto thyroiditis), immunodeficiency states such as AIDS or the common variable immunodeficiency, and HCV infection could also present [9].

Radiological findings of pulmonary lymphoma are heterogeneous; these are characterized by consolidations with well-defined mass or reticulonodular pattern [3]. Computed tomography usually shows findings in the parenchyma or on the peripheral zone especially in the lower lobes. Between 60 and 70% of the cases show bilateral involvement, while between 70 and 77% of the cases have got single or multiple nodules with consolidated areas or cysts. The commonest

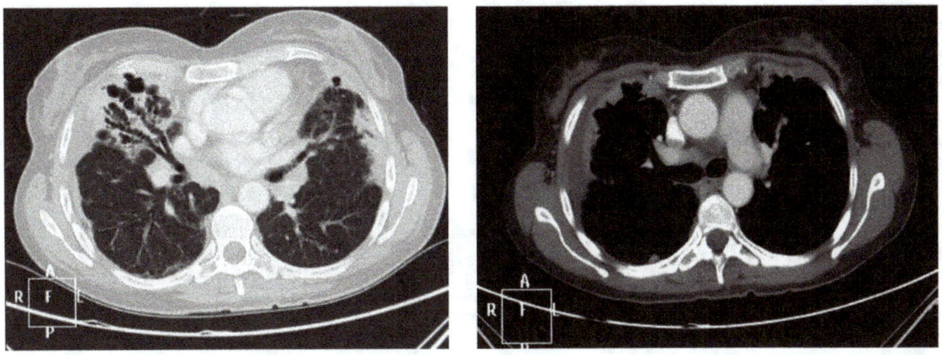

(a) (b)

FIGURE 2: CT scan showing bronchiectasis in the medium and lower lobule and bilateral pleural thickening (a), without adenomegalies (b).

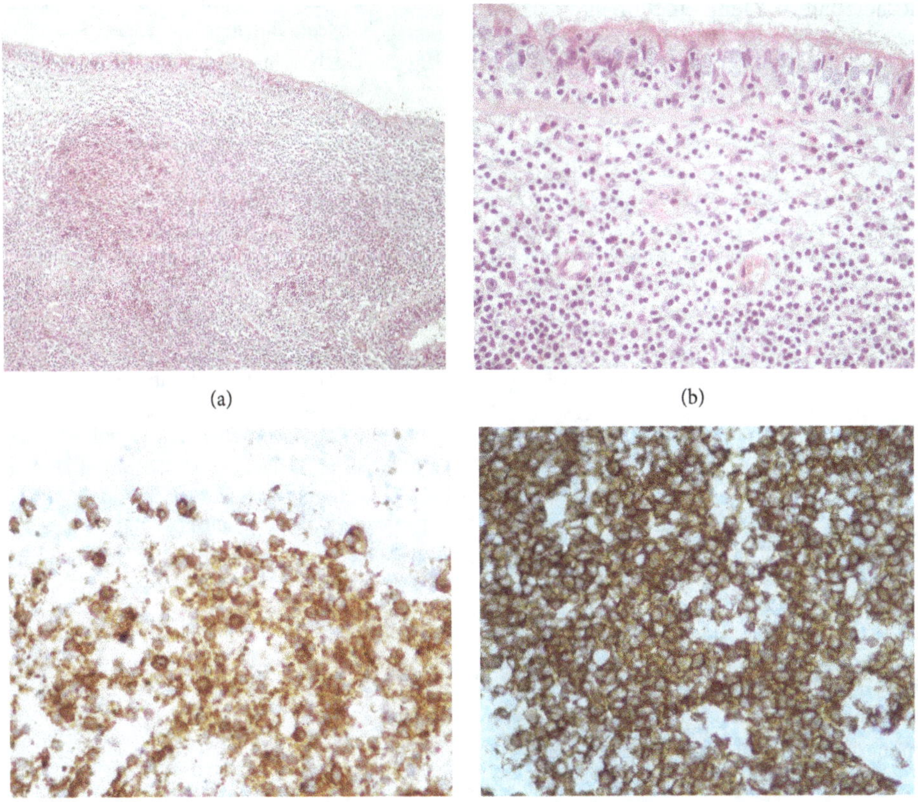

(a) (b) (c) (d)

FIGURE 3: Lung biopsies. (a) Bronchial mucosa with lymphoid infiltration by small cells with germinal center formation. (40x-HE). (b) Lymphoepithelial lesions (100x-HE). Immune-histochemical demonstrating that lymphocytes were positive for BCL-2 (c) and CD20 (d).

presentation includes findings such as masses with well-defined margins or with air bronchogram. For this reason, the main proposed differential diagnosis would be the bronchoalveolar carcinoma [10, 11].

Only one patient with bronchiectasis and bilateral hilar and mediastinal lymph node enlargement has been previously described. However, the physicians initially suspected in the diagnosis of sarcoidosis [10]. According to this case, our patient showed bronchiectasis in the medium lobule, lingula, and pleural bilateral thickening but without adenomegalies to support another differential diagnosis.

Other associated features include angiogram sign and ground glass halo in thickening peribronchovascular area, especially in the margins of the tumor [12].

Hilar or mediastinal lymphadenopathies are less common and their presence would be suggesting dissemination of the disease and would be associated with bad prognosis. Nevertheless, pleural and vascular involvements have not been associated with poor prognosis. The cavitation of nodules is extremely rare [4, 13]. Bronchoalveolar lavage contributes to finding lymphoid infiltration in about 65% of cases [5], although the immunohistochemistry to diagnose such illness is necessary. These cells express B-cell markers, such as CD20 and CD79a, and are negative for CD5, CD10, CD23, and cyclin-D1 [14].

Therapeutic strategies include surgical resection followed by chemotherapy and/or radiotherapy. The choice will depend on the stage of the tumor; however, treatment in patients with limited disease remains not well established. It has been suggested that patient coursing the initial diagnosis of BALT without symptoms could be observed and followed up without treatment [15]. However, this indication is controversial [16]. The benefits of lung surgery and radiation therapy are questionable because some patients have presented with complications as thoracic pain and lung function impairment [17]. Until now, chemotherapy with chlorambucil would be the best treatment option for cases with disseminated disease [18]; however, another option is treatment with rituximab in patients with cells CD20+ [19].

To conclude, pulmonary BALT lymphoma is a rare tumor with a variety of radiological manifestations. The consolidation and multiple pulmonary nodules are the most frequent; however, we have presented this rare case, with bronchiectasis, as unique radiological finding.

References

[1] J. Cadranel, M. Wislez, and M. Antoine, "Primary pulmonary lymphoma," *European Respiratory Journal*, vol. 20, no. 3, pp. 750–762, 2002.

[2] P. Isaacson and D. H. Wright, "Malignant lymphoma of mucosa-associated lymphoid tissue. A distinctive type of B-cell lymphoma," *Cancer*, vol. 52, no. 8, pp. 1410–1416, 1983.

[3] S. Hare, C. A. Souza, G. Bain et al., "The radiological spectrum of pulmonary lymphoproliferative disease," *The British Journal of Radiology*, vol. 85, no. 1015, pp. 848–864, 2012.

[4] L. J. King, S. P. G. Padley, A. C. Wotherspoon, and A. G. Nicholson, "Pulmonary MALT lymphoma: imaging findings in 24 cases," *European Radiology*, vol. 10, no. 12, pp. 1932–1938, 2000.

[5] J. H. Kim, S. H. Lee, J. Park et al., "Primary pulmonary non-Hodgkin's lymphoma," *Japanese Journal of Clinical Oncology* vol. 34, no. 9, pp. 510–514, 2004.

[6] S. L. Saltzstein, "Pulmonary malignant lymphomas and pseudolymphomas: classification, therapy and prognosis," *Cancer* vol. 16, pp. 928–955, 1963.

[7] V. J. Verma, S. Jain, S. Singhal et al., "Primary pulmonary mucosa-associated lymphoid tissue lymphoma in a patient with acquired immune deficiency syndrome," *Respiratory Care*, vol. 56, no. 7, pp. 1046–1049, 2011.

[8] P. G. Isaacson, "Mucosa-associated lymphoid tissue lymphoma," *Seminars in Hematology*, vol. 36, no. 2, pp. 139–147, 1999.

[9] M. I. Ramos Cancelo, "Patrón intersticial como manifestación de linfoma MALT con afectación pulmonar y gástrica," *Revista de Patología Respiratoria*, vol. 10, no. 4, pp. 191–193, 2007.

[10] Y. A. Bae, K. S. Lee, J. Han et al., "Marginal zone B-cell lymphoma of bronchus-associated lymphoid tissue: imaging findings in 21 patients," *Chest*, vol. 133, no. 2, pp. 433–440, 2008.

[11] R. G. Yoon, M. Y. Kim, J. W. Song, E. J. Chae, C. M. Choi, and S. Jang, "Primary endobronchial marginal zone B-cell lymphoma of bronchus-associated lymphoid tissue: CT findings in 7 patients," *Korean Journal of Radiology*, vol. 14, no. 2, pp. 366–374, 2013.

[12] K. Mucha, B. Foroncewicz, P. Palczewski et al., "Pulmonary post-transplant lymphoproliferative disorder with a CT halo sign," *Annals of Transplantation*, vol. 18, no. 1, pp. 482–487, 2013.

[13] M. Wislez, J. Cadranel, M. Antoine et al., "Lymphoma of pulmonary mucosa-associated lymphoid tissue: CT scan findings and pathological correlations," *European Respiratory Journal*, vol. 14, no. 2, pp. 423–429, 1999.

[14] P. J. Kurtin, J. L. Myers, H. Adlakha et al., "Pathologic and clinical features of primary pulmonary extranodal marginal zone B-cell lymphoma of MALT type," *The American Journal of Surgical Pathology*, vol. 25, no. 8, pp. 997–1008, 2001.

[15] M. Troch, B. Streubel, V. Petkov, K. Turetschek, A. Chott, and M. Raderer, "Does MALT lymphoma of the lung require immediate treatment? An analysis of 11 untreated cases with long-term follow-up," *Anticancer Research*, vol. 27, no. 5, pp. 3633–3637, 2007.

[16] S. Ahmed, S. J. Kussick, A. K. Siddiqui et al., "Bronchial-associated lymphoid tissue lymphoma: a clinical study of a rare disease," *European Journal of Cancer*, vol. 40, no. 9, pp. 1320–1326, 2004.

[17] S. Y. Oh, W. S. Kim, J. S. Kim et al., "Pulmonary marginal zone B-cell lymphoma of MALT type—what is a prognostic factor and which is the optimal treatment, operation, or chemotherapy?: Consortium for Improving Survival of Lymphoma (CISL) study," *Annals of Hematology*, vol. 89, no. 6, pp. 563–568, 2010.

[18] R. Borie, M. Wislez, G. Thabut et al., "Clinical characteristics and prognostic factors of pulmonary MALT lymphoma," *European Respiratory Journal*, vol. 34, no. 6, pp. 1408–1416, 2009.

[19] A. Conconi, G. Martinelli, C. Thiéblemont et al., "Clinical activity of rituximab in extranodal marginal zone B-cell lymphoma of MALT type," *Blood*, vol. 102, no. 8, pp. 2741–2745, 2003.

17

Metastatic Recurrence of Typical Pulmonary Carcinoid Accompanied by Carcinoid Syndrome, Successfully Treated with Octreotide LAR

Asako Yanagisawa,[1] Satoshi Hirano,[2] Shinichiro Shimizu,[3] Takuma Hiroishi,[1] Kohei Shikano,[1] Noriko Hayama,[1] Tetsuo Fujita,[1] Hiroyuki Amano,[1] Makoto Nakamura,[1] Sukeyuki Nakamura,[1] and Hiroshi Tabeta[1]

[1]*Department of Respiratory Medicine, Funabashi Municipal Medical Center, Chiba, Japan*
[2]*Department of Medical Oncology, Funabashi Municipal Medical Center, Chiba, Japan*
[3]*Department of Pathology, Funabashi Municipal Medical Center, Chiba, Japan*

Correspondence should be addressed to Satoshi Hirano; shirano@mmc.funabashi.chiba.jp

Academic Editor: Jeanine M. Buchanich

We present a case of metastatic recurrence of carcinoid tumor accompanied by carcinoid syndrome in a 68-year-old Japanese man, 12 years after resection of typical pulmonary carcinoid. Histopathologic examination from percutaneous liver biopsy revealed metastatic typical carcinoid. Clinical symptoms gradually improved after administration of octreotide LAR. Two years after starting treatment, the disease remains well controlled. This case report illustrates the possibility of antiproliferative effects of octreotide LAR on typical pulmonary carcinoid.

1. Introduction

Typical pulmonary carcinoid is known as a low-grade subtype of lung neuroendocrine tumor (NET) and is characterized by an indolent nature. Recurrence of typical pulmonary carcinoid after complete resection is very rare (3–5%) [1]. The frequency of carcinoid syndrome among lung NETs is also very low [2]. Somatostatin analogues such as octreotide have been reported to improve the symptoms of carcinoid syndrome [3]. Furthermore, octreotide long-acting repeatable (LAR) has shown antitumor activity against midgut NETs [4].

2. Case

A 68-year-old Japanese man was referred to our hospital because of multiple hyperechoic lesions in the liver without any symptoms. The patient was a former smoker with a 45-pack-year history. Twelve years prior to this presentation, he had undergone thoracoscopic left upper lobectomy for typical pulmonary carcinoid (pT1N0M0, stage I). Histopathologic examination of the surgical specimen revealed finely granular nuclear chromatin, eosinophilic cytoplasm, and rosette formation (Figure 1(a)). The immunohistology was positive for synaptophysin, chromogranin A, and CD56 (Figure 1(b)). The presence of 1 mitosis per $2\,mm^2$ and absence of necrosis were consistent with typical carcinoid. The hilar and mediastinal lymph nodes were negative for any tumor, and the surgical margins as well were free of any tumor.

The patient had a history of atrial fibrillation. Physical examination revealed no abnormalities. Computed tomography (CT) with intravenous contrast of the abdomen revealed multiple low-density areas. Percutaneous liver biopsy of one of the lesions demonstrated well-differentiated tumor with positive expressions of chromogranin A, synaptophysin, and CD56 (Figure 2). The presence of 1 mitosis per $2\,mm^2$ and no necrosis were also demonstrated, which

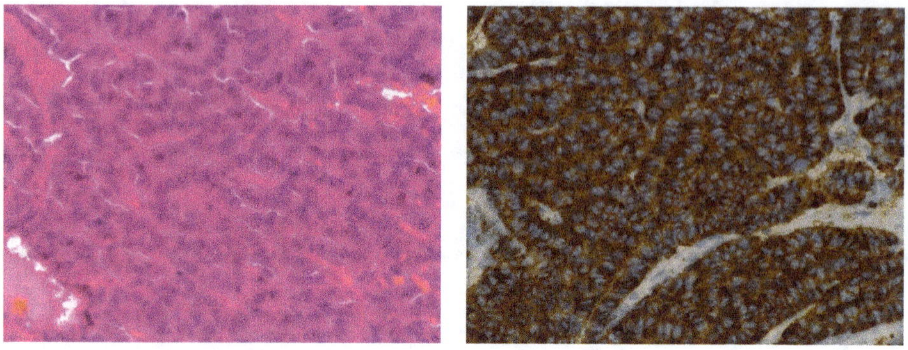

(a) (b)

Figure 1: Histologic examination of surgically resected pulmonary carcinoid tumor shows finely granular nuclear chromatin, eosinophilic cytoplasm, and rosette formation (a) and positive expression of chromogranin A (b).

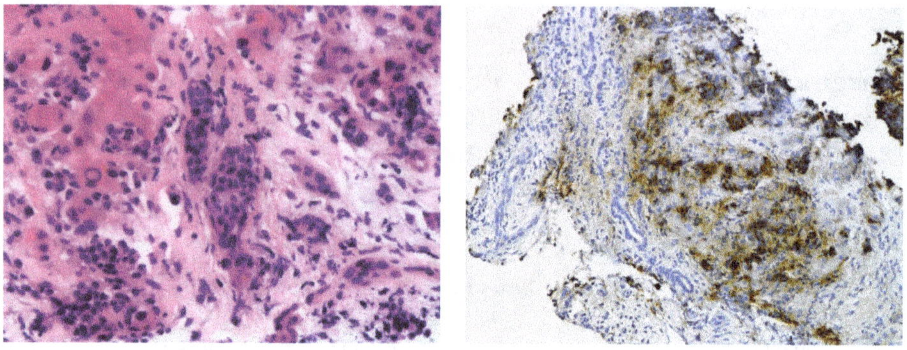

(a) (b)

Figure 2: Histologic examination of a liver biopsy specimen shows a well-differentiated tumor (a) with positive expression of chromogranin A (b).

was compatible for metastatic typical carcinoid. During 6 months of close observation, the patient developed chronic diarrhea resulting in 12 kg of weight loss. His general condition worsened, and he was hospitalized.

Physical examination showed hepatomegaly and wheezing. Levels of neuron-specific enolase and α-fetoprotein were both elevated, at 24.7 ng/ml (normal range (NR) < 16.3 ng/ml) and 56 ng/ml (NR < 10 ng/ml), respectively. Blood 5-hydroxyindole acetate (5-HIAA), urine 5-HIAA, and serotonin degradation metabolite levels were elevated at 1121 ng/ml (NR 57–230 ng/ml), 472 ng/ml (NR 1.8–6.1 ng/ml), and 86.9 mg/13 h (NR 1–6 mg/24 h), respectively, confirming the diagnosis of carcinoid syndrome. Chest CT showed no abnormalities. Abdominal contrast-enhanced CT revealed multiple tumors in the liver and spleen, as well as hepatomegaly (Figure 3). Magnetic resonance imaging (MRI) of the brain revealed an enhanced nodular lesion in the right occipital lobe, compatible with a brain metastasis.

Considering that immunostaining for somatostatin receptor 2 antibody was scored as 3 (circumferential membranous reactivity in >50% of tumor cells), subcutaneous octreotide therapy was started at a dose of 100 μg/day (Figure 4). Blood serotonin, blood 5-HIAA, and neuron-specific enolase levels decreased markedly and diarrhea gradually improved. Following 20 mg of LAR octreotide via intramuscular injections every 4 weeks, the dose was increased to 30 mg every 4 weeks because of persistent diarrhea. Two years after starting octreotide therapy, the disease is well controlled with almost no symptoms, except for transient ischemic attack.

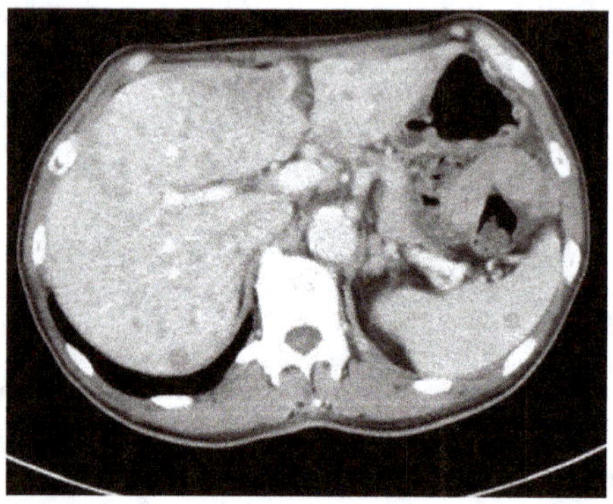

Figure 3: Abdominal contrast-enhanced CT shows multiple low-density areas, hepatomegaly, and metastasis to the spleen.

3. Discussion

Pulmonary carcinoid tumor is a rare NET that accounts for less than 2% of all lung tumors. Good prognosis can be expected following complete surgical resection of

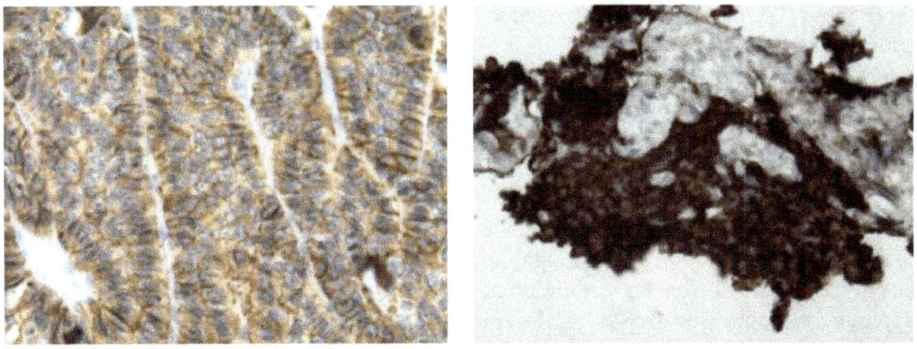

(a) (b)

FIGURE 4: Immunohistochemical analysis demonstrates immunoreactivity for somatostatin receptor 2 antibody immunostaining in most tumor cells in the lung (a) and liver (b).

pulmonary carcinoid tumor. The recurrence rate for typical carcinoid is lower (3.6%) than that of atypical carcinoid (33.3%) [5]. Histological subtype, staging, and nodal status are reported to be significant predictors of disease-free survival [6]. In contrast, Maurizi showed that only histological subtype (and not nodal status) can influence disease-free survival, with a statistically significant advantage for typical carcinoid [7]. The distinction between typical and atypical carcinoid is thus very important in the determination of prognosis. The WHO 2015 classification for lung NETs states that the defining features of atypical carcinoid are the presence of 2–10 mitoses per 2 mm^2 and/or the presence of necrosis [8]. As for atypical carcinoid, Arrigoni et al. [9] first described the histological criteria for atypical bronchopulmonary carcinoid tumors in 1972, namely, increased mitotic activity with 5–10 mitoses per 2 mm^2 (10 high-power field (HPF)), nuclear pleomorphism, and irregularity with hyperchromatism and prominent nucleoli, areas of increased cellularity with disorganization, and necrosis. Travis et al. reported increased mitotic activity as the only independent predictor of prognosis in the criteria described by Arrigoni [10]. He proposed that either a mitotic count ≥ 2 and <10 per 2 mm^2 (10 HPF) in viable tumor or the presence of necrosis should be the histologic criterion for atypical carcinoid, because atypical carcinoid would be underestimated if the mitotic range is set between 5 and 10 mitoses (10 high-powered fields), and the presence of necrosis is indicative of poor prognosis.

Only a small number of patients with typical carcinoid experience recurrences, with a median time to recurrence of 4 years (range, 0.8–12 years), longer than that for atypical carcinoid [11]. As a result, few case reports have addressed the late recurrence of typical carcinoid tumors. Our case was valuable in that liver metastases occurred more than 10 years after complete resection of the primary tumor.

The primary lesion was diagnosed as typical carcinoid. However, part of the primary lesion showed conspicuous nucleoli and high cellularity, consistent with atypical carcinoid according to the former criteria [9]. These features may indicate the potential for recurrence or metastasis of typical carcinoid. Arrigoni et al. reported that 70% of 23 carcinoids with such histologic features exhibited metastasis, as compared to 5.6% of histologically typical carcinoid [9]. Atypical features including high cellularity and prominent nucleoli could be assumed to be related to metastasis to the liver, and the low mitotic count was associated with late recurrence in our case.

Whether liver metastases originated from the lung in our case represents an important issue, because there is a possibility of the presence of another primary site. When liver metastases are demonstrated, CT of the chest and abdomen, abdominal ultrasonography, upper gastrointestinal endoscopy, and colonoscopy are performed to exclude primary tumors other than those of the lung, but no other gastroenteropancreatic neuroendocrine tumors were found in our case. Brain metastasis without pulmonary lesions is not common for primary sites other than the lung.

Patients with carcinoid syndrome display a shorter overall survival (median, 5 years) than patients without carcinoid syndrome (5.6 years) [2]. Patients with NETs and carcinoid syndrome show marked impairments in multiple areas. Carcinoid syndrome also affects patients' quality of life. Although the frequency of carcinoid syndrome in lung NETs is very low, our patient was diagnosed with typical pulmonary carcinoid and carcinoid syndrome.

Somatostatin receptor scintigraphy (SRS) is useful for the diagnosis of neuroendocrine tumors [12]. Accumulations on SRS reflect the degree of tumor differentiation, and SRS shows high sensitivity for the detection of low-grade neuroendocrine tumors. SRS is a helpful option for detecting metastatic lesions that are hard to find by other imaging modalities and for predicting the outcomes of octreotide treatment [13]. Although we did not perform SRS, strongly positive results for somatostatin receptor 2 were seen on immunohistochemical staining [14]. Octreotide suppresses the production of physiologically active substances through binding to somatostatin receptors on tumor cells [15]. Octreotide can be expected to have somatostatin receptor-mediated and antiangiogenic antiproliferative effects [16].

The LAR formulation of octreotide inhibits tumor growth in patients with metastatic midgut neuroendocrine tumors [4]. Octreotide treatment resulted in control of carcinoid syndrome and tumor reduction or complete regression in 43% of patients with liver metastases of pulmonary atypical carcinoid [17]. An antiproliferative effect of octreotide on pulmonary carcinoid tumor can be expected. However, few case reports have addressed the antiproliferative effects of octreotide LAR on typical pulmonary carcinoid. An antiproliferative effect of another long-acting somatostatin analogue lanreotide was demonstrated in a study of more than 200 patients with somatostatin receptor-positive enteropancreatic neuroendocrine tumors with Ki-67 values of less than 10% [18]. Although the patients in this study were thought to have more indolent tumors, the estimated rates of progression-free survival were 65.1% in the lanreotide group and 33.0% in the placebo group. In our case, carcinoid syndrome was well controlled after administration of octreotide LAR, which also resulted in a long period of disease stabilization. Considering the median PFS of 11.3 months in the placebo plus octreotide LAR group in the RADIANT-2 trial [3], our case may indicate that treatment with octreotide LAR is associated with longer tumor stabilization in typical carcinoid, which has the lower mitotic rate.

In summary, this case report illustrates the possibility of antiproliferative effects of octreotide LAR on typical pulmonary carcinoid.

Ethical Approval

The study design was exempt from ethics review board approval.

Consent

The patient provided informed consent.

Acknowledgments

The authors thank Dr. Robert Yoshiyuki Osamura from Diagnostic Pathology Center at International University of Health and Welfare (IUHW) Mita Hospital in Tokyo for somatostatin receptor 2 immunohistochemical staining.

References

[1] E. M. Wolin, "Challenges in the diagnosis and management of well-differentiated neuroendocrine tumors of the lung (typical and atypical carcinoid): current status and future considerations," *Oncologist*, vol. 20, no. 10, pp. 1123–1131, 2015.

[2] D. M. Halperin, C. Shen, A. Dasari et al., "Frequency of carcinoid syndrome at neuroendocrine tumour diagnosis: a population-based study," *Lancet Oncology*, vol. 18, no. 4, pp. 525–534, 2017.

[3] M. E. Pavel, J. D. Hainsworth, E. Baudin et al., "Everolimus plus octreotide long-acting repeatable for the treatment of advanced neuroendocrine tumours associated with carcinoid syndrome (RADIANT-2): a randomised, placebo-controlled, phase 3 study," *The Lancet*, vol. 378, no. 9808, pp. 2005–2012, 2011.

[4] A. Rinke, H. H. Müller, C. Schade-Brittinger et al., "Placebo-controlled, double-blind, prospective, randomized study on the effect of octreotide LAR in the control of tumor growth in patients with metastatic neuroendocrine midgut tumors: a report from the PROMID Study Group," *Journal of Clinical Oncology*, vol. 27, no. 28, pp. 4656–4663, 2009.

[5] H. Asamura, T. Kameya, Y. Matsuno et al., "Neuroendocrine neoplasms of the lung: a prognostic spectrum," *Journal of Clinical Oncology*, vol. 24, no. 1, pp. 70–76, 2006.

[6] P. C. Lee, N. C. Osakwe, N. Narula et al., "Predictors of disease-free survival and recurrence in patients with resected bronchial carcinoid tumors," *Thoracic and Cardiovascular Surgeon*, vol. 64, no. 2, pp. 159–165, 2016.

[7] G. Maurizi, M. Ibrahim, C. Andreetti et al., "Long-term results after resection of bronchial carcinoid tumour: evaluation of survival and prognostic factors," *Interactive Cardio Vascular and Thoracic Surgery*, vol. 19, no. 2, pp. 239–244, 2014.

[8] W. D. Travis, E. Brambilla, A. P. Burke et al., *WHO Classification of Tumours of the Lung, Pleura, Thymus and Heart*, International Agency for Research on Cancer, Lyon, France, 2015.

[9] M. G. Arrigoni, L. B. Woolner, and P. E. Bernatz, "A typical carcinoid tumors of the lung," *Journal of Thoracic and Cardiovascular Surgery*, vol. 64, no. 3, pp. 413–421, 1972.

[10] W. D. Travis, W. Rush, D. B. Flieder et al., "Survival analysis of 200 pulmonary neuroendocrine tumors with clarification of criteria for atypical carcinoid and its separation from typical carcinoid," *American Journal of Surgical Pathology*, vol. 22, no. 8, pp. 934–944, 1998.

[11] F. Lou, I. Sarkaria, C. Pietanza et al., "Recurrence of pulmonary carcinoid tumors after resection: implications for postoperative surveillance," *Annals of Thoracic Surgery*, vol. 96, no. 4, pp. 1156–1162, 2013.

[12] F. Gibril, J. C. Reynolds, J. L. Doppman et al., "Somatostatin receptor scintigraphy: its sensitivity compared with that of other imaging methods in detecting primary and metastatic gastrinomas. A prospective study," *Annals of Internal Medicine*, vol. 125, no. 1, pp. 26–34, 1996.

[13] G. D. Slooter, A. Mearadji, W. A. Breeman et al., "Somatostatin receptor imaging, therapy and new strategies in patients with neuroendocrine tumours," *British Journal of Surgery*, vol. 88, no. 1, pp. 31–40, 2001.

[14] G. D. Slooter, A. Mearadji, W. A. Breeman et al., "Somatostatin receptor type 2A immunohistochemistry in neuroendocrine tumors: a proposal of scoring system correlated with somatostatin receptor scintigraphy," *Modern Pathology*, vol. 20, no. 11, pp. 1172–1182, 2007.

[15] M. E. Caplin, E. Baudin, P. Ferolla et al., "Pulmonary neuroendocrine (carcinoid) tumors: European Neuroendocrine Tumor Society expert consensus and recommendations for best practice for typical and atypical pulmonary carcinoids," *Annals of Oncology*, vol. 26, no. 8, pp. 1604–1620, 2015.

[16] K. Oberg, "Cancer: antitumor effects of octreotide LAR, a somatostatin analog," *Nature Reviews Endocrinology*, vol. 6, no. 4, pp. 188-189, 2010.

[17] P. L. Filosso, E. Ruffini, A. Oliaro et al., "Long-term survival of atypical bronchial carcinoids with liver metastases, treated with octreotide," *European Journal of Cardio-Thoracic Surgery*, vol. 21, no. 5, pp. 913–917, 2002.

[18] M. E. Caplin, M. Pavel, J. B. Ćwikła et al., "Lanreotide in metastatic enteropancreatic neuroendocrine tumors," *New England Journal of Medicine*, vol. 371, no. 3, pp. 224–233, 2014.

18

Craniofacial Brown Tumor in Patients with Secondary Hyperparathyroidism to Chronic Renal Failure: Report of Two Cases in Cipto Mangunkusumo Hospital

Diani Kartini, Maria K. Siswiandari, Gunawan Wibisana, Erwin D. Yulian, Ahmad Kurnia, Sonar S. Panigoro, Azdi Z. Albar, and Muchlis Ramli

Oncology Division, Department of Surgery, Dr. Cipto Mangunkusumo General Hospital, Faculty of Medicine, Universitas Indonesia, Jakarta, Indonesia

Correspondence should be addressed to Diani Kartini; d.kartini@gmail.com

Academic Editor: Jeanine M. Buchanich

Brown tumor is a bone lesion that arises in the setting of excess osteoclast activity in hyperparathyroidism. It consists of fibrous tissue, woven bone, and supporting vasculature, while contains no matrix. The characteristic of brown-colored lesion is a result of hemosiderin deposition into the osteolytic cysts. Two cases of young women aged 26 and 29 years old, respectively, are known with a history of end-stage renal disease (ESRD). Dialysis is performed two times/week over the last 7 years. Our patients presented with an intraoral mass of the hard palate since 12 months ago and decreased body height of 10 cm. The lesion causes difficulties in swallowing and talking. Laboratory workup showed elevated parathormone or PTH (3.391 pg/mL and >5.000 pg/mL). Neck ultrasound showed enlargement of the parathyroid glands. Supporting examination to diagnose brown tumor are neck ultrasound, CT of the neck, and parathyroid sestamibi scan. We performed parathyroidectomy. Pathology revealed hyperplasia of the parathyroid. The tumor regressed significantly within 2 weeks following the surgery, and we still observe tumor regression as well as reduction in PTH level. As clinicians, we should be alert to other possible causes of bony lesions. Clinical examination, laboratory finding, and imaging present important information to diagnose brown tumor.

1. Introduction

Secondary hyperparathyroidism is a complication of renal failure, developed from many factors such as calcitriol deficiency, vitamin D deficiency, and the increased retention of phosphorus [1, 2]. These conditions cause hypocalcemia and trigger the production of PTH and hyperplasia of the parathyroid gland. The increase of fibroblast growth factor 23 (FGF-23) from renal failure also has a role in the development of secondary hyperparathyroidism [3]. The impacts of secondary hyperparathyroidism are bone resorption caused by the increased osteoclast activity, soft tissue calcification (calciphylaxis), cardiovascular events, pruritus, calcific uremic arteriolopathy, and many other [4].

Another complication of hyperparathyroidism is brown tumor, with incidence rate of 0.1%. Brown tumor is a giant cell granuloma which appears as a result of the imbalanced osteoclast activity and peritrabecular fibrosis [5]. It consists of fibrous tissue, woven bone, and supporting vasculature, while contains no matrix. Brown tumor histologically appears similar to giant cell tumor [6, 7]. The characteristic of brown-colored lesion is as a result of hemosiderin deposition into the osteolytic cysts [7]. This lesion rarely involves the craniofacial region, while it more commonly occurs in the mandible than in the maxilla [5]. It is also common in the long bones, ribs, and the pelvis. The lesion could be located in any part of the bones [8, 9].

Brown tumor presents as a fixated growing mass with bony consistency. The tumor itself is usually asymptomatic but causes disability in chewing, talking, and breathing if it occurs in the craniofacial region [8]. It may also cause secondary back pain or acute spinal compression if it occurs in the spinal cord [7]. Radiographic findings present the single or multiple osteolytic (radiolucent) lesion as well as the

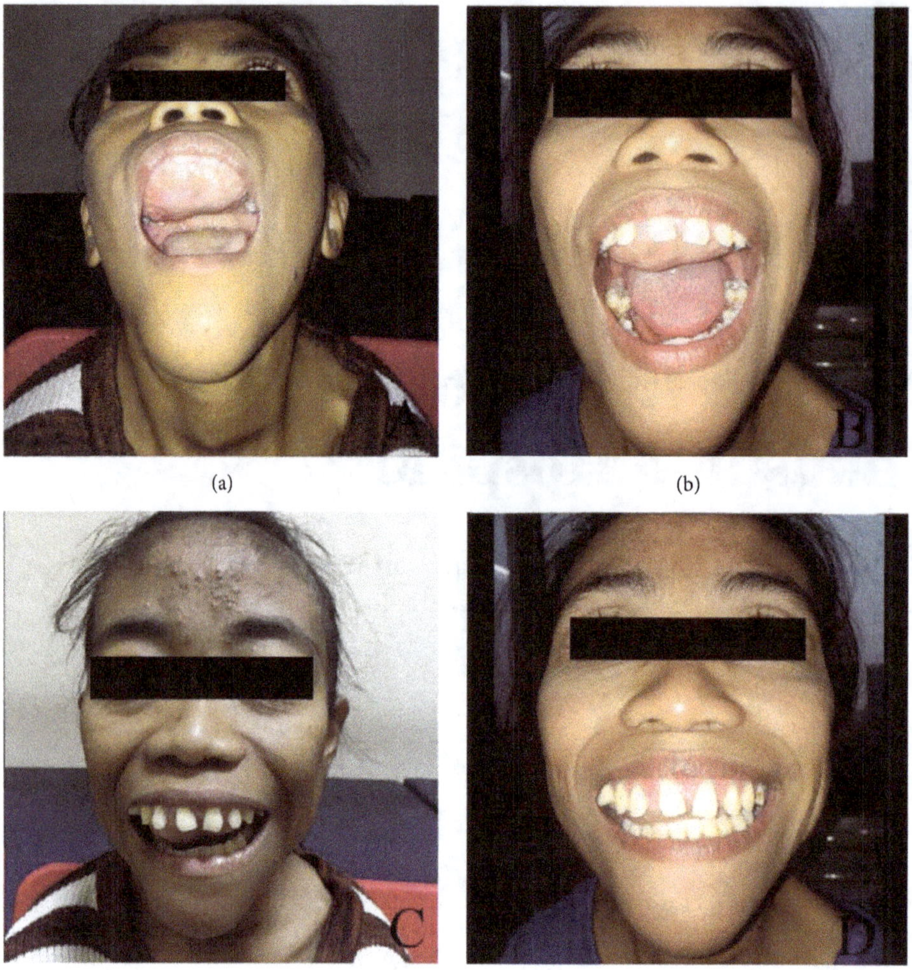

(a) (b) (c) (d)

FIGURE 1: Case 1. (a) Hard palate mass. (b) Facial asymmetry due to the mass. (c, d) Regressed mass after parathyroidectomy.

decreased density of the bones and a change in normal trabecular pattern [6].

1.1. Case 1. A 26-year-old female patient complained a growing mass in the hard palate since 12 months ago. This mass causes swallowing and closing mouth difficulty. She also complained about changes in the shape of her finger bones, mandible, and ribs. The decrease in height of 9 cm and weight loss of 10 kg were observed within 2 years. The patient experienced end stage of renal failure and has been treated with hemodialysis 2 times per week for seven years since 2009.

The physical examination showed a mass in the palatum durum and mandible, measured $4 \times 6 \times 2$ cm and 3×4 cm in size, respectively. The mass has rough surface, hard-solid consistency, with no tenderness. A mass in the right neck was measured 3×5 cm in size. The mass has smooth surface and solid consistency (Figure 1).

The result of the palatum and mandible biopsy was compatible with ossifying fibroma or fibrous dysplasia. Neck ultrasonography showed a solid mass in the right thyroid, bilateral cystic nodule in the thyroid lobes, and small cystic nodule in the thyroid isthmus. Bone survey showed the diffused decreasing bone density, fractured right clavicle, multiple lytic lesions among the cranium, humerus, clavicle, iliac, and pubic bone (Figure 2 and Figure 3). Paranasal sinus CT showed a decreased bone density in the cranial, facial, and cervicothoracic bones; lytic lesion in the maxilla bone extended to the palatum durum and shifted the tongue inferiorly, with the measurement of $5.2 \times 4.6 \times 3.7$ cm (Figure 4). Similar lytic lesions were also found in the midline and right mandible, measured $3.8 \times 3.2 \times 2.8$ and $2 \times 2.3 \times 2.1$ in size, respectively. Workup laboratory examination showed the elevated intact parathyroid hormone level (PTH) (3.391 pg/mL), ureum (124 mg/dL), and creatinine (6.60 mg/dL) and normal range of calcium level (9.5 mg/dL) and phosphate (3.6 mg/dL). Histopathologic findings suggest ossifying fibroma with a differential diagnosis of fibrous dysplasia. No signs of malignancies were revealed in the histopathologic examination.

Based on the physical examination and laboratory findings, we concluded brown tumor as the diagnosis due to secondary hyperparathyroidism. The treatment for this patient was right parathyroidectomy and right isthmulobectomy with frozen section. The right isthmulobectomy was chosen because the patient has secondary diagnosis which was right nontoxic nodular enlargement of the thyroid gland. In

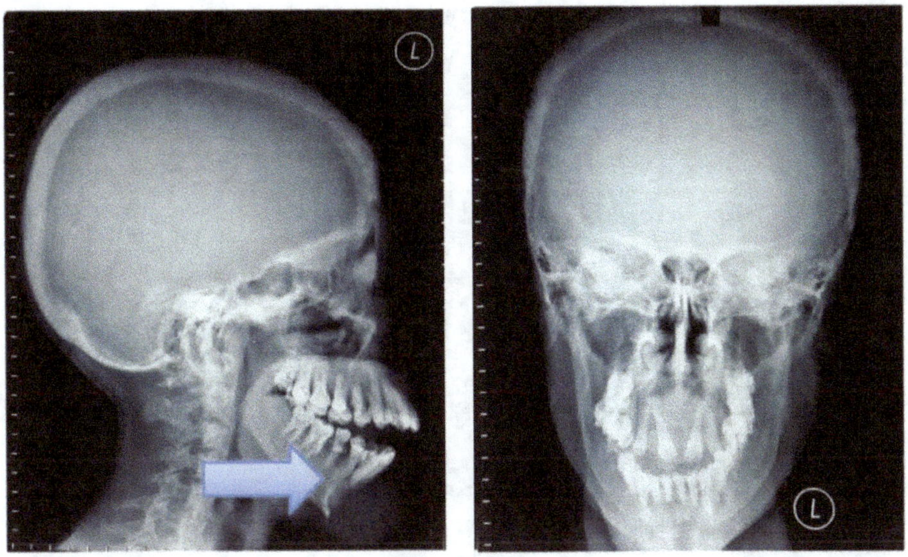

(a) (b)

FIGURE 2: Case 1. (a) Bone survey radiographic examination of the cranium. (b) Multiple lytic lesion with well-defined border in the cranium. Arrow shows bone resorption activity in lower alveolar area.

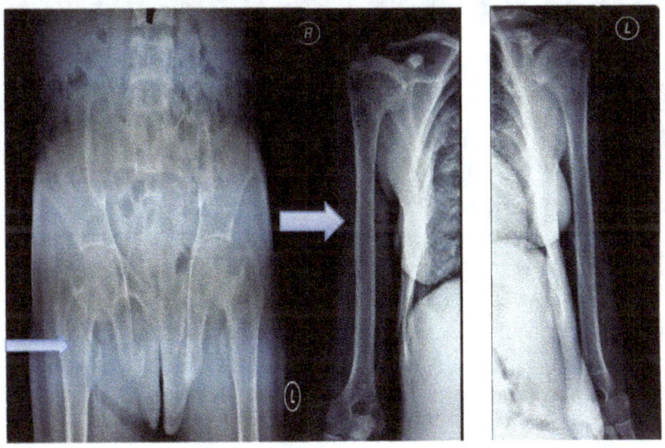

(a) (b)

FIGURE 3: Case 1. Bone survey radiographic examination of the (a) pelvis showing multiple lytic lesion along the bilateral iliac bone and pubic bone and the (b) humerus and clavicle showing multiple lytic lesion along the lateral edge of the humerus. Pathologic fractures of the distal part of the left clavicle are observed, increased bone resorption among the bilateral clavicle.

addition, the technique was considered to be appropriate to access the parathyroid gland with the antecedent removal of the thyroid gland. Frozen section revealed hyperplasia of the right parathyroid. Three days following the surgery, PTH level was significantly decreased from the initial preoperative level (851.10 pg/mL). Result from definitive pathology anatomy was hyperplasia of the parathyroid gland.

One month following the surgery, the patient felt regression among her hard palate and mandible mass and ease in swallowing. During follow-up, we performed additional evaluative examination. Neck 4D CT was done 2 times at the 2nd and 5th month of follow-up. The first one showed multiple lymphadenopathy around the neck and left supraclavicle, no residual mass in the right thyroid, no abnormality in the left thyroid, and no ectopic parathyroid gland was found. While the second Neck 4D CT found a single solid lesion in the left thyroid and 2 solid lesions in aortopulmonary window, suggestive of parathyroid nodes. At the 6th month of follow-up, sestamibi parathyroid scan showed no abnormality and no residual mass in the right thyroid lobe. PTH level evaluation performed in the 4th and 7th month showed an elevation to 909.7 pg/mL and 1.137 pg/mL, respectively.

Patient complained pain in all her bones and started walking with a cane. Seven months following the first surgery, we decided to perform left parathyroidectomy and left lobectomy with frozen section and intraoperative PTH evaluation. Thirty minutes following parathyroidectomy, the PTH level decreased significantly to 76.95 pg/mL. Frozen section result revealed hyperplasia of the left parathyroid.

Two weeks following the second surgery, the mass regressed significantly, and symptoms were much reduced.

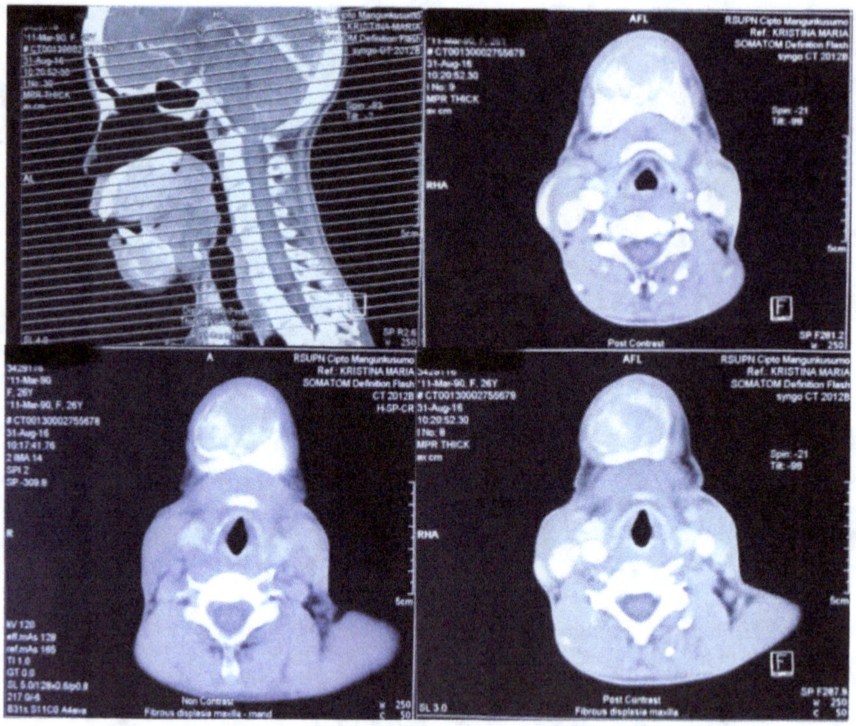

Figure 4: Case 1. Paranasal CT scan. Decreased diffuse with ground glass appearance among the cranium, facial, and cervicothoracic bones. Multiple lytic lesion in the maxillary bones.

1.2. Case 2. A 31-year-old female patient complained a mass in her maxilla and mandible. The mass was gradually increasing in size over the last 6 months. The mass caused talking disturbances, swallowing difficulty, dilating gap between upper teeth, and narrowing gap between lower teeth. She also complained hard masses in her fingers and the middle of chest. There was a decrease in height (15 cm in 8 years) and weight (19 kg in 8 years). The patient was on end stage of renal failure and has been treated with hemodialysis 2 times per week for eight years since 2008. The patient was planned to be performed renal transplantation. Comorbidities were reported among this patient, which are chronic heart failure, grade II hypertension, lung tuberculosis on therapy, and hepatitis C. The physical examination showed facial asymmetry with mass in the palatum durum, measured 4×3 cm in size (Figure 5). Palpation revealed hard consistency originated from the bone, smooth surface, and no tenderness.

X-ray of the maxilla and mandible showed diffused decreasing bone density and multiple lytic lesion, which suggest metabolic bone disease or renal osteodystrophy or hyperparathyroidism (Figure 6). BNO showed compression fracture in thoracolumbar vertebrae and multiple calcification in soft tissue abdominal and pelvic region compatible with renal osteodystrophy. Bone survey also showed the decreased bone density. Facial CT with contrast showed diffuse hyperostosis, lytic lesion in the mandible bone, maxillary bone, cranium, and multiple calcification in the soft tissue which is compatible with osteorenal dystrophy (Figure 7). Thyroid ultrasonography showed bilateral multiple cysts in the thyroid, a firm lesion with calcification in the left parathyroid fossa, and oval lesion in the left pericarotid. Parathyroid scan showed an increased activity in the inferior aspect of left thyroid which was suggestive of parathyroid adenoma.

Laboratory examination showed the elevated ureum (202 mg/dL), creatinine (11.1 mg/dL), and normal calcium level (9.7 mg/dL). In November 2016, PTH level was >5000 pg/mL and phosphate level was 6.1 mg/dL.

Physical examination and laboratory examination lead us to brown tumor as the diagnosis due to secondary hyperparathyroidism. The treatment for this patient was subtotal parathyroidectomy with frozen section and intraoperative PTH evaluation. Intraoperative parathyroid hormone level was evaluated following subtotal parathyroidectomy. The result decreased to normal range 10.37 pg/mL (normal range: 10–65 pg/mL). Frozen section revealed hyperplasia of the parathyroid. Calcium level was evaluated every day for 7 days, and the result ranged from 5.0 mg/dL to 7.4 mg/dL. The parathyroid hormone on the 3rd month following the surgery was 4.31 pg/mL. Definitive pathology anatomy result revealed hyperplasia of the parathyroid with water clear cell parathyroid adenoma.

The masses in the maxilla, mandible, and sternum were observed to be significantly regressed. This patient then underwent renal transplantation approximately 4 months following parathyroidectomy. One month following the renal transplantation, PTH level was 6 pg/mL.

2. Discussion

There are numerous options for hyperparathyroidism treatment such as dietary modification, pharmacological therapy (e.g., vitamin D receptor activator, non-calcium-

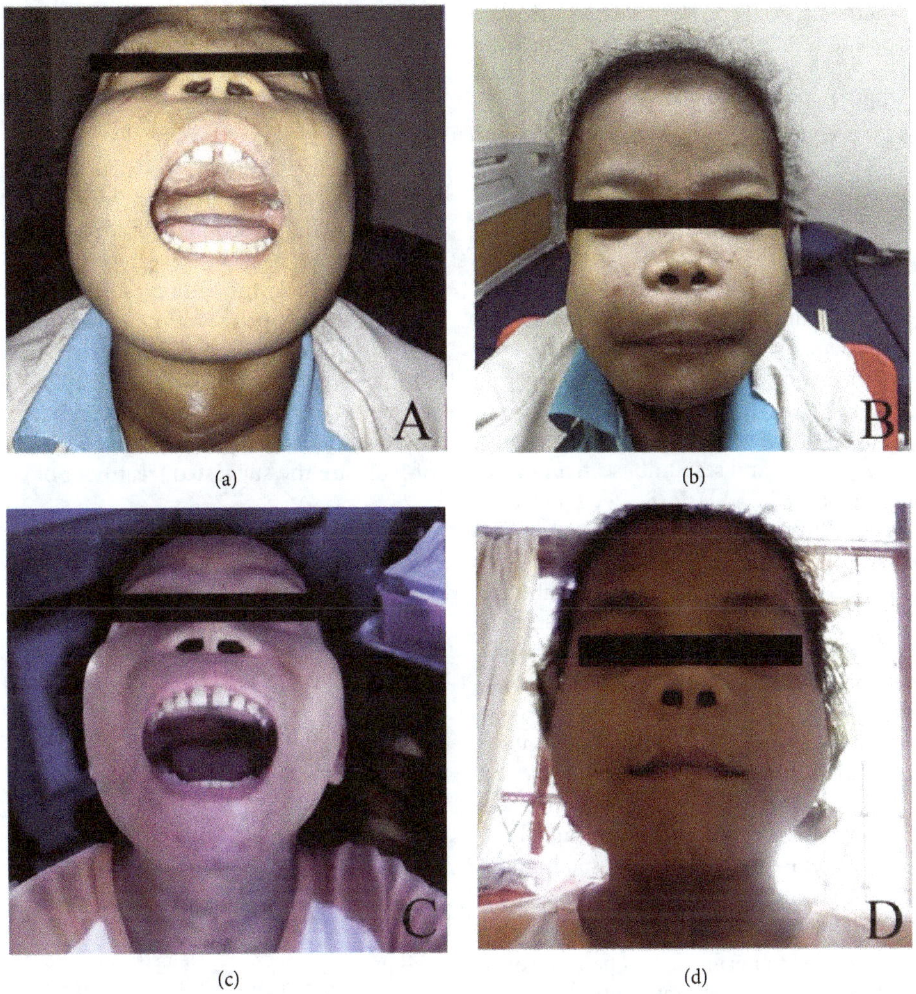

FIGURE 5: Case 2. (a) Hard palate mass. (b) Swelling in the bilateral maxilla and mandible. (c, d): Regressed mass after parathyroidectomy.

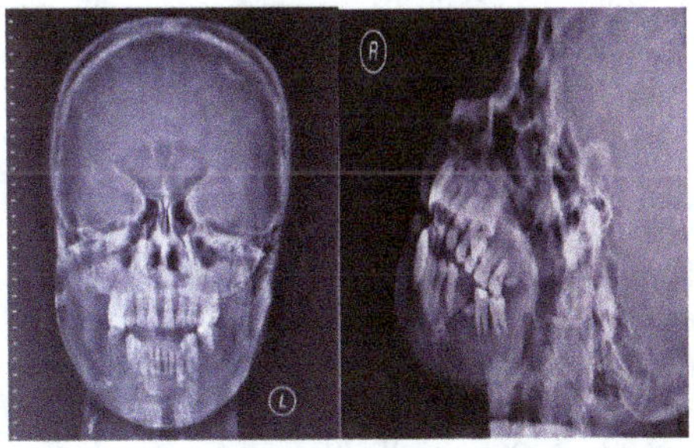

FIGURE 6: Case 2. Bone radiographic examination of the skull showing multiple lytic lesion among the calvaria, decreased diffuse bone density among the calvaria, and multiple lytic lesion in the calvaria, maxilla, and mandible. Salt and pepper appearance in the calvaria.

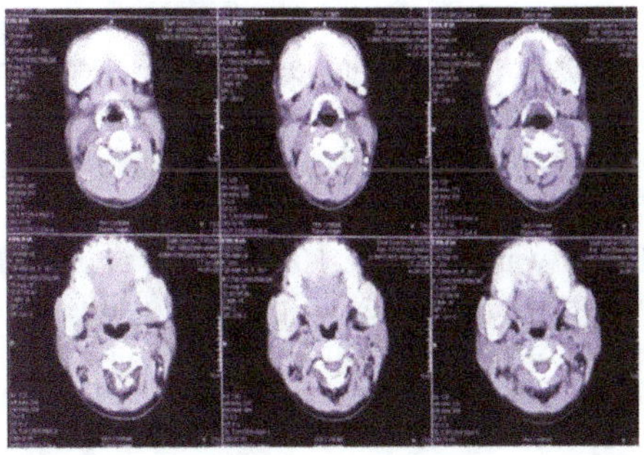

FIGURE 7: Case 2. Head CT scan showing diffused hyperostosis with multiple lytic lesion among the bones of maxilla, mandible, and the skull.

based phosphate binders, calcimimetics, and paricalcitol), and parathyroidectomy [10]. The indication for surgical intervention are PTH level > 800 pg/mL, hypercalcemia, hyperphosphataemia, hypercalciuria, and severe symptom of hyperparathyroidism including unbearable bone pain, osteoporosis/osteopenia, and severe pruritus [11, 12]. Failure to maintain normal level of phosphate, calcium, and PTH among patients with chronic kidney disease promotes to the higher mortality rate due to cardiovascular complication related to ectopic calcification [13]. Therefore, the parathyroid intervention should be considered to replace pharmacological treatment [14].

It is very important to determine the extent of parathyroidectomy prior to surgery to prevent recurrent or persistent disease and avoidance of permanent hypoparathyroidism

[12, 15]. Therefore, there is a need for further investigations such as neck ultrasound, sestamibi scan, CT imaging, 4D CT, and MRI [15, 16]. Selection of imaging depends on surgeons' preference and the available facilities.

The first choices for preoperative examination are combination of ultrasonography and technetium Tc99m sestamibi scan, with the sensitivity of 74%–95% for single gland disease. Whereas for multigland disease and multiple adenomata, the sensitivity of ultrasonography is 15%–35% and sestamibi scan is 30%–44% [17]. 4D CT may be useful for preoperative evaluation in patients with multigland disease, reoperative parathyroid patients, patients with mild hypercalcemia, and patients with negative or inconclusive ultrasound and sestamibi scan results [16]. With sensitivity ranges from 85.7 to 89.4% for localization, 4D CT provides greater sensitivity compared with ultrasonography and sestamibi scan and able to predict multigland disease (85.7%) [16, 18, 19]. The localization result from 4D CT would be superior if combined with intraoperative parathyroid measurement [20].

There are three methods of surgical treatment: subtotal parathyroidectomy, total parathyroidectomy with autotransplantation, and total parathyroidectomy without autotransplantation [10]. Selection of surgical method may be based on the expected survival after procedure and surgeon's preference. Subtotal parathyroidectomy is suitable for dialysis patients with kidney transplantation and younger patients, while total parathyroidectomy with autotransplantation is recommended for dialysis patients without kidney transplantation. Total parathyroidectomy without autotransplantation is recommended for enlarged parathyroid glands revealed at surgery or reoperation patient [21].

In the first case, we decided to perform right parathyroidectomy and right isthmulobectomy without intraoperative PTH examination due to limited facilities. The isthmulobectomy was chosen because the patient has secondary diagnosis which was nontoxic nodular enlargement of the thyroid gland. In addition, the technique was considered to be appropriate to access the parathyroid gland with the antecedent removal of the thyroid gland.

In the 4th and 7th month of follow-up, it is found that the PTH level was still high, 909.7 pg/mL and 1.137 pg/mL, respectively. 4D CT revealed single solid lesion in the left thyroid and 2 solid lesions in the aortopulmonary window, suggestive of parathyroid nodes. Therefore, 7 months after the first operation, we performed excision of superior part of the left parathyroid and left lobectomy with intraoperative PTH examination, and the result was 76.95 pg/mL. In the second case, we performed subtotal parathyroidectomy with intraoperative PTH examination, and the result was 10.37 pg/mL. In the 3rd month of follow-up, PTH level was 4.31 pg/mL. This patient underwent renal transplantation approximately 7 months after subtotal parathyroidectomy. PTH level one month after follow-up was 6 pg/mL.

Our delay in the PTH examination is due to the fact that this examination is not covered by the national health insurance. PTH examination is considerably expensive in Indonesia, which costs approximately 60 USD. Therefore, the PTH examination is not a routine test for this patient.

3. Conclusion

Brown tumor is one of the escalating problems due to secondary hyperparathyroidism because of ESRD. The clinical presentation of secondary hyperparathyroidism should be integrally assessed to reveal the possibility of developing brown tumor in the future, especially for patients who present with mass in the maxilla and mandible. A significant increase in the level of PTH and decreased bone density lead to the diagnosis of brown tumor. 4D CT and sestamibi are suggested to be the preferable examination to reveal the parathyroid abnormalities. Surgery and intraoperative assessment of PTH are the suggested treatment of choice.

Disclosure

This study was presented as a poster presentation at the "5th Congress of Asian Society of Head and Neck Oncology (ASHNO) 2017."

References

[1] T. B. Drüeke, "Hyperparathyroidism in chronic kidney disease," in *Endotext [Internet]*, L. J. Groot, G. Chrousos, and K. Dungan, Eds., MDText.com, Inc., South Dartmouth, MA, USA, 2000, https://www.ncbi.nlm.nih.gov/books/NBK278975/.

[2] M. Rodriguez, E. Nemeth, and D. Martin, "The calcium-sensing receptor: a key factor in the pathogenesis of secondary hyperparathyroidism," *American Journal of Physiology-Renal Physiology*, vol. 288, no. 2, pp. F253–F264, 2005.

[3] M. Koizumi, H. Komaba, and M. Fukagawa, "Parathyroid function in chronic kidney disease: role of FGF23-klotho axis," *Contributions to nephrology*, vol. 180, pp. 110–123, 2013.

[4] W. G. Goodman, "The consequences of uncontrolled secondary hyperparathyroidism and its treatment in chronic kidney disease," *Seminars in Dialysis*, vol. 17, no. 3, pp. 209–216, 2004.

[5] N. Soundarya, P. Sharada, N. Prakash, and G. Pradeep, "Bilateral maxillary brown tumors in a patient with primary hyperparathyroidism: report of a rare entity and review of literature," *Journal of Oral and Maxillofacial. Pathology*, vol. 15, no. 1, pp. 56–59, 2011.

[6] J. M. Jakubowski, I. Velez, and S. A. McClure, "Brown tumor as a result of hyperparathyroidism in an end-stage renal disease patient," *Case Reports in Radiology*, vol. 2011, Article ID 415476, 3 pages, 2011.

[7] S. M. H. A. Araújo, V. M. S. Bruin, A. S. Nunes et al., "Multiple brown tumors causing spinal cord compression in association with secondary hyperparathyroidism," *International Urology and Nephrology*, vol. 45, no. 3, pp. 913–916, 2013.

[8] Ö. Can, B. Boynueğri, A. M. Gökçe et al., "Brown tumors: a case report and review of the literature," *Case Reports in Nephrology and Dialysis*, vol. 6, no. 1, pp. 46–52, 2016.

[9] K. V. Arunkumar, S. Kumar, and D. Deepa, "Brown tumor in mandible as a first sign of vitamin D deficiency: a rare case

report and review," *Indian Journal of Endocrinology and Metabolism*, vol. 16, no. 2, pp. 310–315, 2012.

[10] S. C. Pitt, R. S. Sippel, and H. Chen, "Secondary and tertiary hyperparathyroidism, state of the art surgical management," *The Surgical clinics of North America*, vol. 89, no. 5, pp. 1227–1239, 2009.

[11] V. Lorenzoni, L. Trieste, and G. Turchetti, "The cost-effectiveness of drug therapies to treat secondary hyperparathyroidism in renal failure: a focus on evidence regarding paricalcitol and cinacalcet," *Expert review of pharmacoeconomics & outcomes research*, vol. 15, no. 4, pp. 611–624, 2015.

[12] K. Lorenz, D. K. Bartsch, J. J. Sancho, S. Guigard, and F. Triponez, "Surgical management of secondary hyperparathyroidism in chronic kidney disease—a consensus report of the European Society of Endocrine Surgeons," *Langenbeck's Archives of Surgery*, vol. 400, no. 8, pp. 907–927, 2015.

[13] G. A. Block, P. S. Klassen, J. M. Lazarus, N. Ofsthun, E. G. Lowrie, and G. M. Chertow, "Mineral metabolism, mortality, and morbidity in maintenance hemodialysis," *Journal of the American Society of Nephrology*, vol. 15, no. 8, pp. 2208–2218, 2004.

[14] Y. Tominaga, "Current status of parathyroidectomy for secondary hyperparathyroidism in Japan," *NDT Plus*, vol. 1, Supplement 3, pp. iii35–iii38, 2008.

[15] J. B. Lee, W. Y. Kim, and Y.-M. Lee, "The role of preoperative ultrasonography, computed tomography, and sestamibi scintigraphy localization in secondary hyperparathyroidism," *Annals of Surgical Treatment and Research*, vol. 89, no. 6, pp. 300–305, 2015.

[16] M. M. Mortenson, D. B. Evans, J. E. Lee et al., "Parathyroid exploration in the reoperative neck: improved preoperative localization with 4D-computed tomography," *Journal of the American College of Surgeons*, vol. 206, no. 5, pp. 888–895, 2008.

[17] N. A. Johnson, S. E. Carty, and M. E. Tublin, "Parathyroid imaging," *Radiologic Clinics of North America*, vol. 49, no. 3, pp. 489–509, 2011.

[18] L. F. Starker, A. Mahajan, P. Bjorklund, G. Sze, R. Udelsman, and T. Carling, "4D parathyroid CT as the initial localization study for patients with de novo primary hyperparathyroidism," *Annals of Surgical Oncology*, vol. 18, no. 6, pp. 1723–1728, 2011.

[19] K. Cheung, T. S. Wang, F. Farrokhyar, S. A. Roman, and J. A. Sosa, "A meta-analysis of preoperative localization techniques for patients with primary hyperparathyroidism," *Annals of Surgical Oncology*, vol. 19, no. 2, pp. 577–583, 2012.

[20] A. K. Lundstroem, W. Trolle, C. H. Soerensen, and P. S. Myschetzky, "Preoperative localization of hyperfunctioning parathyroid glands with 4D-CT," *European Archives of Oto-Rhino-Laryngology*, vol. 273, no. 5, pp. 1253–1259, 2016.

[21] Y. Tominaga, S. Matsuoka, and N. Uno, "Surgical and medical treatment of secondary hyperparathyroidism in patients on continuous dialysis," *World Journal of Surgery*, vol. 33, no. 11, pp. 2335–2342, 2009.

19

Refractory IgD Multiple Myeloma Treated with Daratumumab

Muhammad Husnain,[1] Sandra Kurtin,[2] Nikki Barkett,[2] Irbaz Bin Riaz,[1] and Amit Agarwal[1,2]

[1] *Department of Medicine, University of Arizona, Tucson, AZ, USA*
[2] *Banner University Medical Center Tucson, Department of Hematology Oncology, University of Arizona, Tucson, AZ, USA*

Correspondence should be addressed to Amit Agarwal; aagarwal@uacc.arizona.edu

Academic Editor: Josep M. Ribera

Patients with relapsed and refractory multiple myeloma have poor prognosis. A recent analysis of patients with relapsed and refractory multiple myeloma who were refractory to both proteasome inhibitors and immunomodulatory drugs showed the median overall survival of 9 months only. Daratumumab is the first-in-class human monoclonal antibody against CD38 cells which was studied in phase I/II trials for treatment of these patients with relapsed refractory multiple myeloma. It showed an overall response rate of 36% and a median overall survival (OS) of 17 months in these patients. We report a case of 40-year-old man with immunoglobulin D (IgD) multiple myeloma whose disease was refractory to at least 5 different chemotherapy regimens including proteasome inhibitors and immunomodulatory drugs. The clinical studies assessing daratumumab did not include any patients with IgD myeloma which is a rare form of multiple myeloma and to our knowledge is the first study reporting use of daratumumab in IgD myeloma.

1. Introduction

The conventional treatment options in relapsed multiple myeloma include hematopoietic cell transplantation (HCT) or trial of the previously tried chemotherapy regimens. Several new drugs such as Panobinostat (first-in-class histone deacetylase inhibitor), daratumumab (the first monoclonal antibody), ixazomib (the first oral proteasome inhibitor), and Elotuzumab (the first-in-class immunostimulatory agent) have been approved in the past year [1–4]. However, there is limited experience with the use of these novel drugs in the real life clinical setting and there are no published reports of real life experience with these drugs since their approval. Daratumumab has shown promising results in clinical trials in the setting of relapsed refractory multiple myeloma but most of the patients in clinical trials were IgG, IgA, or Bence Jones proteins multiple myeloma. There is little data regarding daratumumab role in the setting of IgD multiple myeloma. We present a case of Immunoglobulin D (IgD) multiple myeloma which was refractory to at least five different regimens and finally responded when treated with daratumumab.

2. Case Presentation

A 40-year-old man with a known diagnosis of Immunoglobulin D (IgD) lambda multiple myeloma presented with relapsed multiple myeloma (MM). He first presented in September 2007 with the chief complaint of cough and left sided abdominal pain. Physical examination was significant for splenomegaly. His labs were significant for pancytopenia. A bone marrow biopsy in September 2007 was significant for 100% cellularity and sheets of atypical cells positive for CD138 and lambda light chains consistent with multiple myeloma. Protein electrophoresis showed a monoclonal spike (M spike) and an elevated IgD level of 190 mg/L. A diagnosis of IgD multiple myeloma was made and he was initially started on dexamethasone and later in October 2007 thalidomide

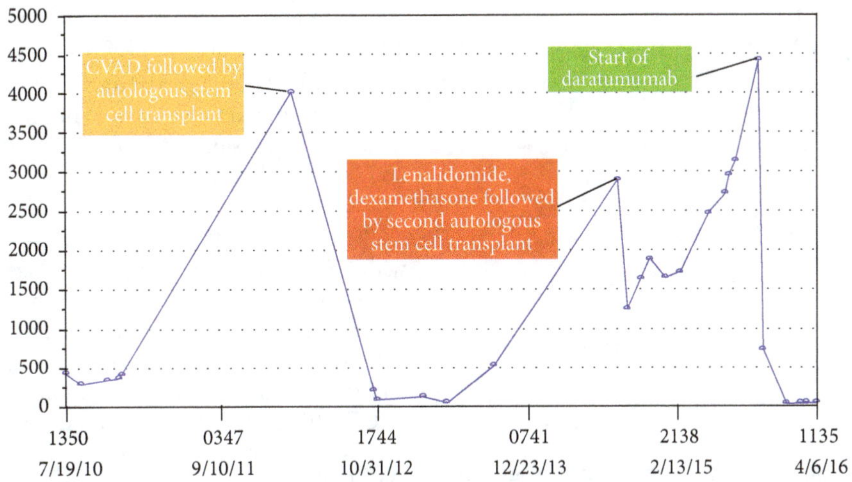

FIGURE 1: IgD levels over the course of 6 years of treatment.

was added to his regimen. Patient had intermittent lapses in his thalidomide treatment because of his insurance issues and his IgD level slowly kept rising. In July 2008 his IgD level was found to be 293 mg/L. A bone marrow biopsy performed in July 2008 was significant for 5% plasma cells by immunohistochemistry. He was continued on dexamethasone and thalidomide. A repeat bone marrow biopsy in July 2009 showed 40% plasma cells. At that point bortezomib was added to his regimen to reduce his tumor burden and he was referred for autologous peripheral blood stem cell transplantation (PBSCT). Patient only took 50 mg of thalidomide instead of usual 100 mg. His repeat bone marrow biopsy in February 2010 showed persistent multiple myeloma with 20% monoclonal plasma cells with overall cellularity of 60%. In March 2010 his IgD level increased up to 531 mg/L. At that point his thalidomide dose was increased to 200 mg daily. Patient was having issues with compliance. Eventually, he underwent autologous peripheral blood stem cell transplant (PBSCT) on January 2011 after 6 cycles of salvage CVAD (cyclophosphamide, vincristine, doxorubicin, and dexamethasone) chemotherapy. He was transplanted with stable disease with his pretransplant IgD level of 112 mg/L. He did not receive maintenance therapy and only 10 months after transplant there was evidence of myeloma progression with IgD level increasing to over 500 mg/L in October 2011. Patient at that point chose to pursue alternative therapies and was lost to follow-up. He presented again in April 2012 with severe lower back pain and an IgD level of 4020 mg/L. He was immediately started on pulse dose dexamethasone and lenalidomide was added in May 2012 (25 mg daily for 21 of 28 days). His IgD level decreased to 60 mg/L in November 2012 consistent with a very good partial response (VGPR) and he underwent a second autologous PBSCT in January 2013. His posttransplant course was complicated by some chemotherapy associated nausea, diarrhea, and neutropenic fever. He recovered well and was discharged home in stable condition. His day 100 bone marrow biopsy in April 2013 showed 20–40% plasma cells and an IgD level of 107 mg/L consistent with disease progression. Patient was restarted on lenalidomide 25 mg daily and had an initial response with a decrease in his IgD, which nadired at about 23.9 mg/L in June 2013 but his IgD quickly began to rise again.

Despite lenalidomide and dexamethasone, his IgD continued to rise to as high as 500 mg/L and at that point he was started on Pomalidomide in December 2013. He completed 2 cycles of Pomalidomide and dexamethasone but his disease continued to progress so he was switched to bortezomib, Pomalidomide, and dexamethasone in September 2014 for about 4-5 months and later carfilzomib, Pomalidomide, and dexamethasone for an additional 5 months from January 2015 to May 2015 without much improvement. He was started on bortezomib, Panobinostat, and dexamethasone in July 2015 but could not tolerate this regimen. He was deemed to be unsuitable for allogeneic stem cell transplant by his insurance. He was requiring PRBC transfusion twice a week to maintain his hemoglobin to >7. He was not a candidate for clinical trials because of his cytopenias. At that point we decided to treat him with daratumumab. His pretreatment IgD levels in December 2015 were 4000 mg/L and came down drastically to 5 mg/L in May 2016 after 5 cycles of daratumumab showing very good partial response (Figure 1). During his first infusion, he developed a grade 3 infusion reaction. His other side effects to medication were transient neutropenia and *E. coli* and *Giardia* diarrhea for which he was treated with antibiotics. His transfusion requirements which had been very high throughout his disease course requiring multiple transfusions with packed red blood cells (PRBCs) also came down dramatically with stable hemoglobin levels after the start of daratumumab (Figure 2). Patient continues on daratumumab, with his last IgD level at 12 mg/L in June 2016.

3. Discussion

Multiple myeloma is a plasma cell neoplasm with an incidence of 6.3 cases per 100,000 persons per year in United States [5, 6]. The treatment outcome and overall survival have significantly improved after the use of novel agents and autologous stem cell transplant for multiple myeloma [1]. However,

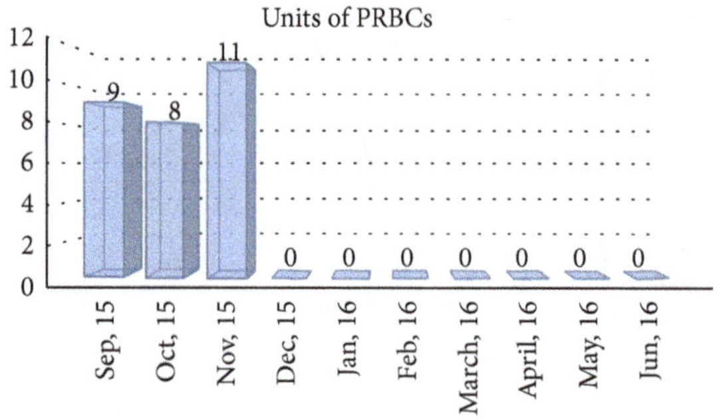

Figure 2: Transfusion requirements prior to starting daratumumab and after daratumumab.

for patients who are refractory to these agents, the prognosis remains poor with overall survival (OS) of 9 months only [7]. This clearly demonstrates the need for additional agents with novel mechanisms of actions. In the past decade, many new potential therapeutic targets have been identified, including histone deacetylation, proteasome activity, mammalian target of rapamycin, and targetable surface receptors such as SLAMF-7, CD38, and CD40 [1, 2, 8]. Monoclonal antibodies in particular present a new exciting approach. Two new monoclonal antibodies daratumumab (anti-CD38) and Elotuzumab (anti-SLAMF-7) have been approved by FDA for relapsed refractory multiple myeloma [9].

CD38 is a transmembrane glycoprotein that is highly expressed on multiple myeloma cells and at low levels on normal lymphoid and myeloid cells [10, 11]. It functions as an ectoenzyme involved in regulating intracytoplasmic concentration of calcium and the catabolism of extracellular nucleotides. Daratumumab, an IgG1-k fully human anti-CD38 monoclonal antibody, exerts its cytotoxic effect through a number of mechanisms after binding to CD38, including antibody-dependent cell-mediated cytotoxicity (ADCC), complement-dependent cytotoxicity (CDC), antibody-dependent cell-mediated phagocytosis (ADCP), and the direct induction of apoptosis [12, 13]. Moreover, an immunomodulatory effect of daratumumab was also recently described [14]. The safety of daratumumab was investigated in a dose-escalation phase I/II trial of 104 patients with relapsed or refractory multiple myeloma. The most common adverse events were grade 3 or 4 pneumonia and thrombocytopenia. The overall response rate was 36% in the cohort that received 16 mg per kilogram and 10% in the cohort that received 8 mg per kilogram. In the cohort that received 16 mg per kilogram, the median progression-free survival was 5.6 months [11]. In another open label phase II trial (SIRIUS) 106 patients with multiple myeloma who had failed at least three lines of treatment including a proteasome inhibitor and immunomodulatory drugs were treated with daratumumab [15]. Two dose levels 8 mg/kg and 16 mg/kg were evaluated. Daratumumab was well tolerated and there were no discontinuations due to drug-related treatment emergent adverse effects. Infusion reactions were seen in 45 (42%) patients but these were mostly grades 1 and 2 with five patients reporting grade 3 and none with grade 4 infusion reaction. Other side effects included fatigue (40%) and anemia (33%). Patients treated with daratumumab showed 29% overall response with a median time to first response of one month. The estimated median progression-free and overall survival rates were 3.7 and 17.5 months, respectively [15].

Two phase III trials [16] are evaluating patients with relapsed or refractory disease; one is comparing daratumumab plus bortezomib and dexamethasone with bortezomib and dexamethasone (NCT02136134) [16], and the other is comparing daratumumab plus lenalidomide and dexamethasone with lenalidomide and dexamethasone (NCT02076009) [16]. The final results of these studies are awaited but the CASTOR trial (Velcade/dex versus Dara/Velcade/dex) was stopped early because at an interim analysis the study met its end point with a very impressive hazard ratio of 0.39 favoring the daratumumab arm. The POLLUX study (Rev/dex versus Dara/Rev/dex) has also shown similarly impressive results with a hazard ratio of 0.37 favoring the Dara arm. Two additional phase III studies are being performed in patients with previously untreated multiple myeloma; one is comparing daratumumab plus bortezomib, melphalan, and prednisone with bortezomib, melphalan, and prednisone (NCT02195479), and the other is evaluating daratumumab plus lenalidomide and dexamethasone with lenalidomide and dexamethasone (NCT02252172) [17].

4. Conclusions

Despite significant progress in the treatment of multiple myeloma, the disease remains incurable in a vast majority of patients. The approval of promising new agents will undoubtedly improve outcomes for myeloma patients. Daratumumab is a monoclonal antibody that is now approved for treatment of multiple myeloma patients and has shown significant response in the real world setting. Our case illustrates the potential of a dramatic response using monoclonal antibodies in patients that are heavily pretreated and having a very meaningful impact towards their outcome.

References

[1] S. Ito, "Novel agents in multiple myeloma treatment," *Rinsho Ketsueki*, vol. 56, no. 10, pp. 2066–2073, 2015.

[2] J. El-Amm and I. A. Tabbara, "Emerging therapies in multiple myeloma," *American Journal of Clinical Oncology*, vol. 38, no. 3, pp. 315–321, 2015.

[3] S. Afifi, A. Michael, and A. Lesokhin, "Immunotherapy: a new approach to treating multiple myeloma with daratumumab and elotuzumab," *Annals of Pharmacotherapy*, vol. 50, no. 7, pp. 555–568, 2016.

[4] A. Poh, "Multiple myeloma gets three new drugs," *Cancer Discovery*, vol. 6, no. 1, p. 4, 2016.

[5] A. Smith, D. Howell, R. Patmore, A. Jack, and E. Roman, "Incidence of haematological malignancy by sub-type: a report from the Haematological Malignancy Research Network," *British Journal of Cancer*, vol. 105, no. 11, pp. 1684–1692, 2011.

[6] R. L. Siegel, K. D. Miller, and A. Jemal, "Cancer statistics, 2016," *CA: A Cancer Journal for Clinicians*, vol. 66, no. 1, pp. 7–30, 2016.

[7] "Daratumumab improves overall survival in multiple myeloma," *American Health & Drug Benefits*, vol. 9, article 14, 2016.

[8] E. M. Ocio, P. G. Richardson, S. V. Rajkumar et al., "New drugs and novel mechanisms of action in multiple myeloma in 2013: a report from the International Myeloma Working Group (IMWG)," *Leukemia*, vol. 28, no. 3, pp. 525–542, 2014.

[9] J. Kuroda, H. Nagoshi, Y. Shimura, and M. Taniwaki, "Elotuzumab and daratumumab: emerging new monoclonal antibodies for multiple myeloma," *Expert Review of Anticancer Therapy*, vol. 13, no. 9, pp. 1081–1088, 2013.

[10] J. P. Laubach and P. G. Richardson, "CD38-targeted immunochemotherapy in refractory multiple myeloma: a new horizon," *Clinical Cancer Research*, vol. 21, no. 12, pp. 2660–2662, 2015.

[11] H. M. Lokhorst, T. Plesner, J. P. Laubach et al., "Targeting CD38 with daratumumab monotherapy in multiple myeloma," *The New England Journal of Medicine*, vol. 373, no. 13, pp. 1207–1219, 2015.

[12] M. S. Van Der Veer, M. De Weers, B. Van Kessel et al., "The therapeutic human CD38 antibody daratumumab improves the anti-myeloma effect of newly emerging multi-drug therapies," *Blood Cancer Journal*, vol. 1, no. 10, article e41, 2011.

[13] M. B. Overdijk, S. Verploegen, M. Bögels et al., "Antibody-mediated phagocytosis contributes to the anti-tumor activity of the therapeutic antibody daratumumab in lymphoma and multiple myeloma," *mAbs*, vol. 7, no. 2, pp. 311–321, 2015.

[14] Y. Khagi and T. M. Mark, "Potential role of daratumumab in the treatment of multiple myeloma," *OncoTargets and Therapy*, vol. 7, pp. 1095–1100, 2014.

[15] S. Lonial, B. M. Weiss, S. Z. Usmani et al., "Daratumumab monotherapy in patients with treatment-refractory multiple myeloma (SIRIUS): an open-label, randomised, phase 2 trial," *The Lancet*, vol. 387, no. 10027, pp. 1551–1560, 2016.

[16] A. Palumbo, M. A. Dimopoulos, D. E. Reece et al., "Twin randomized studies of daratumumab (DARA; D) plus standard of care (lenalidomide/dexamethasone or bortezomib/dexamethasone [DRd or DVd]) versus Rd or Vd alone in relapsed or refractory multiple myeloma (MM): 54767414MMY3003 (Pollux) and 54767414MMY3004 (Castor)," in *Proceedings of the 2015 ASCO Annual Meeting*, 2015.

[17] M.-V. Mateos, M. Cavo, A. J. Jakubowiak et al., "A randomized open-label study of bortezomib, melphalan, and prednisone (VMP) versus daratumumab (DARA) plus VMP in patients with previously untreated multiple myeloma (MM) who are ineligible for high-dose therapy: 54767414MMY3007 (Alcyone)," *Journal of Clinical Oncology*, vol. 33, supplement, abstract TPS8608, 2015, Proceedings of the ASCO Annual Meeting.

20

A Hormonally Active Malignant Struma Ovarii

**Carolina Lara,[1] Dalia Cuenca,[1] Latife Salame,[2]
Rafael Padilla-Longoria,[3] and Moisés Mercado[1,2]**

[1]*Department of Medicine, ABC Medical Center, Mexico City 01120, Mexico*
[2]*Neurological Center, ABC Medical Center, Mexico City 01120, Mexico*
[3]*Department of Surgical Oncology, Hospital Angeles de Interlomas, Huixquilucan 52763, Mexico*

Correspondence should be addressed to Moisés Mercado; mmercadoa@yahoo.com

Academic Editor: Annekathryn Goodman

Struma ovarii is a rare monodermal variant of ovarian teratoma that contains at least 50% thyroid tissue. Less than 8% of struma ovarii cases present with clinical and biochemical evidence of thyrotoxicosis due to ectopic production of thyroid hormone and only 5% undergo malignant transformation into a papillary thyroid carcinoma. Only isolated cases of hormonally active papillary thyroid carcinoma developing within a struma ovarii have been reported in the literature. We report the case of a 36-year-old woman who presented with clinical signs and symptoms of hyperthyroidism as well as a left adnexal mass, which proved to be a thyroid hormone-producing, malignant struma ovarii.

1. Introduction

Germ cell tumors represent 15–20% of all ovarian cancers and most of them are mature cystic teratomas [1]. Struma ovarii (SO) is a monodermal variant of ovarian teratoma that contains at least 50% of thyroid tissue [1]. Initially described by Buttlin in 1888, SO was first recognized to consist of thyroid tissue in 1902 by Pick [2]. In approximately 5% of cases, the thyroid tissue within SO is found to contain areas of well-differentiated carcinoma, most commonly, papillary thyroid carcinoma (PTC) [3, 4]. SO generally occurs in women in the fifth and sixth decades of life, presenting in the majority of cases, as a unilateral adnexal mass, with clear left side predominance [3–5]. Over 92% of the patients are clinically and biochemically euthyroid [5–7]. Thus, the occurrence of hyperfunctioning thyroid tissue within SO is a very rare event and is usually listed in the differential diagnosis of thyrotoxicosis in the setting of a low radioiodine uptake [5–7]. We here in present the case of a woman with a pelvic mass that proved to be a PTC containing, hormonally active SO.

2. Case Report

A previously healthy, 36-year-old woman was admitted to the hospital because of left lower abdominal pain and nausea of 5 days' duration. Pain was referred to as intense, colicky, and located over the left iliac fossa and radiating to her left groin and lower back. She denied fever, chills, genitourinary symptoms, or any changes in her bowel habits but mentioned palpitations, heat intolerance, a 7-Kg unintentional weight loss, insomnia, and tremor over the preceding 6 months. On physical exam, her blood pressure was 105/60 mmHg, heart rate 110 bpm and regular, respiratory rate 20, and temperature 36.5°C. She appeared notoriously anxious but in no acute distress. Cardiopulmonary exam revealed a hyperdynamic precordium. Neck was supple; the thyroid gland was not readily palpable. The abdomen was soft, with no palpable organomegalies; she had pain over the left iliac fossa upon deep palpation with no rebound tenderness and the peristalsis was normal. She has had two previous uneventful pregnancies, the latest one three years prior to admission; her menstrual cycles were regular and she did not use any contraceptive method. She had no allergies, did not use any medications, and regularly abused alcohol on weekends (usually a pint of tequila). Her family history was remarkable for primary hypothyroidism in her maternal grandmother.

Initial laboratory workup showed a normal CBC as well as basic blood chemistry, liver function tests, serum electrolytes, and urinalysis. Thyroid function tests revealed

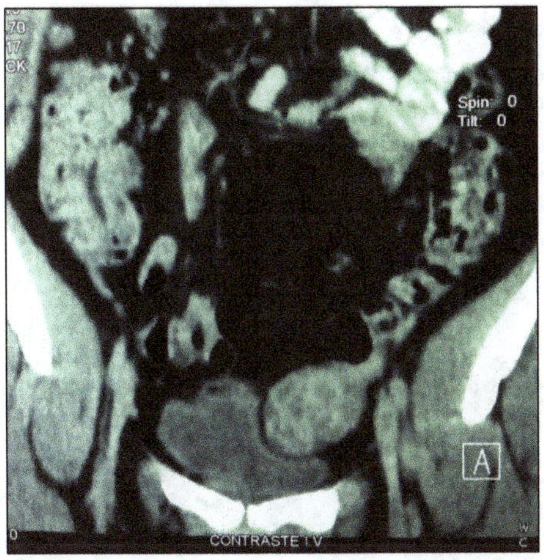

FIGURE 1: Contrast-enhanced abdominal CT revealing tumour on left ovary.

a TSH of <0.01 mIU/mL and a free T4 of 2.6 ng/dL. A solid, left adnexal mass was found on abdominal-pelvic ultrasound and was confirmed by CT scan (Figure 1). A ^{99m}Tc thyroid scan showed a complete absence of uptake. Thyroid ultrasonography was unrevealing.

Upon surgical exploration she was found to have a solid 50 × 40 × 30 mm left ovarian mass and a left salpingo-oophorectomy with omentectomy was performed. On histopathological examination the mass consisted of normal thyroid tissue with several areas of papillary carcinoma with multifocal capsular invasion but without perineural or vascular extension (Figure 2). Immunohistochemistry was strongly positive for both thyroid transcription factor-1 (TTF-1) and thyroglobulin (Figure 3).

In view of these findings, it was decided to proceed with a total thyroidectomy. On histopathological examination the thyroid gland appeared completely normal. Four weeks later she received a 75 mCi, ablative radioactive iodine dose. Thyroid bed uptake was documented upon a posttherapeutic total body scan, with no abnormal radioiodine accumulation anywhere else.

The patient is currently asymptomatic on thyroid suppression therapy; her latest recombinant TSH-stimulated thyroglobulin was undetectable one year after initial presentation.

3. Discussion

The most common clinical presentation of SO is that of a pelvic mass, which can either be incidentally found on pelvic ultrasound or manifest as lower abdominal pain [3–5]. Less than 8% of the patients with SO present with hyperthyroidism and when they do, it is usually mild and subclinical [5–7]. Our patient presented with lower abdominal pain and clinical signs and symptoms, as well as biochemical evidence of thyrotoxicosis. In fact, a hormonally active SO should be considered in the differential diagnosis of thyrotoxicosis in the setting of a low or absent radioiodine or tecnetium thyroid uptake [5–7]. The pathogenesis of thyrotoxicosis in patients with SO is incompletely understood. There have been several case reports of patients with preexisting or concomitant Graves' disease in whom anti-TSH receptor autoantibodies stimulate thyroid hormone production in both the eutopic and ectopic thyroid tissues; in these cases the diagnosis of SO has been made only after an apparently successful thyroid ablation fails to normalize thyroid hormone levels [8, 9]. Unfortunately thyroid autoantibodies were not available in our patient, although she did not have any features suggestive of autoimmune thyroid disease such as Graves' ophthalmopathy. Somatic, activating mutations of the TSH receptor explain the hyperthyroidism in the majority of autonomous thyroid nodules and such mutations have been sought but not found in patients with thyrotoxicosis associated with SO [7]. Thus, it appears that in most patients with hyperthyroidism due to SO the autonomous production of thyroid hormone by the ectopic tissue is not related to the presence of TSH receptor antibodies or to gain-of-function mutations of the TSH receptor but to mechanisms more closely resembling those involved in Plummer's disease or toxic multinodular goiter.

The emergence of a well-differentiated carcinoma arising in these ectopically located thyroid tissues is an infrequent event, occurring in about 5% of all SO cases [3, 10, 11]. Although all the variants of well-differentiated thyroid cancer have been reported, in over 70% of the cases the histopathology is that of a typical papillary thyroid carcinoma [3, 10–12]. Immunohistochemically these tumors stain positive for both thyroglobulin and TTF-1 [10]. The possibility of a primary papillary thyroid carcinoma with ovarian metastases needs to be ruled out, which is achieved by demonstrating the absence of thyroid lesions by means of high-resolution ultrasonography, CT, or even MRI. Multiple molecular abnormalities have been described in thyroid cancers arising from ovarian teratomas, including point mutations in *BRAF* (V600E and K601E) 67% of cases [13] and *KRAS* and *NRAS* [13] as well as loss of heterozigocity in the PTEN region and *ret/PTC* rearrangements [12, 13].

There are no consensus guidelines for the management of malignant SO. In patients who wish to preserve fertility and provided the disease burden is confined to the ovary the recommended approach consists of unilateral salpingo-oophorectomy, along with near-total thyroidectomy and radioactive iodine ablation [10, 14]. When fertility is not an issue and/or in cases with more invasive tumors, a total abdominal hysterectomy with bilateral salpingo-oophorectomy is the usual course of action; adjunctive systemic chemotherapy has been used in patients with distant metastasis. As was done in our case, some authors recommend thyroidectomy and ^{131}I ablation as the first-line of treatment in order to be able to use the measurement of thyroglobulin as a tumor marker [3, 15, 16].

4. Conclusion

Struma ovarii is a monodermal variant of ovarian teratoma, defined by the presence of >50% thyroid tissue that generally occurs in women between the ages of 40 and 60 and usually presents as a unilateral adnexal mass. The occurrence of hyperfunctioning thyroid tissue within struma ovarii is a very rare event. When fertility is not a concern and in patients with

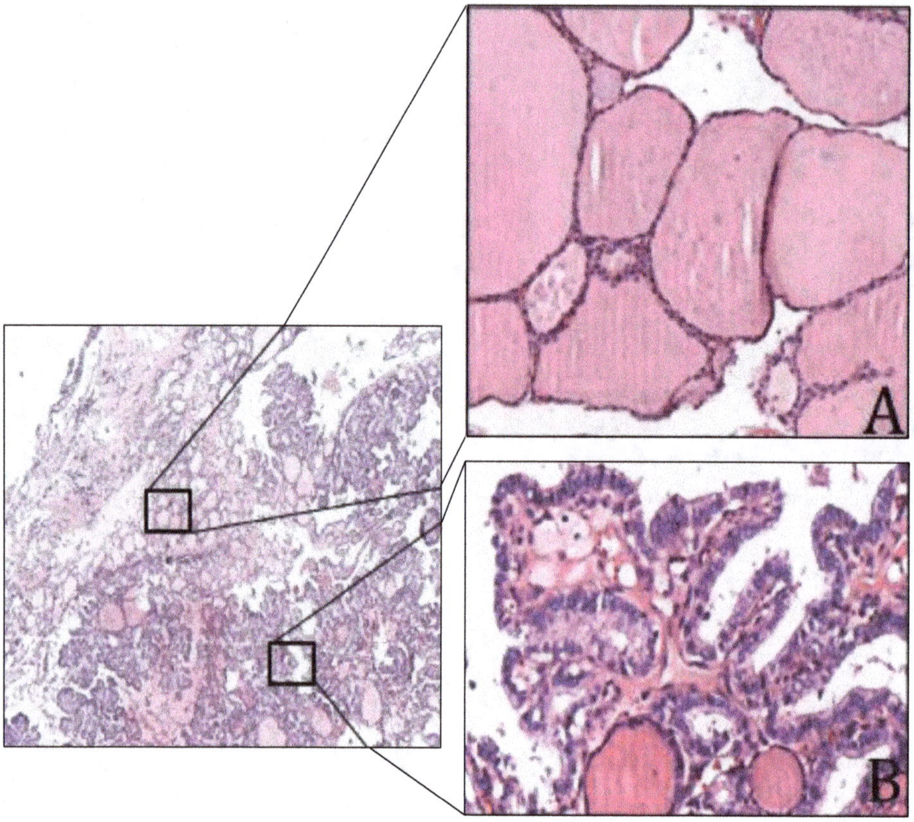

FIGURE 2: Malignant struma ovarii with classic variant papillary thyroid cancer. On (A) normal thyroid tissue and (B) areas with papillary thyroid cancer.

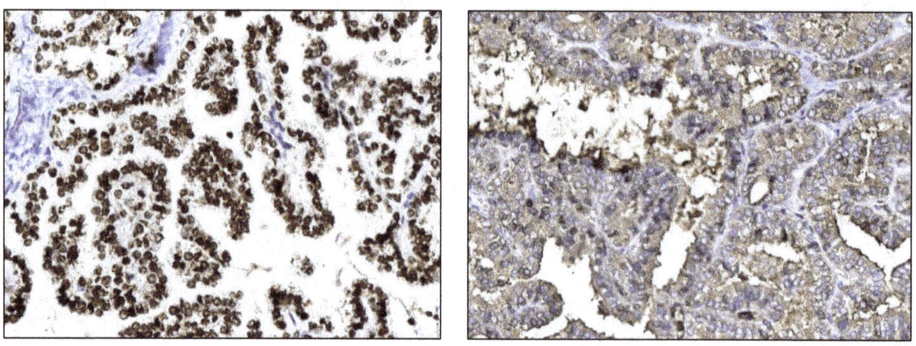

(a) (b)

FIGURE 3: Positive immunohistochemical stain for TTF-1 (a) and thyroglobulin (b).

invasive tumors, treatment consists of total abdominal hysterectomy with bilateral salpingo-oophorectomy; adjuvant chemotherapy is recommended when distant metastasis is present. In patients who wish to preserve fertility and provided the tumor is confined to one ovary, the recommended treatment is unilateral salpingo-oophprectomy, along with total thyroidectomy and radioactive iodine ablation.

Competing Interests

The authors have no conflict of interests to declare.

References

[1] L. M. Roth and A. Talerman, "The enigma of struma ovarii," *Pathology*, vol. 39, no. 1, pp. 139–146, 2007.

[2] L. Pick, "Beitrag zur Lehre von den Greschwülsten über struma thyroidaea ovarii aberrata," *Verhandlungen der Berliner Medizinischen Geselschaft*, vol. 33, pp. 139–146, 1903.

[3] L. Yassa, P. Sadow, and E. Marqusee, "Malignant struma ovarii," *Nature Clinical Practice Endocrinology and Metabolism*, vol. 4, no. 8, pp. 469–472, 2008.

[4] P. Goffredo, A. M. Sawka, J. Pura, M. A. Adam, S. A. Roman, and J. A. Sosa, "Malignant struma ovarii: a population-level analysis

of a large series of 68 patients," *Thyroid*, vol. 25, no. 2, pp. 211–215, 2015.

[5] S. C. Yoo, K. H. Chang, M. O. Lyu, S. J. Chang, H. S. Ryu, and H. S. Kim, "Clinical characteristics of struma ovarii," *Journal of Gynecologic Oncology*, vol. 19, no. 2, pp. 135–138, 2008.

[6] K. Matsuda, T. Maehama, and K. Kanazawa, "Malignant struma ovarii with thyrotoxicosis," *Gynecologic Oncology*, vol. 82, no. 3, pp. 575–577, 2001.

[7] A. Ciccarelli, H. Valdes-Socin, J. Parma et al., "Thyrotoxic adenoma followed by atypical hyperthyroidism due to struma ovarii: clinical and genetic studies," *European Journal of Endocrinology*, vol. 150, no. 4, pp. 431–437, 2004.

[8] Y. Mimura, M. Kishida, H. Masuyama et al., "Coexistence of Graves' disease and struma ovarii: case report and literature review," *Endocrine Journal*, vol. 48, no. 2, pp. 255–260, 2001.

[9] T. Sitasuwan, S. Hanamornroongruang, T. Peerapatdit, and N. Thongtang, "Coexistence of Graves' disease and unilateral functioning struma ovarii: a case report," *BMC Endocrine Disorders*, vol. 15, no. 1, article 68, 2015.

[10] X. Zhang and C. Axiotis, "Thyroid-type carcinoma of struma ovarii," *Archives of Pathology and Laboratory Medicine*, vol. 134, no. 5, pp. 786–791, 2010.

[11] L. M. Roth, A. W. Miller III, and A. Talerman, "Typical thyroid-type carcinoma arising in struma ovarii: a report of 4 cases and review of the literature," *International Journal of Gynecological Pathology*, vol. 27, no. 4, pp. 496–506, 2008.

[12] O. Boutross-Tadross, R. Saleh, and S. L. Asa, "Follicular variant papillary thyroid carcinoma arising in struma ovarii," *Endocrine Pathology*, vol. 18, no. 3, pp. 182–186, 2007.

[13] J. Schmidt, V. Derr, M. C. Heinrich et al., "BRAF in papillary thyroid carcinoma of ovary (struma ovarii)," *The American Journal of Surgical Pathology*, vol. 31, no. 9, pp. 1337–1343, 2007.

[14] S. Jean, J. L. Tanyi, K. Montone, C. McGrath, M. M. Lage-Alvarez, and C. S. Chu, "Papillary thyroid cancer arising in struma ovarii," *Journal of Obstetrics and Gynaecology*, vol. 32, no. 3, pp. 222–226, 2012.

[15] C. P. DeSimone, S. M. Lele, and S. C. Modesitt, "Malignant struma ovarii: a case report and analysis of cases reported in the literature with focus on survival and I131 therapy," *Gynecologic Oncology*, vol. 89, no. 3, pp. 543–548, 2003.

[16] F. Pacini, M. Schlumberger, C. Harmer et al., "Post-surgical use of radioiodine (^{131}I) in patients with papillary and follicular thyroid cancer and the issue of remnant ablation: a consensus report," *European Journal of Endocrinology*, vol. 153, no. 5, pp. 651–659, 2005.

21

Pneumocephalus after the Treatment of an Inoperable Superior Sulcus Tumor with Chemoradiation

Ashley Albert,[1] Robert Allbright,[1] Todd Nichols,[2] Edward Farley,[2] and Srinivasan Vijayakumar[1]

[1]*Department of Radiation Oncology, University of Mississippi Medical Center, Jackson, MS, USA*
[2]*Department of Radiology, University of Mississippi Medical Center, Jackson, MS, USA*

Correspondence should be addressed to Ashley Albert; aalbert@umc.edu

Academic Editor: Didier Frappaz

Background. Pneumocephalus is a rare phenomenon that can occur as a complication after operations involving the thoracic discs, following thoracotomy for tumor resection, and after an intracranial operation or cranial trauma. This complication frequently occurs when a tumor is located in the costovertebral angle and an operative intervention creates a tear in the dura resulting in a pleural-dural fistula. *Case Presentation.* We describe the case of a 58-year-old man with an inoperable superior sulcus tumor who developed pneumocephalus after the initiation of chemoradiation secondary to a pleural-dural fistula. *Conclusions.* Although a rare occurrence, pneumocephalus should be considered when patients with tumors in the superior sulcus treated with radiation develop neurologic symptoms characteristic of increased intracranial pressure.

1. Background

Pneumocephalus is an uncommon phenomenon, and most cases occur after resection of lung tumors as a result of the formation of an iatrogenic subarachnoid pleural fistula (ISPF). This type of fistula occurs when there is a disruption of both the dura and the parietal pleura which allows intradural air to accumulate [1]. Symptoms of pneumocephalus include headaches, altered mental status, focal deficits, seizures, and stroke. A characteristic finding of pneumocephalus is a subjective "splashing" sound induced by a rapid change in head position which is referred to as *bruit hydro aerique* [2].

The spinal nerves are formed by the dorsal and ventral roots, and these roots exit the dura through separate fenestrations [1]. Dural defects affecting these nerve roots can occur during a thoracotomy in which there is traction on a tumor adherent to the nerve and the nerve root is sacrificed intentionally or due to forceful rib retraction. Such disruptions can lead to the formation of an ISPF. During the respiratory cycle, inspiration results in negative intrathoracic pressure, and CSF is drawn into the pleural space. With expiration, positive intrathoracic pressure drives air in the subarachnoid space resulting in pneumocephalus. The combination of these pressure changes, and a valve-like mechanism can lead to a tension pneumocephalus which can be life threatening [3]. Pneumocephalus as a sequela of an ISPF usually leads to air with the ventricles and basilar cisterns, whereas head trauma or craniotomy may result in air located over the cerebral convexities [4].

Approximately half of the reported cases of pneumocephalus as a result of a pleural-dural fistula after a thoracotomy received neoadjuvant radiotherapy [5]. Pneumocephalus after radiation alone is rare and has been described in cases of definitive radiation for treatment of nasopharyngeal carcinoma. The authors of one such case report proposed that radiation resulted in the destruction of a tumor invading the base of the skull that then created a defect through which air entered the intracranial cavity resulting in pneumocephalus [6].

2. Case Presentation

A 58-year-old man initially presented with a 3-month history of cough, hemoptysis, right-sided chest and back

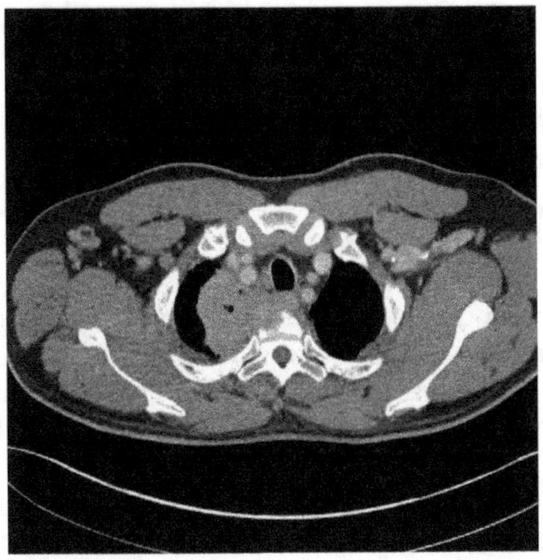

FIGURE 1: Computed tomography scan of the chest showing right superior sulcus mass invading a vertebral body.

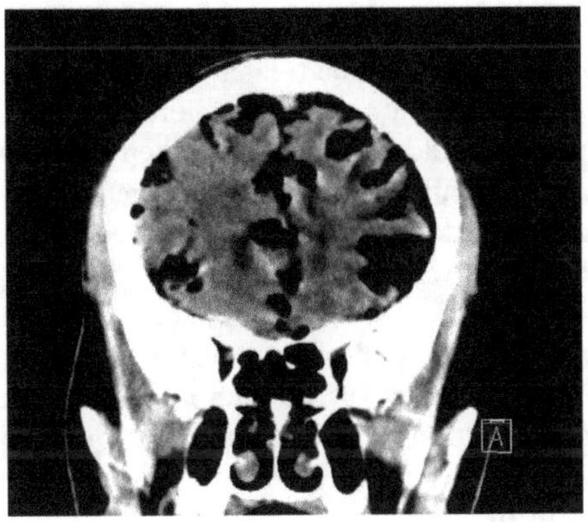

FIGURE 2: CT head with extensive pneumocephalus within the sulci and cisterns.

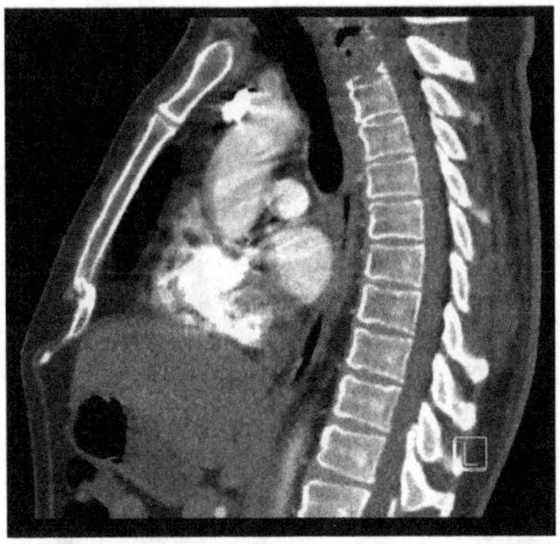

FIGURE 3: CT spine demonstrating local invasion of the tumor and air within the vertebral bodies.

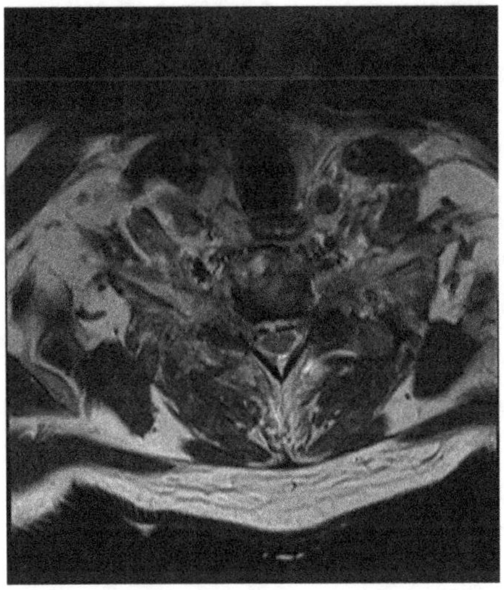

FIGURE 4: MRI thoracic spine showing local invasion of tumor.

pain, and progressive right-sided arm numbness and right-sided face weakness. A computed tomography (CT) scan revealed a large lung mass in the right superior sulcus with invasion of the C7 through T2 vertebral bodies, encasement of the right subclavian artery, compression of the right brachiocephalic vein, and possible invasion of the upper esophagus (Figure 1). Enlarged mediastinal, right hilar, and right supraclavicular lymph nodes concerning metastatic lymphadenopathy were also present. Magnetic resonance imaging (MRI) of the brain was negative for metastases. Bronchoscopy with a transbronchial biopsy was performed, and pathology was consistent with squamous cell carcinoma. The tumor was deemed inoperable due to extensive local invasion and lymph node involvement. Concurrent chemoradiation with carboplatin and Taxol was initiated. Given the concern for possible spinal cord compression, conformal radiation therapy was started emergently using AP/PA technique planned to a dose of 40 gray (Gy).

After 32 Gy and 2 cycles of carboplatin and paclitaxel, the patient reported a severe headache that had been present for two days. CT scan of the head demonstrated interval development of extensive pneumocephalus tracking along the sulci and within the cisterns with mass effect on the frontal lobes (Figure 2). Foci of gas were also noted within the lower spinal canal. CT and MRI of the spine demonstrated air within the T1 vertebral body extending into the right facet of T1 and T2 (Figures 3 and 4). There was also a minimal amount of air in the central canal at the C5 and C6 vertebral bodies.

He was admitted due to these findings and followed by neurosurgery. Radiation and chemotherapy were discontinued. He was kept in a recumbent position while admitted and treated empirically for meningitis. Serial CT imaging showed resolving pneumocephalus over the course of five days. The patient's headache resolved and he did not require any other interventions. He was subsequently discharged. He was then readmitted on two more occasions for treatment of bacteremia. Completion of treatment was subsequently delayed due to additional hospital admissions. He then received one additional cycle of carboplatin and Taxol as an outpatient. Prior to being able to restart radiation, the patient was admitted again for uncontrolled pain in his shoulders and arms. MRI brain at this point showed complete resolution of the pneumocephalus. During the course of his admission, he was transferred to the medical

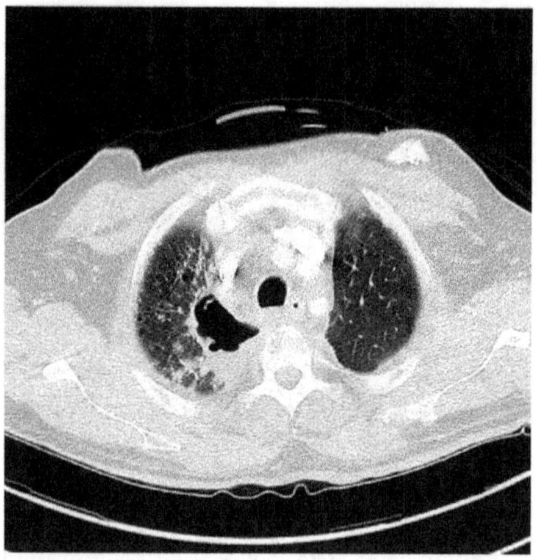

Figure 5: CT chest showing air-fluid levels within chest after initiation of chemoradiation.

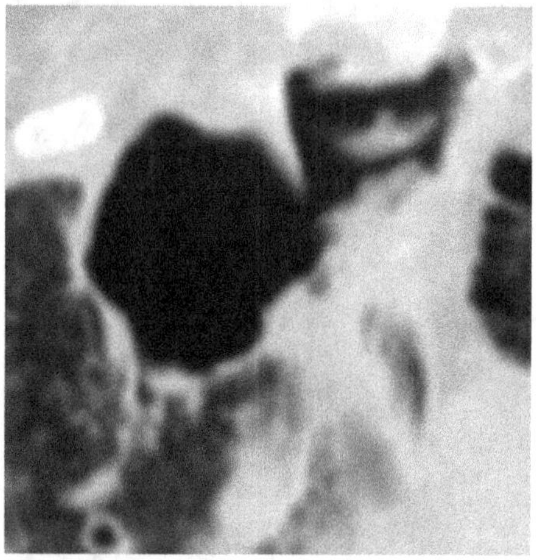

Figure 6: CT chest demonstrating contiguity of mass with bronchus.

intensive care unit due to the development of sepsis which was attributed to his immunosuppressed status secondary to chemotherapy. He also began experiencing respiratory distress. Findings on chest X-rays at that time were consistent with acute respiratory distress syndrome (ARDS) which was felt to be caused by his sepsis. No pleural effusions were noted on imaging. The patient's respiratory status continued to deteriorate despite treatment of his sepsis with antibiotics. His family declined intubation, and the patient was transferred to hospice with comfort care and expired shortly thereafter.

In this case, the tumor invaded the C7 through T2 vertebral bodies at diagnosis. After the initiation of treatment, air was found to be present within the T1 vertebral body and extended into the right facet of T1 and T2. Additionally, air was noted in the central canal at C5-C6. Air-fluid levels within the tumor cavity were also present, indicating rapid necrosis of the mass (Figure 5). Furthermore, the air-fluid levels within the mass were contiguous with a bronchus providing an entry for air (Figure 6). Although involvement of the bronchus in a pleural-dural fistula is not described in the literature as a necessary component for the development of pneumocephalus, we believe it was a contributing factor in this patient.

3. Conclusions

To our knowledge, this is the first case of pneumocephalus secondary to a pleural-dural fistula described in a patient with a superior sulcus tumor who did not undergo a thoracotomy or any other operative intervention. Radiation and concurrent chemotherapy likely resulted in cell killing and necrosis and therefore may have contributed to the disruptions in the dura near the vertebral bodies in the same way that the dura could be violated in an operation. We therefore propose that the destruction of tumor cells during treatment led to the formation of a bronchopleural-dural fistula involving the lung mass, a bronchus, vertebral bodies, and central canal.

Pneumocephalus can be treated conservatively with bed rest, low head position, and antibiotic prophylaxis, and surgical repair should be considered when pneumocephalus does not resolve with conservative management [3]. Repairs have been reported using placement of a free muscle flap, fat, and omentum as well as with synthetic plugs and surgical adhesive [1, 5]. Repeat imaging of the brain of the patient in this case showed resolution of the pneumocephalus, and operative intervention was therefore deemed unnecessary. Furthermore, as in this case, patients with pneumocephalus should be treated empirically with antibiotics to prevent the development of meningitis.

In conclusion, although a potentially rare complication, pneumocephalus should be considered when patients with tumors in the superior sulcus treated with radiation then develop neurologic symptoms. Due to the devastating sequelae of pneumocephalus secondary to intracranial hypertension including seizure and stroke, prompt identification is crucial and radiation and chemotherapy should be discontinued. Operative intervention for the treatment of pneumocephalus may not be necessary in all instances if pneumocephalus resolves with conservative treatment. Supportive care, monitoring for resolution of the fistula, and antibiotics for empiric treatment of meningitis are all necessary components of care.

Abbreviations

ISPF: iatrogenic subarachnoid pleural fistula
CT: computed tomography
MRI: magnetic resonance imaging.

Authors' Contributions

Ashley Albert made substantial contributions to conception and design, acquisition of data, and analysis and interpretation of data. Robert Allbright was involved in drafting the manuscript and revising it critically for important intellectual content.

Todd Nichols made substantial contributions to analysis and interpretation of data. Edward Farley made substantial contributions to analysis and interpretation of data. Srinivasan Vijayakumar has given final approval of the version to be published.

References

[1] M. F. Shamji, S. Sundaresan, V. Da silva, J. Seely, and F. M. Shamji, "Subarachnoid-pleural fistula: applied anatomy of the thoracic spinal nerve root," *ISRN Surgery*, vol. 2011, Article ID 168959, 8 pages, 2011.

[2] W. M. Brown and P. N. Symbas, "Pneumocephalus complicating routine thoracotomy: symptoms, diagnosis and management," *Annals of Thoracic Surgery*, vol. 59, no. 1, pp. 234–236, 1995.

[3] M. Ladehoff, D. Zachow, C. Koch et al., "Cerebellar haemorrhage and tension pneumocephalus after resection of a Pancoast tumour," *Acta Neurochirurgica*, vol. 147, no. 5, pp. 561–564, 2005.

[4] M. H. Bilsky, R. J. Downey, M. G. Kaplitt, E. H. Elowitz, and V. W. Rusch, "Tension pneumocephalus resulting from iatrogenic subarachnoid-pleural fistulae: report of three cases," *Annals of Thoracic Surgery*, vol. 71, no. 2, pp. 455–457, 2001.

[5] B. De olaiz navarro, P. León atance, and A. Alix trueba, "Pneumocephalus and cerebrospinal fluid fistula following removal of a superior sulcus tumor (pancoast tumor)," *Archivos de Bronconeumología*, vol. 40, no. 9, pp. 422–425, 2004.

[6] E. Jimenez-jimenez, S. S. Martí, and M. V. Villas, "Tension pneumocephalus related to radiotherapy for nasopharyngeal carcinoma," *Case Reports in Oncological Medicine*, vol. 2014, Article ID 327380, 4 pages, 2014.

22

Squamous Cell Carcinoma in a Calyceal Diverticulum Detected by Percutaneous Nephroscopic Biopsy

Taku Mitome,[1] **Tadashi Tabei**,[1] **Yukio Tsuura**,[2] **and Kazuki Kobayashi**[1]

[1] *Department of Urology, Yokosuka Kyosai Hospital, 1-16 Yonegahamadori, Yokosuka, Kanagawa, Japan*
[2] *Department of Pathology, Yokosuka Kyousai Hospital, 1-16 Yonegahamadori, Yokosuka, Kanagawa, Japan*

Correspondence should be addressed to Taku Mitome; e053053a@yahoo.co.jp

Academic Editor: Jose I. Mayordomo

A 73-year-old woman was referred to our department with a complaint of asymptomatic gross hematuria. Dynamic computed tomography revealed a complicated (Bosniak type IIF) cyst in the upper pole of her right kidney, which was diagnosed as a calyceal diverticulum. The diagnosis was confirmed by ureteroscopy. The diverticulum was filled with a soft protein matrix that was difficult to completely remove from the inner surface of the calyceal diverticulum. Endoscopy combined with intrarenal surgery (ECIRS) was performed to completely remove the matrix. Percutaneous nephroscopy further revealed papillary lesions on the surface of the diverticulum, confirmed as squamous cell carcinoma on pathological assessment. A laparoscopic right radical nephroureterectomy was performed, with curative intent. Pathological assessment confirmed a high-grade squamous cell carcinoma with renal parenchymal invasion (pT3). Although carcinomas in a calyceal diverticulum are highly uncommon, when present, these tend to be high-grade neoplasms that deeply invade the parenchymal wall. As the effective management of these lesions is difficult, early-stage diagnosis is required for curative treatment. We report the case of squamous cell carcinoma in a calyceal diverticulum that was difficult to diagnose on preoperative computed tomography, urinal cytology examination, and ureteroscopy but was found during ECIRS.

1. Introduction

Carcinoma in a calyceal diverticulum is largely uncommon. Although in most previous cases, the diagnosis was established on preoperative imaging, in one of these cases, the lesion was identified during percutaneous nephrolithotripsy [1]. We report a case of squamous cell carcinoma in a calyceal diverticulum that we identified using percutaneous biopsy and pathological analysis. Preoperative findings on computed tomography (CT), urinal cytology examination, and ureteroscopy were negative.

2. Case Presentation

A 73-year-old woman was referred to our department with a complaint of asymptomatic gross hematuria. She had experienced a urinary tract infection and urolithiasis several years ago. On cystoscopy, we identified a gross hematuria from the right ureteral orifice. Noncontrast enhanced CT revealed a right renal stone and a complicated cyst in the upper pole of her right kidney, which was categorized as a Bosniak type IIF cyst on dynamic CT, with a maximum diameter of 58 mm (Figure 1).

The renal stone was removed using flexible ureteroscopic lithotripsy. The calyceal diverticulum, which had been diagnosed preoperatively as a complicated cyst, was confirmed by ureteroscopy and retrograde pyelogram (Figure 2). As the diverticulum was filled with a soft protein matrix that was adherent to its wall, it was difficult to remove all the contents of the diverticulum while preserving the inner surface of the calyceal. With many fragments of the soft protein matrix floating in the calyceal diverticulum, renal pelvis, and ureter, obstruction of the ureter and ureteropelvic junction were predicted. Therefore, it was necessary to fully remove the matrix. Considering Bosniak type IIF classification of the cyst and the class II classification of the

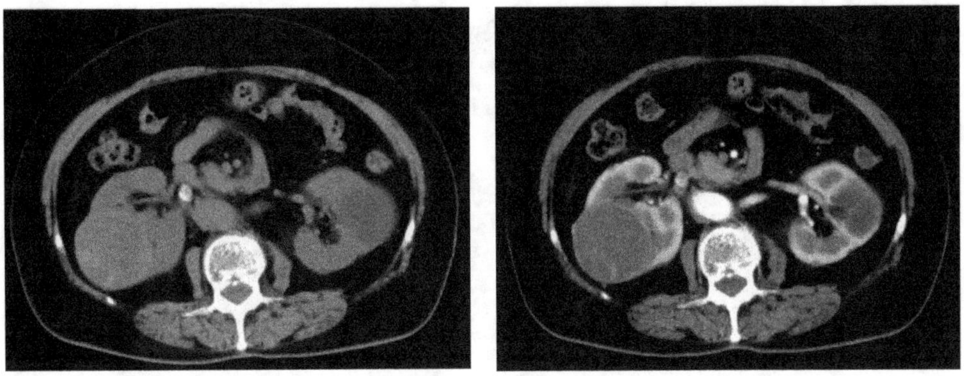

(a) (b)

FIGURE 1: (a) Plain computed tomography image, showing a stone in the right upper urinary tract, but with no indication of the soft protein matrix in the right renal pelvis and calyceal diverticulum, which is radiolucent. (b) Dynamic computed tomography image, showing a complicated cyst, classified as a Bosniak type IIF cyst, arising from the right side of the kidney.

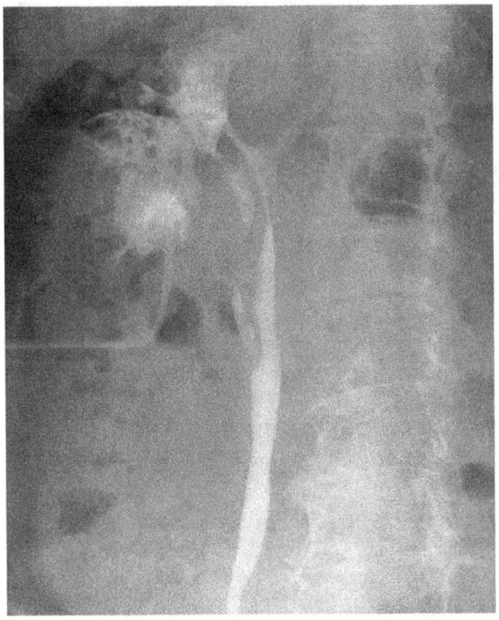

FIGURE 2: Retrograde pyelogram image, showing a duplex collecting system in the right kidney and calyceal diverticulum connected to the upper renal calyx. Defect sign of retrograde pyelogram, caused by filling of the diverticulum by the soft protein matrix, is observable. A percutaneous nephrostomy tube in the diverticulum was placed prior to ECIRS to remove the contents completely.

urine cytology examination, we proceeded with endoscopy combined with intrarenal surgery (ECIRS) to remove the contents completely, without follow-up observation.

We punctured the diverticulum and dilated it using a 24 Fr balloon catheter (X-Force N30 Nephrostomy Balloon Dilation Catheter; Bard, New Providence, NJ, USA), under ultrasound guidance and ureteroscopy, with a working sheath placed at the edge of the diverticular cavity. After the soft protein matrix was completely removed, papillary lesions were observed on the surface of the diverticulum using percutaneous nephroscopy (Figure 3), and a biopsy was performed. Pathological analysis confirmed the diagnosis of squamous cell carcinoma, with the upper urinary tract stone composed of unspecified protein.

A right radical nephroureterectomy was performed using a laparoscopic approach, with curative intent. Pathological analysis confirmed a high-grade squamous cell carcinoma with renal parenchymal invasion (pT3) (Figure 4). Local recurrence was confirmed by CT imaging performed 2 months after that surgery, and the patient was treated with adjuvant systemic chemotherapy, using cisplatin and gemcitabine. The patient went into septic shock during the first course of chemotherapy, requiring cessation of systemic therapy, with her general condition worsening thereafter. At that point, the patient opted for palliative care only and she passed away 4 months after the radical nephroureterectomy was performed.

3. Discussion

Carcinoma in a calyceal diverticulum is extremely rare, with only 16 cases reported in the literature, to our knowledge. Moreover, only one case of primary squamous cell carcinoma in a calyceal diverticulum has previously been reported [1–7]. Among these 17 cases, including ours, the pathological findings included an urothelial carcinoma in 13 cases, urothelial carcinoma with squamous metaplasia in 2 cases, and squamous cell carcinoma in 2 cases [2]. In 11 of the 17 cases (64.7%), the tumor was classified as a high-grade carcinoma. In brief, the histological grade of carcinoma in calyceal diverticula tends to be high. Deep invasion in carcinoma into the wall of parenchyma is a notable clinical problem of these tumors, with a pT3 invasion of the carcinoma reported in 5 of the 17 cases (29.4%), including our case.

There is no consensus on the cause of calyceal diverticula. Dysfunction of the sphincters surrounding the calyces, which facilitate synchronized filling and emptying [3], has been proposed as one possible cause. Such calyceal achalasia results in chronic inefficient emptying, leading to progressive dilation proximal to the sphincter and subsequent formation of a diverticulum [3]. In this situation, the possible thinness or loss of the sphincter surrounding the mucosa of the

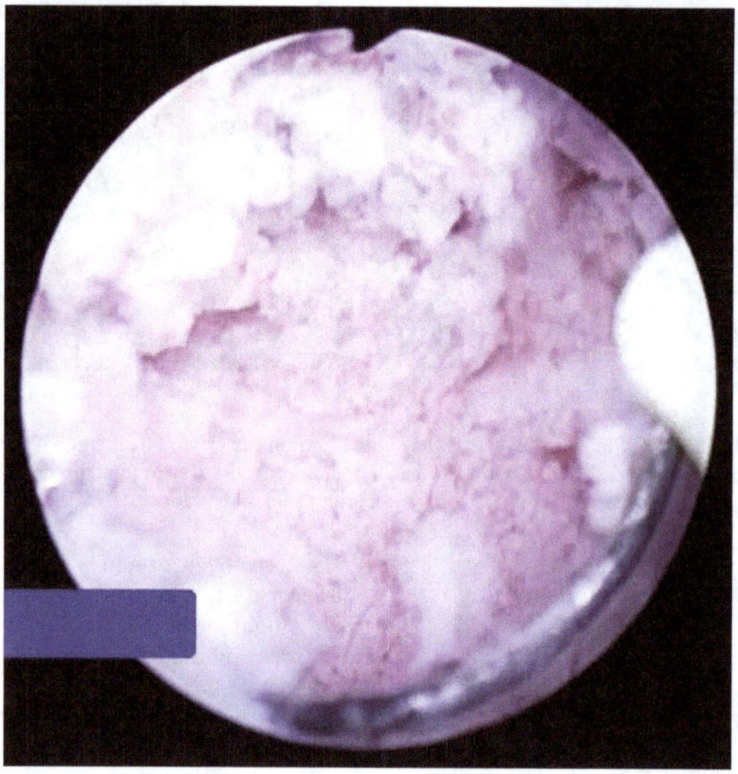

Figure 3: Percutaneous nephroscopic examination, showing papillary lesions in the calyceal diverticulum.

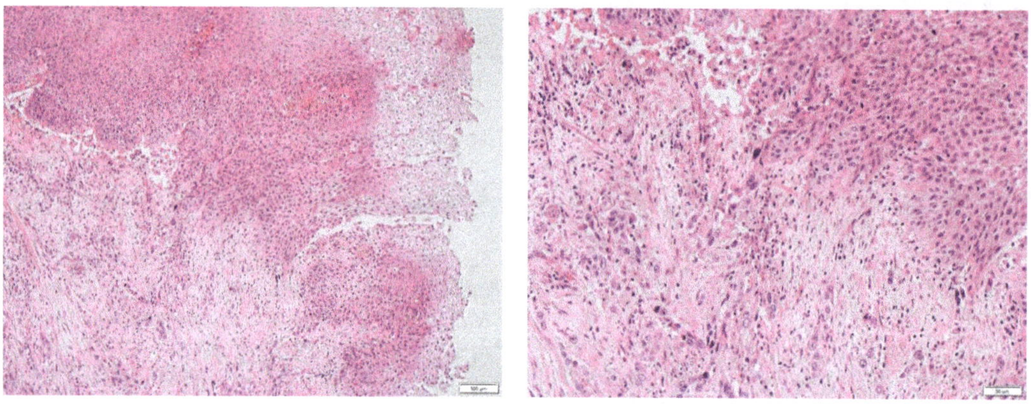

(a) (b)

Figure 4: Histopathological examination. (a) An area of verrucous squamous cell carcinoma, connected to a high-grade squamous cell carcinoma, identified on the inner surface of the calyceal diverticulum. (b) Under magnification, the high-grade squamous cell carcinoma was shown to invade the renal parenchyma.

calyceal diverticula may result in tumor invasion across the muscle layer of the sphincter [3]. Because of the risk of tumor invasion, any case of malignancy in a calyceal diverticulum should be carefully observed, with surgical treatment, with curative intent, performed as early as possible.

Calyceal diverticula often contain stones, and therefore, urolithiasis for stone removal should be performed in patients presenting with chronic pain, recurrent urinary tract infection, gross hematuria, or a decline in renal function [3]. Carcinoma in a calyceal diverticulum is also often associated with calculi, which were evident in 9 of the 17 cases reported (52.9%), including ours. Therefore, a possible diagnosis of malignancy should be considered in patients with calyceal diverticula. In cases of stone-related urothelial malignancy, chronic irritation and infection may play a significant role in the development of renal pelvis/ureter or bladder cancer [8].

In our case, pathological examination revealed a high-grade invasive squamous cell carcinoma, with squamous cell hyperplasia and verrucous carcinoma. There have been several studies on the correlation between squamous cell carcinoma and stones in the urinary tract [8]. Those pathological findings suggested that chronic irritation due to infection and the stones caused a transformation of the urothelium to squamous cell hyperplasia, accelerating the differentiation of squamous cell carcinoma.

In previously reported cases, the clinical diagnosis was exclusively based on preoperative imaging, with only one case identified during percutaneous nephrolithotripsy. Because in our case the diverticulum was classified as a Bosniak type IIF cyst and that the calyceal diverticulum was filled with a soft protein matrix, the diagnosis was difficult to make based on CT images and retrograde ureteroscopy. The decision to fully remove the soft protein matrix was made to prevent obstruction of the ureter and uteropelvic junction by the multiple fragments that were floating in the calyceal diverticulum, renal pelvis, and ureter. It was only after the matrix was completely removed, and the diverticular cavity was cleared that papillary lesions were observable, with a definitive diagnosis confirmed by percutaneous nephroscopic biopsy.

Naturally, seeding of carcinoma cells in the percutaneous tract during the percutaneous is of concern. However, a previous study reported a low incidence of seeding of urothelial carcinoma in the percutaneous tract, 0.3% overall and 0.75% (1/133) in the most experienced center [9]. Previous studies have reported the incidence of seeding of urothelial carcinoma in the percutaneous tract to be relatively low. Precautions to prevent seeding include the use of a large diameter sheath or low-pressure resection with continuous flow and avoiding the long-term implantation of a nephrostomy tube [10, 11]. Considering the low risk of seeding, we proceeded with percutaneous lithotripsy with all precautionary measures, although the presence of malignancy in the diverticulum could not be completely denied. As it is occasionally difficult to approach a calyceal diverticulum and observe its inner surface in detail, even with flexible ureteroscopy, we support the use of percutaneous nephroscopic biopsy as an option in patients with negative findings on preoperative CT and urinal cytology examination.

In summary, we report an extremely rare case of squamous cell carcinoma in a calyceal diverticulum that was diagnosed by percutaneous nephrosopic examination. The definitive diagnosis of carcinoma in a calyceal diverticulum can be difficult to confirm by imaging, urinal cytology examination, and ureteroscopy. In our case, the diagnosis was made during the percutaneous endoscopic procedure.

Acknowledgments

The authors would like to thank Editage (http://www.editage.jp) for English language editing.

References

[1] J. M. Zuckerman, C. Passman, and D. G. Assimos, "Transitional cell carcinoma within a calyceal diverticulum associated with stone disease," *Reviews in Urology*, vol. 12, no. 1, pp. 52–55, 2010.

[2] Y. W. Chen, S. H. Shen, Y. H. Chang, and C. C. Pan, "Squamous cell carcinoma arising from a renal calyceal diverticulum," *Urology*, vol. 95, pp. e5–e6, 2016.

[3] T. Nakano, Y. Kitagawa, K. Izumi, H. Ikeda, and M. Namiki, "Invasive urothelial carcinoma within a calyceal diverticulum associated with renal stones: a case report," *Oncology Letters*, vol. 10, no. 4, pp. 2439–2441, 2015.

[4] T. Adachi, K. Ezaki, and K. Funai, "A case of transitional cell carcinoma in a pyelocaliceal diverticulum," *Hinyokika Kiyo. Acta Urologica Japonica*, vol. 35, no. 8, pp. 1383–1386, 1989.

[5] K. Yoshimura, H. Yoshida, N. Kawase, and Y. Taki, "A case of transitional cell carcinoma and milk of calcium in a pyelocalyceal diverticulum," *Hinyokika Kiyo. Acta Urologica Japonica*, vol. 44, no. 9, pp. 649–652, 1998.

[6] C. C. Roberts, J. M. Collins, T. K. Lidner, and T. R. Larson, "Transitional cell carcinoma obstructing a calyceal diverticulum: unusual presentation as a peripheral cystic mass," *Journal of Ultrasound in Medicine*, vol. 18, no. 1, pp. 19–21, 1999.

[7] J. Akatsuka, Y. Suzuki, T. Hamasaki, G. Kimura, and Y. Kondo, "Urothelial carcinoma in a pyelocaliceal diverticulum discovered by magnetic resonance urography," *International Brazilian Journal of Urology*, vol. 40, no. 2, pp. 274–276, 2014.

[8] W. H. Chow, G. Gridley, M. S. Linet et al., "Risk of urinary tract cancers following kidney or ureter stones," *JNCI Journal of the National Cancer Institute*, vol. 89, no. 19, pp. 1453–1457, 1997.

[9] A. R. Rastinehad, M. C. Ost, B. A. VanderBrink et al., "A 20-year experience with percutaneous resection of upper tract transitional carcinoma: is there an oncologic benefit with adjuvant Bacillus Calmette Guérin therapy?," *Urology*, vol. 73, no. 1, pp. 27–31, 2009.

[10] J. Palou, L. F. Piovesan, J. Huguet, J. Salvador, J. Vicente, and H. Villavicencio, "Percutaneous nephroscopic management of upper urinary tract transitional cell carcinoma: recurrence and long-term followup," *The Journal of Urology*, vol. 172, no. 1, pp. 66–69, 2004.

[11] D. W. Soderdahl, M. D. Fabrizio, N. U. Rahman, T. W. Jarrett, and D. H. Bagley, "Endoscopic treatment of upper tract transitional cell carcinoma," *Urologic Oncology: Seminars and Original Investigations*, vol. 23, no. 2, pp. 114–122, 2005.

23

A Rare Case of Sunitinib-Induced Rhabdomyolysis in Renal Cell Carcinoma

Andrew D. Liman,[1] Vida A. Passero,[1] Agnes K. Liman,[2] and Jenna Shields[3]

[1]Hematology and Oncology, VA Pittsburgh Healthcare System, University of Pittsburgh School of Medicine, Pittsburgh, PA 15240, USA
[2]Laboratory and Pathology, VA Pittsburgh Healthcare System, University of Pittsburgh School of Medicine, Pittsburgh, PA 15240, USA
[3]Pharmacy, VA Pittsburgh Healthcare System, Pittsburgh, PA 15240, USA

Correspondence should be addressed to Andrew D. Liman; andrew.liman@va.gov

Academic Editor: Jose I. Mayordomo

We report a rare case of metastatic renal cell carcinoma (RCC) in a patient who developed rhabdomyolysis while on sunitinib. He was admitted to the hospital due to muscle weakness, fatigue, poor oral intake, and difficulty swallowing in March 2017. He was found to have pancytopenia, liver failure, kidney failure, high uric acid, and increased creatine phosphokinase of more than 5000. He quickly developed lactic acidosis and acute respiratory failure. He was transferred to the ICU, but his condition declined rapidly. He died 3 days later. In this article we discussed about sunitinib-mediated inhibition of adenosine monophosphate kinase (AMPK) as a possible pathophysiology of rhabdomyolysis. Our case is the third sunitinib-induced rhabdomyolysis reported in the literature.

1. Introduction

Kidney cancer is among the ten most frequently diagnosed cancers in men and women in the United States, with more than an estimated 62,000 new cases in 2016. The prognosis has historically been poor, with current 5-year survival rates of 74% overall, decreasing to 53% among patients with locoregional (stage III) disease and 8% among patients with metastatic disease. Although more than 14,000 patients die from kidney cancer each year, there has been considerable progress in the systemic treatment of metastatic RCC in the past 20 years. Clear cell RCC makes up approximately 70% of RCCs [1].

In 2005 and 2006, the Food and Drug Administration (FDA) approved multikinase inhibitors sorafenib and sunitinib, respectively. The approval of five other antiangiogenic drugs (pazopanib, axitinib, bevacizumab, cabozantinib, and lenvatinib) followed. Two mTOR inhibitors, temsirolimus and everolimus, were approved in later years. The immune checkpoint inhibitor nivolumab showed benefit in randomized phase 3 trials and was approved by the FDA in 2015. Sunitinib is an oral multitargeted drug against the VEGF receptors (VEGFRs) 1, 2, and 3; platelet-derived growth factor receptors (PDGFRs); and other tyrosine kinases. Sunitinib has been associated with higher response rate, longer progression-free survival, and overall survival than interferon alfa [1].

2. Case Presentation

The patient is a 71-year-old white male who was found to have a 3.5 cm right kidney mass and had been followed by the urology team closely at VA Pittsburgh Healthcare System. Urine cytology was suspicious for malignant cells. He underwent a radical right nephrectomy on February 3, 2014. Pathology showed clear cell RCC. The tumor was located at the lower pole with a size of 4.5 cm (pT1b) and Fuhrman nuclear grade 2. All margins were not involved by carcinoma, and there was no vascular invasion. He had been followed with a regular CT scan every year. He was found to have small bilateral lung metastasis and lymphadenopathy in 2016. The PET scan on April 26, 2016, revealed FDG activity in the lung and hilar and mediastinal lymph nodes. He underwent endobronchial ultrasound biopsy of the mediastinal lymph node which confirmed to be metastatic from clear cell RCC. Due to his comorbidities and mild thrombocytopenia, we started him on lower dose sunitinib at 37.5 mg per oral daily ×4 weeks every 6 weeks in May 2016. In total, he received 7 cycles of sunitinib. He had been followed every 6 weeks in the clinic. He only developed fatigue due to mild hypothyroidism for which he received levothyroxine. During the follow-up, he was found to have worsening thrombocytopenia with platelet counts in the range of 60,000 to 90,000. A follow-up CT scan and PET scan in October 2016 showed improvement of the lung metastasis and lymphadenopathy. He was last seen in the clinic on March 13, 2017.

He was admitted on March 29, 2017, due to muscle weakness, fatigue, poor oral intake, and difficulty swallowing for 2 weeks. During admission, his platelet count was found to be 13,000, serum creatinine 2.3, total bilirubin 4, AST/ALT > 2000, INR 2.9, calcium 7.5, creatine phosphokinase (CPK) > 5000, and uric acid 12 (see Table 1). Sunitinib was discontinued on the first day of admission. CT head revealed no evidence of metastatic disease. Chest X-ray did not show evidence of infiltration or effusion. Echocardiogram showed severe global hypokinesia with LVEF of 30–35%. His LVEF was 55% prior to starting on sunitinib. He quickly developed lactic acidosis and acute respiratory failure. In the intensive care unit, he received bicarbonate, high-dose oxygen, furosemide, and treatment for hyperkalemia. Despite all treatment support, he continued to decline. His family chose to deescalate care, and he died on April 1, 2017.

Table 1

LAB 2017	Day 1 (3/29)	Day 2 (3/30)	Day 3 (3/31)	Day 4 (4/1)
WBC (K/cmm)	5.4	6.4	7.5	5.3
HGB (g/dL)	14.7	14	14	12.6
Platelet (K/cmm)	13	17	18	13
Potassium (mmol/L)	5.8	6.1	4.8	4.0
AST (IU/L)	462	1984	2032	2450
ALT (IU/L)	351	1579	2277	2197
BUN (mg/dL)	29	30	31	31
Creatinine (mg/dL)	2.0	2.0	2.3	2.2
Bilirubin (mg/dL)	4.1	4.7	4.0	4.0
Uric acid (mg/dL)	—	12.1	—	—
Lactic acid (mmol/L)	—	—	9.4	10.5
CPK (IU/L)	1393	3667	5149	3582
Troponin (ng/mL)	0.10	0.11	0.12	—

3. Discussion

Sunitinib is one of the standards of care therapy in patients with metastatic RCC with good or intermediate risk factors based on Memorial Sloan Kettering Cancer Center (MSKCC) risk factor criteria. Our patient had achieved a good response in the lung metastasis and hilar and mediastinal lymphadenopathy; however, after 10 months on sunitinib, he was admitted with anemia, worsening thrombocytopenia, hyperuricemia, acute renal failure, and evidence of myocardial failure. He was found to have severe global myocardial hypokinesia with LVEF decreased from 55% prior to sunitinib to 30% to 35% after initiating treatment with sunitinib. The diagnosis of sunitinib-induced rhabdomyolysis is based on the fact that he developed multiorgan failure and cardiomyopathy with CPK increased to more than 5000. Sunitinib is the only plausible cause to his clinical presentation. Ruggeri et al. reported two cases of rhabdomyolysis while on sunitinib in metastatic RCC [2]. Both patients developed exactly the same clinical and laboratory abnormalities like our patient with high AST/ALT and very high CPK. One patient died three days later, and the other patient survived after emergent hemodialysis for his anuria [2].

Side effects of sunitinib include, but are not limited to, fatigue, nausea, diarrhea, hypertension, hypothyroidism, cardiac toxicity, and skin toxicity. A decrease in the LVEF is one of the main cardiac toxicities of sunitinib. Grade 3 LVEF decline was reported in 3% in phase III first-line clinical sunitinib trial [3, 4]. Sunitinib inhibits VEGFRs 1, 2, and 3; PDGFRs, and other tyrosine kinases. PDGFRs, which are expressed in cardiomyocytes, have been reported to serve a protective role in the heart exposed to ischemic injury. However, the study by Edelberg et al. employed exogenous administration of PDGF to the heart [5]. But it was unclear whether the inhibition of endogenous PDGFRs by sunitinib would induce cardiotoxicity.

Kerkela et al. obtained an endomyocardial biopsy in a patient with RCC who developed acute decompensated systolic heart failure after 11 months of sunitinib treatment (37.5 mg daily dose) [6]. Prior to therapy, the LVEF was 65%. When the patient presented with heart failure, the LVEF had decreased to 20–25%. Transmission electron microscopy revealed widespread and severe structural alterations in mitochondria which included markedly swollen mitochondria. The authors identified in the human heart biopsy that off-target inhibition by sunitinib demonstrated disruption of the mitochondrial architecture and an IC50 for adenosine monophosphate kinase (AMPK) inhibition as low as 0.2 mM [6].

AMPK is a critical kinase in times of energy depletion when adenosine triphosphate (ATP) levels decline and adenosine monophosphate (AMP) levels increase. AMPK activation blocks energy-consuming pathways, including protein translation/synthesis and fatty acid synthesis. AMPK activates energy-generating pathways by increasing fatty acid oxidation via phosphorylation of acetyl-coA carboxylase 2 (ACC2) and glycolysis via activation of phosphofructo-2-kinase (PFK) (Figure 1(a)). Sunitinib-mediated inhibition of AMPK could release these energy-consuming pathways and prevent activation of energy-generating pathways, exacerbating the energy rundown in the cell (Figure 1(b)) [6, 7]. It has been suggested that modification or reduction of sunitinib dose to no longer target AMPK might reduce cardiotoxicity.

Hohenegger also proposed the same mechanism that suggests sunitinib could interfere with fatty acid oxidation and glycolysis. Under stress, AMPK activity usually acts as a rescue pathway. Sunitinib inhibits AMPK thus causing a

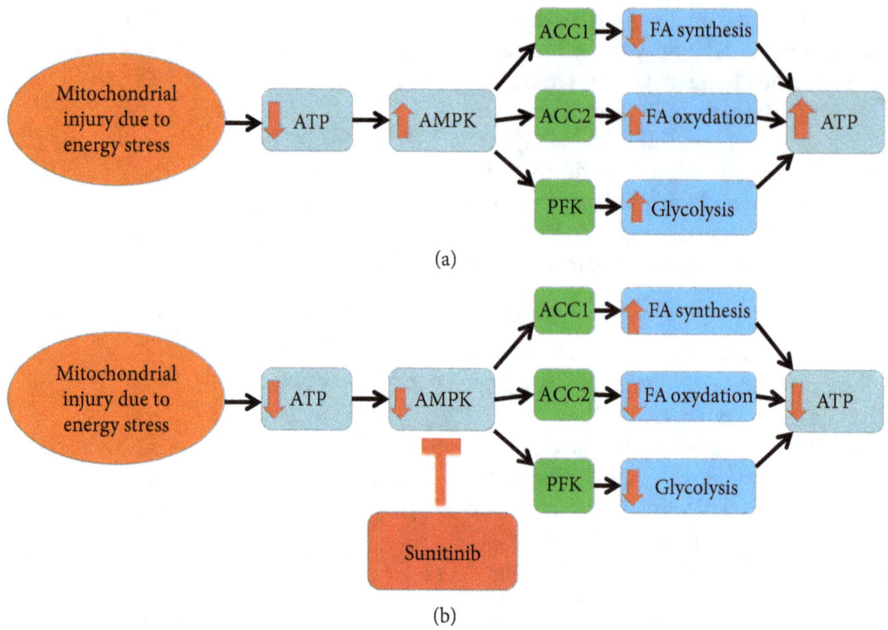

FIGURE 1: (a) Activation of AMP-kinase leads to the increase in ATP. Energy stress causes a decrease in ATP and in turn leads to activation of AMP-kinase. This will induce energy-generating pathways by rapid phosphorylation of acetyl coA carboxylases 1 and 2 (ACC1 and ACC2) and phosphofructokinase (PFK), which lead to decreased fatty acid synthesis, increased fatty acid oxidation, and increased glycolysis. This mechanism is to restore energy homeostasis. (b) Inhibition of AMP-kinase by sunitinib leads to a decrease in ATP. In the presence of sunitinib, ATP cannot bind to AMPK. This will prevent the activation of energy generating pathways and exacerbate energy-consuming pathways.

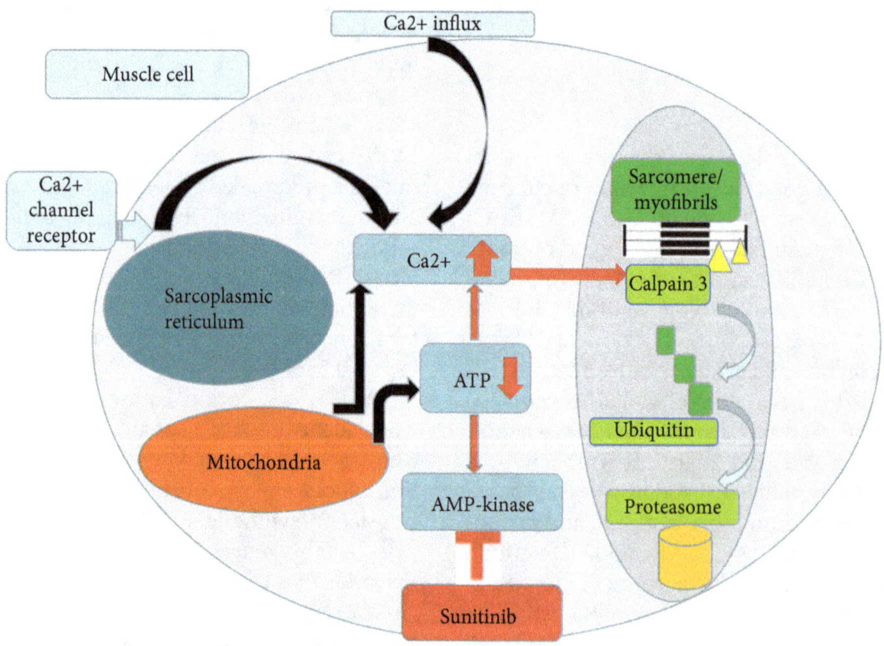

FIGURE 2: Sunitinib inhibits intracellular AMP-kinase and increase myoplasmic Ca2+. Accumulation of Ca2+ will activate calpain 3 kinase that in turn cause degradation of myofibrils. Ubiquitin ligases will ubiquitinate the peptides and target them for degradation in the proteasome.

decline in intracellular ATP and elevation in myoplasmic Ca2+. Sufficient ATP supply by mitochondrial respiratory chain fails, and as a consequence, extrusion of Ca2+ to the extracellular space is reduced [8, 9]. Long-lasting Ca2+ elevations activate calpain proteases, which further degrade proteins that participate in Ca2+ homeostasis and thereby aggravate myoplasmic Ca2+ overload. The skeletal muscle-specific calpain 3 protease may contribute a further mechanism helping to explain the destruction of the myofibrils [10]. Calpain 3 is anchored to the sarcomere which performs the initial proteolytic cleavage that allows ubiquitin ligases to ubiquitinate the peptides and target them for degradation in the proteasome (Figure 2) [11].

Severe global myocardial hypokinesia and increase in CPK due to destruction in myofibrils are the most important clinical presentation of sunitinib-induced rhabdomyolysis. As reported in the two other cases by Ruggeri et al., CPK could be as high as 3000 to 5000. Myoglobin can be found in urine, but with a short half-life (about two to three hours). Serum CPK is a better marker for the diagnosis of rhabdomyolysis. CPK is active in skeletal muscles (CPK-MM) and catalyzes the transportation of one phosphate group from creatinine (C) to ADP, resulting in ATP. CPK is elevated in the first 12 hours after the onset of rhabdomyolysis, peaks within the first three days, and returns to the baseline level at three to five days after the injury. The half-life of CPK is 1.5 days. Therefore, CPK is a more reliable marker than myoglobin in the diagnosis of muscular damage [12].

4. Conclusion

Sunitinib-induced rhabdomyolysis is a very rare occurrence. Rhabdomyolysis presents with rapid deterioration of clinical condition due to liver failure, kidney failure, global hypokinesia of myocardium, very high CPK, hyperuricemia, and lactic acidosis that could lead to death. Inhibition of AMPK has been reported as the possible pathophysiology of this toxicity. Initial recognition of this toxicity is critical to ensure timely management.

Consent

Verbal consent was obtained from the patient's family.

Disclosure

This abstract was presented as a Poster Presentation at the 13th Annual Meeting of Association of Veteran Affairs Hematology and Oncology (AVAHO) in Denver, Colorado, USA, on September 14–17, 2017.

References

[1] T. K. Choueiri and R. J. Motzer, "Systemic therapy for metastatic renal-cell carcinoma," *The New England Journal of Medicine*, vol. 376, no. 4, pp. 354–366, 2017.

[2] E. M. Ruggeri, F. L. Cecere, L. Moscetti, L. Doni, D. Padalino, and F. Di Costanzo, "Severe rhabdomyolysis during sunitinib treatment of metastatic renal cell carcinoma. A report of two cases," *Annals of Oncology*, vol. 21, no. 9, pp. 1926-1927, 2010.

[3] T. F. Chu, M. A. Rupnick, R. Kerkela et al., "Cardiotoxicity associated with tyrosine kinase inhibitor sunitinib," *The Lancet*, vol. 370, no. 9604, pp. 2011–2019, 2007.

[4] T. A. Schmid and M. E. Gore, "Sunitinib in the treatment of metastatic renal cell carcinoma," *Therapeutic Advances in Urology*, vol. 8, no. 6, pp. 348–371, 2016.

[5] J. M. Edelberg, S. H. Lee, M. Kaur et al., "Platelet-derived growth factor-AB limits the extent of myocardial infarction in a rat model: feasibility of restoring impaired angiogenic capacity in the aging heart," *Circulation*, vol. 105, no. 5, pp. 608–613, 2002.

[6] R. Kerkela, K. C. Woulfe, J. B. Durand et al., "Sunitinib-induced cardiotoxicity is mediated by off-target inhibition of AMP-activated protein kinase," *Clinical and Translational Science*, vol. 2, no. 1, pp. 15–25, 2009.

[7] M. C. Towler and D. G. Hardie, "AMP-activated protein kinase in metabolic control and insulin signaling," *Circulation Research*, vol. 100, no. 3, pp. 328–341, 2007.

[8] J. R. López, M. A. Gonzalez, B. Rojas, J. R. López, and A. Terzic, "Myoplasmic Ca^{2+} concentration during exertional rhabdomyolysis," *The Lancet*, vol. 345, no. 8947, pp. 424-425, 1995.

[9] M. Hohenegger, "Drug induced rhabdomyolysis," *Current Opinion in Pharmacology*, vol. 12, no. 3, pp. 335–339, 2012.

[10] R. M. Murphy, "Calpains, skeletal muscle function and exercise," *Clinical and Experimental Pharmacology and Physiology*, vol. 37, no. 3, pp. 385–391, 2010.

[11] J. S. Beckmann and M. Spencer, "Calpain 3, the "gatekeeper" of proper sarcomere assembly, turnover and maintenance," *Neuromuscular Disorders*, vol. 18, no. 12, pp. 913–921, 2008.

[12] M. H. Zhang, "Rhabdomyolosis and its pathogenesis," *World Journal of Emergency Medicine*, vol. 3, no. 1, pp. 11–15, 2012.

24

Unusual Presentation of Follicular Dendritic Cell Sarcoma as a Cystic Neck Swelling

G. Chidananda-Murthy,[1] P. Babu,[2] J. Chandran,[3] and G. Raja[4]

[1]*Sri Venkateshwaraa Medical College Hospital & Research Centre, Department of Surgical Oncology, Puducherry, India*
[2]*Sri Venkateshwaraa Medical College Hospital & Research Centre, Department of Plastic Surgery, Puducherry, India*
[3]*Sri Venkateshwaraa Medical College Hospital & Research Centre, Department of Pathology, Puducherry, India*
[4]*Sri Venkateshwaraa Medical College Hospital & Research Centre, Department of Radiology, Puducherry, India*

Correspondence should be addressed to G. Chidananda-Murthy; cmgiridhar@gmail.com

Academic Editor: Katsuhiro Tanaka

Follicular dendritic cell sarcoma is a very rare neoplasm that most commonly involves cervical lymph nodes and usually presents as a solid mass. Presentation as a cystic neck mass is very rare. Radiological studies and aspiration cytology are often unreliable, and diagnosis is usually made after thorough clinical and pathological examination along with immunohistochemical analysis. In this article, we report a case of a 42-year-old man who presented with right-sided neck swelling of a 2-month duration. Contrast-enhanced CT showed a cystic lesion in the right side of the neck inferomedial to parotid gland located between medial border of sternocleidomastoid muscle and internal jugular vein. Fine needle aspiration cytology was inconclusive. Patient underwent excision biopsy. Histological examination showed a solid-cystic tumor composed of spindle cells arranged in storiform pattern and showed a positive staining for CD23, CD35, and CD21 that confirmed the diagnosis of follicular dendritic cell sarcoma.

1. Introduction

Second branchial cleft cyst (SBCC) is the most common 132#cystic swelling occurring in the neck [1]. Branchial cysts are a developmental anomaly of branchial apparatus that are present usually in the thirties. There are four different types of SBCC based on location. Type II branchial cyst is the commonest. It occurs deep to sternocleidomastoid (SCM) muscle and lies on the great vessels. It is found at the junction of upper and mid-third of SCM muscle and is usually asymptomatic but sometimes may be complicated by infection or hemorrhage [2]. Other neck lesions that present as cystic swellings include cystic lymph node metastases from head and neck squamous cell carcinomas (SCCs) and papillary thyroid carcinomas [3, 4]. Though lymph node metastases from SCC are usually solid, they can undergo cystic degeneration with a reported incidence of 30–60% [3]. Very rarely, it can be lymphoma with cystic degeneration or cystic necrotic schwannoma.

Follicular dendritic cell sarcoma (FDCS) is a very rare neoplasm arising from follicular dendritic cells [5]. It is grouped along with tumors of histiocytes and dendritic cells in the World Health Organization classification of tumors [6]. These tumors commonly occur in lymph nodes of cervical region but can also involve axillary or mediastinal lymph nodes and extranodal sites [5, 7]. They often present as solid painless neck swellings [5, 7]. To the best of the author's knowledge, presentation of FDCS as a cystic swelling has not been reported so far. In this article, the authors describe a case of FDCS presenting as a cystic neck swelling.

2. Case Report

A 42-year-old man presented with swelling on the right side of the neck for two months which was insidious in onset and gradually progressive. He was asymptomatic except for a single episode of fever associated with pain in the swelling which subsided after a course of antibiotics. He was a nonsmoker and had no history of chewing tobacco, consumption of alcohol, or prior radiation exposure. On examination, there was a solitary swelling of 5×3 cm on the right side of the neck, below the angle of

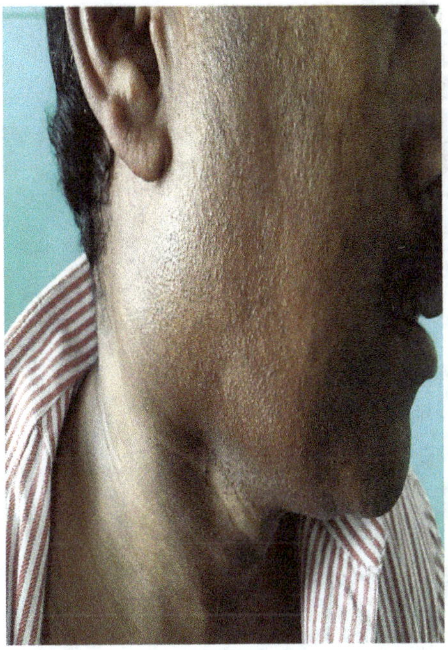

FIGURE 1: Swelling on the right side of the neck below the angle of mandible.

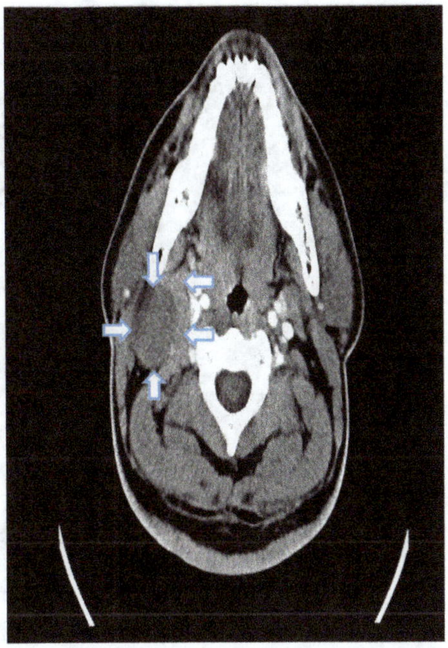

FIGURE 2: CECT neck shows cystic lesion medial to sternocleidomastoid muscle and inferomedial to parotid gland (arrows showing edge of the tumor). Eccentric solid area shows minimal enhancement on contrast administration.

mandible which was deep to sternocleidomastoid muscle at the junction of upper and mid-third of the muscle. It was nontender, firm in consistency, and with well-defined borders and smooth surface. Skin over the swelling was normal and pinchable. It was noncompressible and nonpulsatile (Figure 1). Examination of the oral cavity and other systems was normal. Contrast-enhanced computed tomography (CECT) of the neck was performed which showed a solitary, relatively well-defined predominantly cystic lesion measuring $3.8 \times 3.7 \times 3.9$ cm with smooth margins and minimally enhancing eccentric solid areas in the right side of the neck inferomedial to parotid gland located between sternocleidomastoid muscle laterally and carotid space medially (Figure 2). On magnetic resonance imaging (MRI), cystic component of the lesion showed fluid-fluid level that was hyperintense on both T1- and T2-weighted images suggesting hemorrhagic or proteinaceous component. The eccentric solid component was heterogenous and isointense on T2-weighted images (Figures 3(a) and 3(b)). Fine needle aspiration cytology (FNAC) of the swelling revealed hemorrhagic fluid and inconclusive cytology; hence, excision biopsy of the swelling was performed. A transverse skin incision was placed over the swelling along the upper cervical skin crease. A well-encapsulated $4 \times 3 \times 3$ cm cystic swelling was present in the region of level II between medial border of sternocleidomastoid and internal jugular vein. Superiorly, it extended up to mastoid process. It was excised completely without any spillage. On exploration, there were no significantly enlarged lymph nodes. Postoperative period was uneventful.

Histological examination revealed a globular solid-cystic mass of size $4.5 \times 3.5 \times 2.5$ cm (Figure 4). Cystic area measured 3.5×2.6 cm and was filled with blood while the solid area measured $2 \times 1.1 \times 0.8$ cm. Microscopically, tumor was composed of ovoid to spindle-shaped cells arranged in sheets and focal storiform pattern (Figure 5(a)). Tumor was interspersed with numerous vascular spaces and hyalinized blood vessels. Perivascular cuffing of lymphocytes was present. Individual tumor cells had vesicular nucleus with diffuse fine chromatin (Figure 5(b)). Immunohistochemical analysis showed positive staining for CD23 (Figure 6(a)), CD35 (Figure 6(b)), and vimentin. Tumor cells showed weak staining for CD21 (Figure 6(c)) and negative staining for pan-cytokeratin (panCK) (Figure 6(d)), leukocyte common antigen (LCA), epithelial membrane antigen (EMA), and smooth muscle actin (SMA). Ki67 index was 4–5% (Figure 6(e)). Based on the histologic findings and immunohistochemistry, a diagnosis of FDCS was made. Further staging was done with positron emission tomography-CT (PETCT) that did not show any other site of involvement. The case was discussed in multidisciplinary tumor board, and no further treatment was advised since surgical resection was complete and no adverse prognostic features were present. There is no evidence of recurrence of disease after one year of follow-up.

3. Discussion

Follicular dendritic cell sarcoma is a very rare neoplasm 132#arising from FDCs that was first described by Monda et al. in 1986 [8]. Follicular dendritic cells are components of B cell follicles found in the lymph nodes, spleen, and mucosa-associated lymphoid tissue. These are involved in antigen presentation, germinal center reaction generation, and regulation. Unlike dendritic cells, these are not derived from bone marrow hematopoietic stem cell but are believed

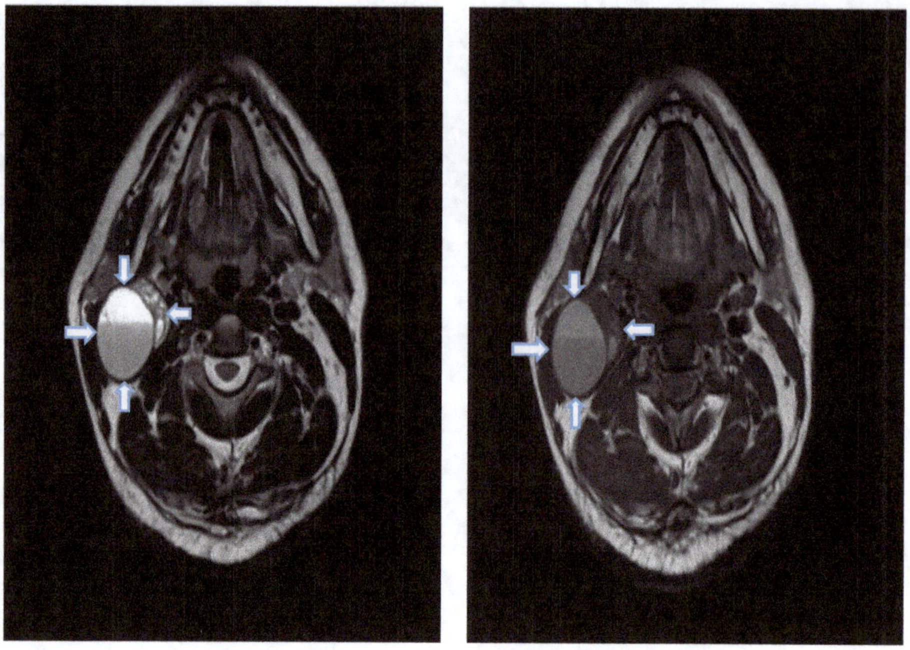

(a) (b)

Figure 3: (a) T2-weighted magnetic resonance imaging shows hyperintense fluid-fluid level and isointense eccentric solid area (arrows showing edge of the tumor). (b) T1-weighted magnetic resonance imaging shows hyperintense fluid-fluid level (arrows showing edge of the tumor).

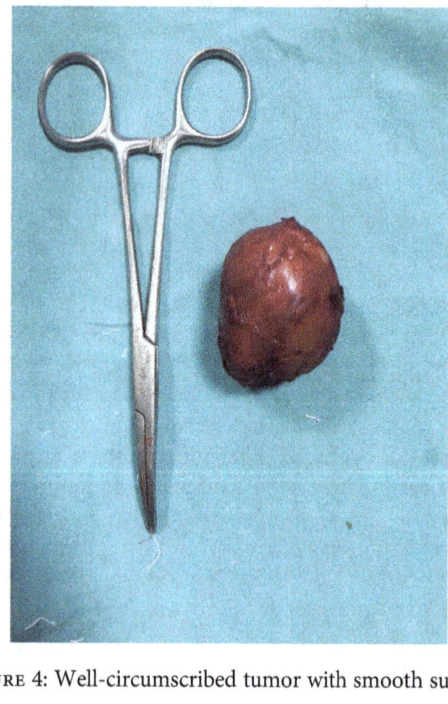

Figure 4: Well-circumscribed tumor with smooth surface.

to develop from a host mesenchymal precursor cell. These present antigens to T lymphocytes mainly on CD21 (CR2) and CD35 (CR1) [9].

The exact etiology of FDCS is not known. Few cases have been shown to be associated with hyalinized vascular Castleman's disease [5, 10]. It is thought that it transforms into FDCS through hyperplasia dysplasia sequence. However, clonal relationship has not been established and further research is needed [10]. A variant of FDCS has been described that resembles inflammatory pseudotumor and it is thought that Epstein-Barr virus (EBV) may have an etiological role in such tumors [5, 11].

Follicular dendritic cell sarcomas commonly occur in lymph nodes of cervical region but also in mediastinal and axillary lymph nodes [5, 7, 12]. The incidence of extranodal site FDCS is around 30–40% and includes sites such as the tonsil, palate, pharynx, mesocolon, pancreas, and small bowel with the most common being tonsils and pancreas [5, 13, 14]. Cases have been reported in the breast, lung, and retroperitoneum also [14]. These tumors occur most commonly between 35 and 45 years and do not show any sex predilection [5, 7, 12]. They usually present as painless enlarging neck swelling without any systemic manifestations [5, 7, 12]. In the present case, patient presented with painless neck mass with progressive increase in size without associated symptoms.

Very less information is available in literature regarding radiological features of FDCS. Long-Hua et al. reported that these tumors have variable and nonspecific features on CECT [15]. According to them, these tumors are usually well defined and homogenous but can have areas of low attenuation due to internal necrosis. In our case, the mass was well defined with smooth rim and no calcification or necrosis. It was predominantly cystic with a small eccentric solid component. Cystic component that was hyperintense on both T1- and T2-weighted MRI images suggested hemorrhagic or proteinaceous component. This correlated with the findings on pathological examination that showed blood-

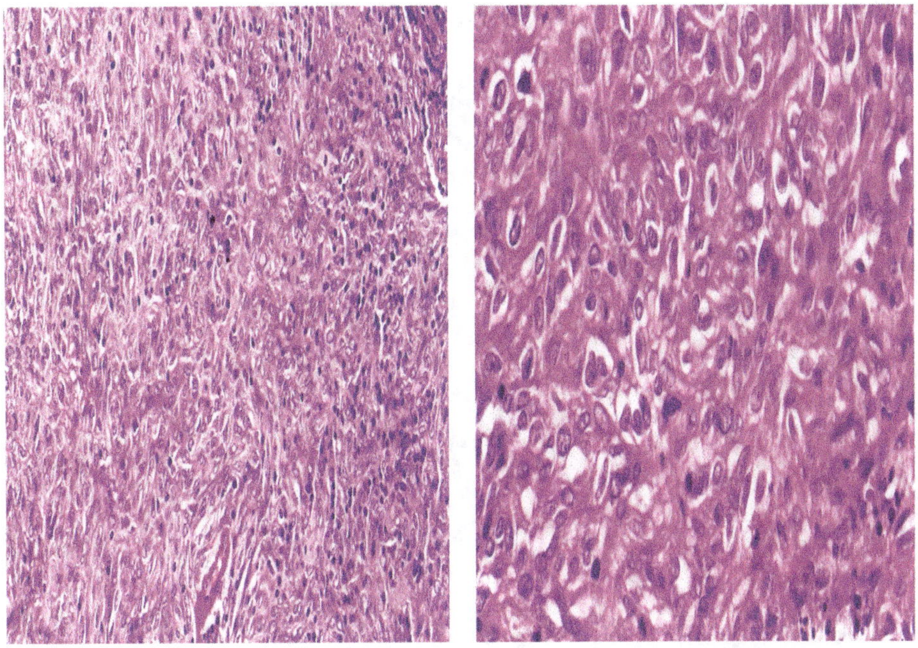

(a) (b)

FIGURE 5: (a) Tumor cells are arranged in storiform pattern and as short fascicles. Tumor cells are intermixed with scattered lymphocytes (hematoxylin and eosin; magnification, 200x). (b) Tumor cells are oval to elongated with indistinct cytoplasmic border and ovoid nucleus with few of them showing prominent nucleoli (hematoxylin and eosin; magnification, 400x).

filled cystic area measuring 3.5 × 2.6 cm. Eccentric solid component showed minimal enhancement on CECT and was isointense on T2-weighted MRI with few hyperintense areas possibly due to hemorrhage. There were no other enlarged regional lymph nodes. Presentation of FDCS as a cystic swelling on CECT/MRI has not been reported till now to the best of our knowledge.

It is difficult to differentiate FDCS from commonly found cystic neck masses such as branchial cyst, cystic lymph node metastases, and neurogenic tumors with cystic degeneration based on imaging alone. Uncomplicated branchial cyst is well circumscribed with smooth rim and nonenhancing on CECT. However, wall thickening and enhancement may occur due to associated inflammation. On MRI, branchial cyst has high-signal intensity on T2-weighted images and low-signal intensity on T1-weighted images depending on protein content [1]. Cystic nodal metastases from squamous cell carcinoma are usually multiple and have focal areas of low attenuation on CECT. They have high-signal intensity on T2-weighted images and low-signal intensity on T1-weighted images on MRI [16]. Neurogenic tumors are located posterior to the neck vessels, whereas paragangliomas are located between external and internal carotid vessels causing splaying. These tumors may have cystic areas secondary to mucinous degeneration, hemorrhage, or necrosis. These tumors have smooth margins, fusiform shape, and nonhomogeneous MR signal intensities with fluid-fluid levels [16].

Diagnostic yield of FNAC of cystic swellings is very low and often this requires excision biopsy for histological confirmation [2, 3]. Grossly, these tumors are well circumscribed with pushing borders. Cut surface is tan colored with areas of hemorrhage and necrosis [5, 6]. Tumor is composed of spindle, ovoid, or polygonal cells arranged in storiform, whorled, fascicular, follicular, or trabecular pattern. Individual tumor cells contain eosinophilic cytoplasm with distinct nucleolus. The borders of tumor cells are indistinct giving a syncytial appearance. Small lymphocytes, T cells more than B cells, are interspersed throughout the tumor and are a characteristic feature of these tumors. Nuclear atypia is usually mild, and proliferation index is between 1 and 20% [5, 6]. Immunohistochemical analysis is absolutely essential for diagnosis. CD21 and CD35 are the most specific antibodies [5, 6]. However, the staining can be focal or patchy. Hence, it is preferred to use these antibodies together [5]. Reactivity for EMA, S100, desmoplakin, and vimentin is variable and not specific. These tumors are always negative for CD3, CD20, cytokeratin, and vascular markers [5, 12]. Diagnosing tumors which arise in lymph nodes is easier as lymph nodes do not contain spindle cells. But high index of suspicion is required in diagnosing those which occur in extranodal sites. Differentiating these tumors from common mesenchymal tumors is difficult and immunohistochemistry (IHC) is mandatory [13]. In our case, tumor cells were ovoid to spindle shaped arranged in storiform pattern with numerous vascular spaces and perivascular lymphocytes. On IHC, tumor cells showed positive staining for CD21, CD23, and CD35.

These tumors have a mortality rate of 15–20% [5, 7, 14]. Incidence of local recurrence is around 30–40%, and distant metastasis is around 20% [5, 7, 14]. Common sites of distant metastases are the lung, peritoneum, or liver [14]. Common prognostic factors are size of the lesion, location, and histological features such as presence of coagulative necrosis,

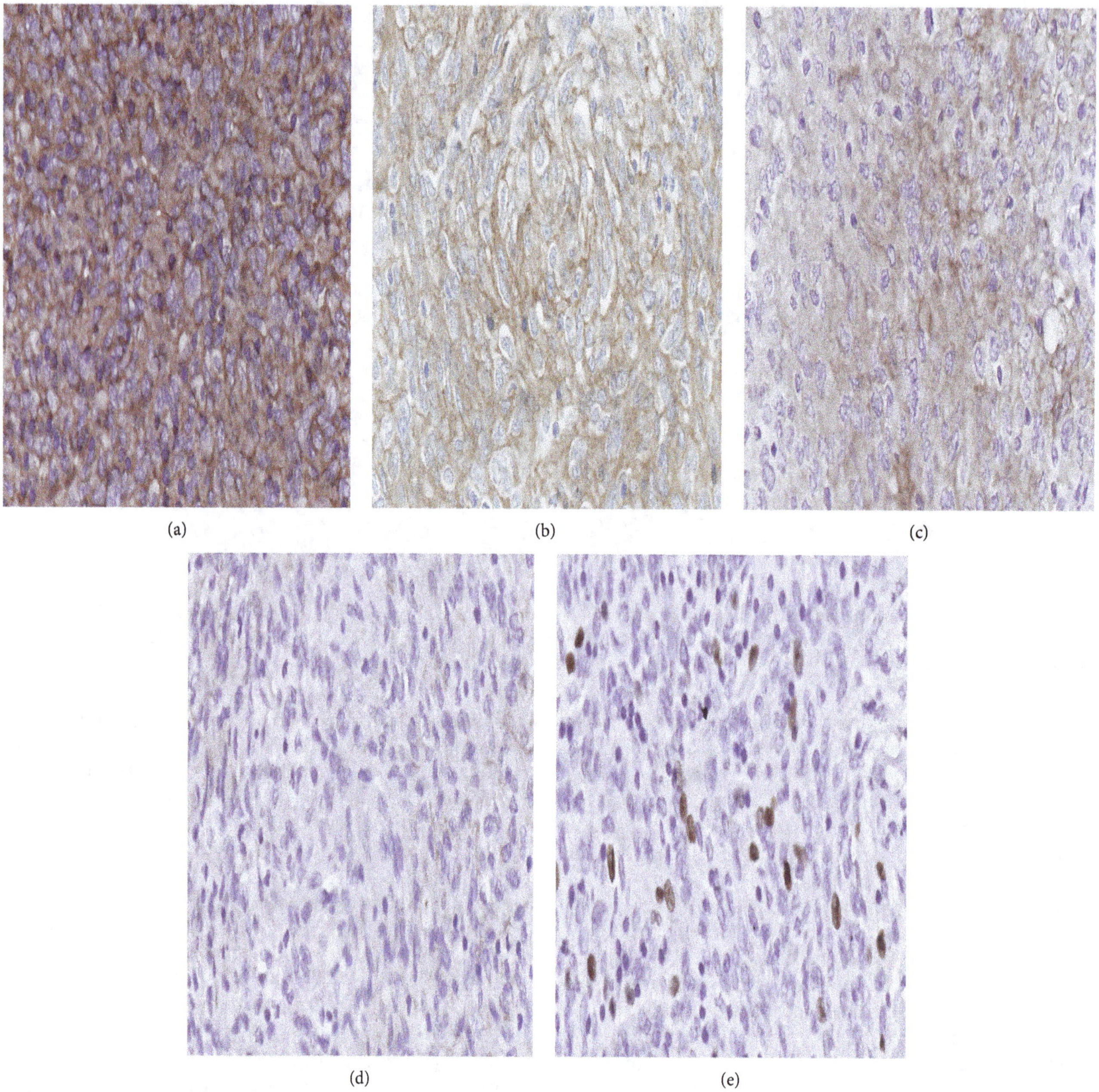

FIGURE 6: (a) Tumor cells show strong membranous staining for CD23 (magnification, 400x). (b) Tumor cells show positive staining for CD35 (magnification, 400x). (c) Tumor cells show weak membranous staining for CD21 (magnification, 400x). (d) Tumor cells show negative staining for panCK (magnification, 400x). (e) Tumor has a low mitotic activity of 4–5% (magnification, 400x).

mitotic count, and nuclear atypia. Intra-abdominal location, size > 6 cm, nuclear atypia, coagulative necrosis, and mitotic count > 5 per 10 high-power field are considered as poor prognostic factors [5, 7].

Due to the rarity of tumor, definitive recommendations regarding optimal treatment are not available. According to Chan et al. and Perez-Ordonez et al., two of the largest series, these tumors should be considered as intermediate-grade sarcoma rather than lymphoma due to their natural history and behavior [5, 7]. In most of the cases, some form of adjuvant therapy has been delivered either chemotherapy (CT) or radiotherapy (RT) or both [5, 7, 12]. Role of RT is not very clear [5]. In a pooled analysis of 97 head and neck cases by Pang et al., patients who received adjuvant RT had lower locoregional recurrence than those who did not ($p = 0.019$) [17]. Adjuvant chemotherapy is considered essential in intra-abdominal tumors and in those with poor prognostic factors [5, 7]. Chemotherapy regimen either similar to that used in high-grade lymphoma (CHOP) or sarcoma (gemcitabine and taxane or doxorubicin and ifosfamide) has been employed [5, 12, 18]. In a study by Gounder et al., there was no significant difference in prognosis in patients who received adjuvant or neoadjuvant therapy ($n = 11$) and those who underwent surgery alone ($n = 12$) [18]. Soriano et al.

studied 14 patients who were treated in MD Anderson Center from 1995 to 2005. Most of the patients received adjuvant therapy, and these authors reported that those who received adjuvant CT in addition to RT had a longer disease free interval (37.6 months) than those who did not receive adjuvant CT (4.6 months) [12]. In the present case, the tumor was localized to the neck and <6 cm in size; surgical excision was complete; histologically, there was no necrosis or atypia and Ki67 index was 4–5%. Since there were no adverse prognostic factors, patient did not receive any adjuvant therapy.

4. Conclusion

Cystic swellings of the neck in adults are commonly 132#presumed to be second branchial cleft cysts. This often results in inadequate evaluation of the patient and delay in surgery as well as definitive management. Radiological studies and aspiration cytology are unreliable in differentiating complicated branchial cysts from FDCS presenting as a cyst. Though such tumors are rare, they should be included in the differential diagnosis of cystic neck masses. A thorough clinical and pathological examination along with immunohistochemical analysis is essential for making a diagnosis of follicular 132#dendritic cell sarcoma.

Ethical Approval

All procedures performed in studies involving human participants were in accordance with the ethical standards of the institutional and/or national research committee and with the 1964 Helsinki declaration and its later amendments or comparable ethical standards.

Consent

Informed consent was obtained from the participant included in the study.

References

[1] P. Pietarinen-Runtti, S. Apajalahti, S. Robinson, F. Passador-Santos, I. Leivo, and A. A. Mäkitie, "Cystic neck lesions: clinical, radiological and differential diagnostic considerations," *Acta Oto-Laryngologica*, vol. 130, no. 2, pp. 300–304, 2010.

[2] B. M. Gold, "Second branchial cleft cyst and fistula," *American Journal of Roentgenology*, vol. 134, no. 5, pp. 1067–1069, 1980.

[3] P. M. Flanagan, N. J. Roland, and A. S. Jones, "Cervical node metastases presenting with features of branchial cysts," *The Journal of Laryngology and Otology*, vol. 108, no. 12, pp. 1068–1071, 1994.

[4] P. Wunderbaldinger, M. G. Harisinghani, P. F. Hahn et al., "Cystic lymph node metastases in papillary thyroid carcinoma," *American Journal of Roentgenology*, vol. 178, no. 3, pp. 693–697, 2002.

[5] J. K. C. Chan, C. D. M. Fletcher, S. J. Nayler, and K. Cooper, "Follicular dendritic cell sarcoma: clinicopathologic analysis of 17 cases suggesting a malignant potential higher than currently recognized," *Cancer*, vol. 79, no. 2, pp. 294–313, 1997.

[6] S. A. Pileri, T. M. Grogan, N. L. Harris et al., "Tumours of histiocytes and accessory dendritic cells: an immunohistochemical approach to classification from the International Lymphoma Study Group based on 61 cases," *Histopathology*, vol. 41, no. 1, pp. 1–29, 2002.

[7] B. Perez-Ordonez, R. A. Erlandson, and J. Rosai, "Follicular dendritic cell tumor: report of 13 additional cases of a distinctive entity," *The American Journal of Surgical Pathology*, vol. 20, no. 8, pp. 944–955, 1996.

[8] L. Monda, R. Warnke, and J. Rosai, "A primary lymph node malignancy with features suggestive of dendritic reticulum cell differentiation. A report of 4 cases," *The American Journal of Pathology*, vol. 122, no. 3, pp. 562–572, 1986.

[9] J. G. Tew, M. H. Kosco, G. F. Burton, and A. K. Szakal, "Follicular dendritic cells as accessory cells," *Immunological Reviews*, vol. 117, no. 1, pp. 185–211, 1990.

[10] A. C. L. Chan, K. W. Chan, J. K. C. Chan, W. Y. Au, W. K. Ho, and W. M. Ng, "Development of follicular dendritic cell sarcoma in hyaline-vascular Castleman's disease of the nasopharynx: tracing its evolution by sequential biopsies," *Histopathology*, vol. 38, no. 6, pp. 510–518, 2001.

[11] R. N. Miranda, J. D. Khoury, and L. J. Medeiros, *Atlas of Lymph Node Pathology*, Springer, New York, NY, USA, 2013.

[12] A. O. Soriano, M. A. Thompson, J. H. Admirand et al., "Follicular dendritic cell sarcoma: a report of 14 cases and a review of the literature," *American Journal of Hematology*, vol. 82, no. 8, pp. 725–728, 2007.

[13] K. Hollowood, G. Stamp, L. Zouvani, and C. D. M. Fletcher, "Extranodal follicular dendritic cell sarcoma of the gastrointestinal tract: morphologic, immunohistochemical and ultrastructural analysis of two cases," *American Journal of Clinical Pathology*, vol. 103, no. 1, pp. 90–97, 1995.

[14] D. A. Biddle, J. Y. Ro, G. S. Yoon, Y. W. Yong, A. G. Ayala, and N. G. Ordonez, "Extranodal follicular dendritic cell sarcoma of the head and neck region: three new cases, with a review of the literature," *Modern Pathology*, vol. 15, no. 1, pp. 50–58, 2002.

[15] Q. Long-Hua, X. Qin, G. Ya-Jia, W. Jian, and F. C. Xiao-Yuan, "Imaging findings of follicular dendritic cell sarcoma: report of four cases," *Korean Journal of Radiology*, vol. 12, no. 1, pp. 122–128, 2011.

[16] M. K. Mittal, A. Malik, B. Sureka, and B. B. Thukral, "Cystic masses of neck: a pictorial review," *Indian Journal of Radiology and Imaging*, vol. 22, no. 4, pp. 334–343, 2012.

[17] J. Pang, W. K. Mydlarz, Z. Gooi et al., "Follicular dendritic cell sarcoma of the head and neck: case report, literature review, and pooled analysis of 97 cases," *Head & Neck*, vol. 38, no. S1, pp. E2241–E2249, 2016.

[18] M. Gounder, V. Desai, D. Kuk et al., "Impact of surgery, radiation and systemic therapy on the outcomes of patients with dendritic cell and histiocytic sarcomas," *European Journal of Cancer*, vol. 51, no. 16, pp. 2413–2422, 2015.

25

Effectiveness of Clavicula Pro Humero Reconstruction for Elderly Patients

Sho Okimatsu,[1,2] Hiroto Kamoda,[1] Tsukasa Yonemoto,[1] Shintaro Iwata,[1] and Takeshi Ishii[1]

[1] *Division of Orthopedic Surgery, Chiba Cancer Center, Chiba 260-8717, Japan*
[2] *Department of Orthopedic Surgery, Chiba University, Chiba 260-8677, Japan*

Correspondence should be addressed to Hiroto Kamoda; kamodahiroto@gmail.com

Academic Editor: Jose I. Mayordomo

Clavicula pro humero (CPH) reconstruction is a method that is used after proximal humeral excision. During CPH reconstruction, the ipsilateral clavicle is rotated downward and connected to the preserved distal humerus by using plates and screws. This method is frequently used for reconstruction surgeries involving young patients and has positive outcomes. In this study, we describe two cases of CPH reconstruction that were performed on elderly individuals after wide resection of the proximal humerus; postoperative results from these surgeries were satisfactory. The average Musculoskeletal Tumor Society (MSTS) functional score after surgery was 68.5%, indicating that CPH reconstruction is suitable for not only younger but also elderly patients, particularly those over the age of 65 years.

1. Introduction

The proximal humerus is a common site of both primary and metastatic bone tumors [1, 2]. Several techniques have been established for the reconstruction of the proximal humerus after resection of malignant tumors. However, as no single approach has been deemed superior, the approach used is determined on a case-by-case basis by the surgeon. One such reconstructive technique is clavicula pro humero (CPH), which was originally described for reconstruction of the upper extremity in children with limb deficiencies [3]. In this study, we describe the outcomes of CPH reconstruction in two elderly patients. The postoperative results from these surgeries were comparable to those of other reconstructive options. We conclude that CPH is a suitable reconstructive technique not only for the young, but also for some elderly patients after tumor resection from the proximal humerus.

2. Case Presentation

Case 1. A 67-year-old man presented with pain and swelling in the right shoulder. He was diagnosed to have metastatic thyroid carcinoma at another facility four years ago and was treated with radioactive iodine.

At initial presentation, he also underwent open reduction and internal fixation of the right proximal humerus for a pathological fracture with the T2 Humeral Nail (Stryker, Kalamazoo, Milwaukee, USA), followed by radiation therapy to the right humerus. He presented to our institution with plain radiographs of his right shoulder showing an osteolytic lesion of the head of the right humerus along with soft tissue swelling of the proximal arm. A computed tomography (CT) scan showed the disappearance of the proximal humeral cortex (Figure 1). Magnetic resonance imaging (MRI) showed the lesion to have mild high signal changes on both T1 and T2 weighted imaging, extending to the surrounding muscles (Figure 2). Needle biopsy confirmed recurrent metastatic thyroid carcinoma. After counseling the patient, a surgical resection and reconstruction were planned. Preoperative embolization of tumor feeding vessels was carried out by interventional radiologists. The surgical incision extended from the medial side of the right clavicle, across the coracoid process, extending to the distal end of the right humerus and included the needle biopsy tract. The tumor and surrounding muscles were carefully resected en bloc with a humeral intramedullary rod. The axillary nerve and posterior humeral circumflex vessels were sacrificed. The right clavicle was

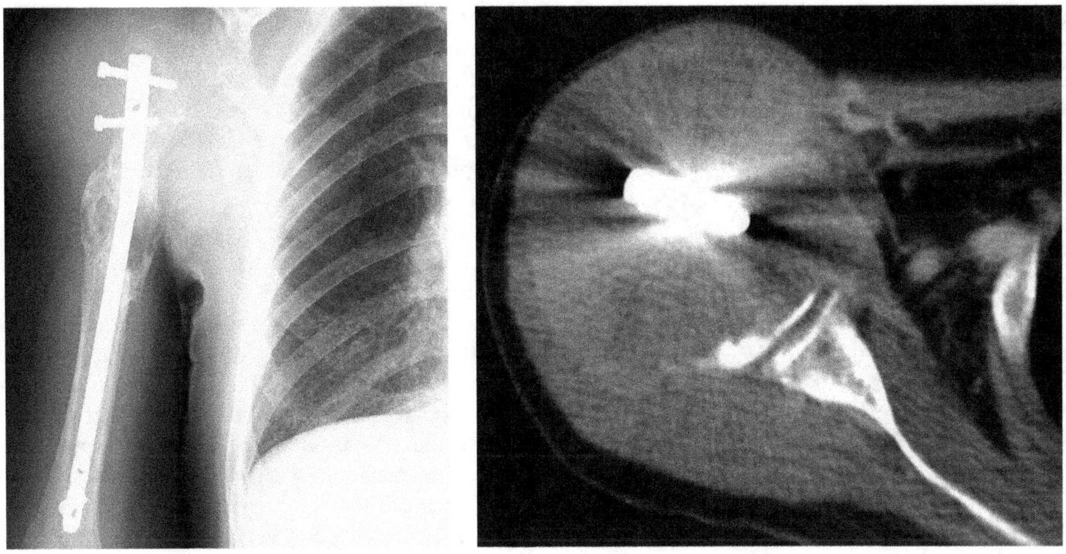

(a) (b)

FIGURE 1: (a) Radiograph and (b) computed tomography (CT) of the right proximal humerus. The lateral cortex of the proximal humerus is absent.

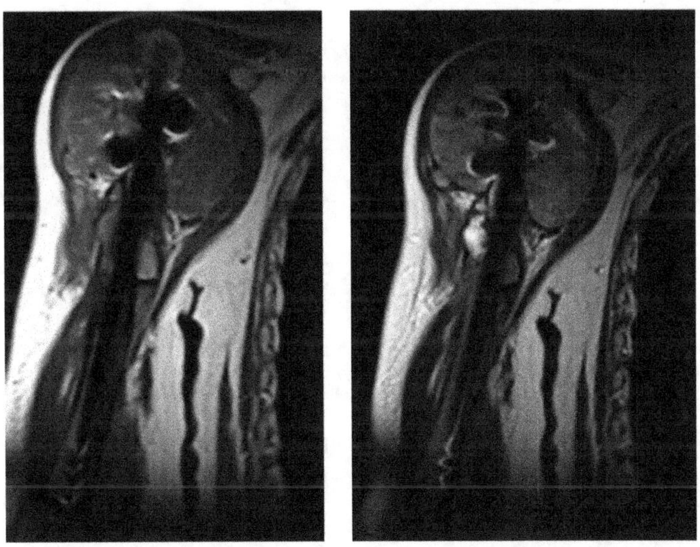

(a) (b)

FIGURE 2: Magnetic resonance imaging (MRI) findings of the right humerus. (a) T1 and (b) T2 weighted imaging show mild high signal changes in the tumor lesion that expanded around the humeral nail.

mobilized by freeing its medial attachments but leaving its attachments to the acromion intact. The floating clavicle was rotated by 90 degrees clockwise and was fixed to the distal humerus with an AO small fragment locking plate.

No postoperative complications were observed after the surgery. Radiographs taken 9 months after the operation showed callus formation between the clavicle and the distal humerus. The postoperative length of the reconstructed upper limb was 28 cm, 1 cm shorter than the preoperative length (Figure 3). The patient had good arm function based on the Musculoskeletal Tumor Society (MSTS) score for limb salvage evaluation with scores of 5 for pain, 3 for function, 3 for emotional acceptance, 2 for positioning of the hand, 5 for manual dexterity, and 2 for lifting ability. The total score was 20 points (67%).

Case 2. A 66-year-old man presented to a nearby hospital, with pain in the left shoulder. He had no history of disease. The range of motion for the left shoulder was normal. Plain radiographs and CT showed intramedullary calcification of the humerus and thinning of the cortex of the proximal humerus (Figure 4). On MRI, the lesion showed low signal change on the T1 weighted image and high signal change on the T2 weighted image that extended into the soft tissue

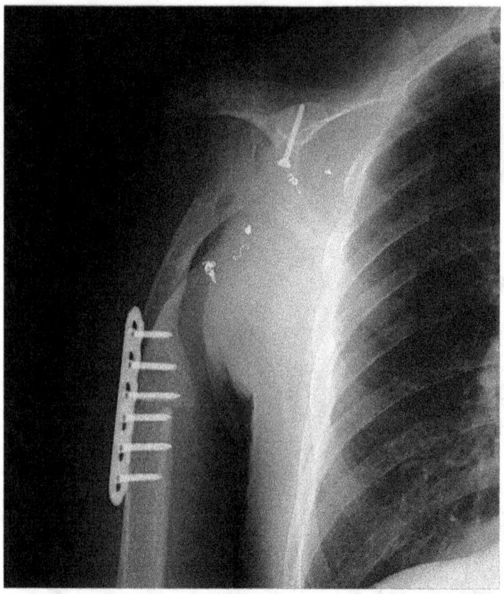

Figure 3: Postoperative XP. The rotated clavicle and distal humerus are fixed with a titanium plate and bony union is observed between them.

around the proximal humerus (Figure 5). Needle biopsy confirmed chondrosarcoma. We performed wide resection of the tumor, followed by a CPH reconstruction.

The length from the head to the distal mineralization was 20 cm; the right humerus was cut 23 cm below the humeral head to obtain an adequate wide margin, together with surrounded muscles of the lesion. In order to maintain the preoperative length of the humerus, we used free fibular bone grafts between the clavicle and distal humerus. No postoperative complications were observed.

Plain radiographs taken 8 months after the operation revealed bony union of the reconstructed upper limb. Its length was 32.5 cm, 0.5 cm shorter than the preoperative length (Figure 6). The patient was in good condition based on the MSTS scores for limb salvage evaluation, with scores of 4 for pain, 3 for function, 2 for emotional acceptance, 3 for positioning of the hand, 5 for manual dexterity, and 4 for lifting ability. The total score was 21 points (70%).

3. Discussion

This study describes two cases of CPH reconstruction that were performed in elderly individuals after wide resection of proximal humeral tumors. The MSTS functional scores after surgery indicated that CPH reconstruction was comparable to other reconstructive techniques for these patients.

The proximal humerus is a common site where bone tumors occur frequently and limb salvage surgery is the preferred surgical option whenever possible [10]. CPH reconstruction was previously performed primarily for the patients with upper extremity phocomelia [3]. Thereafter, Winkelmann began to apply the procedure for malignant tumors of the proximal humerus, as a biologic reconstruction [11]. CPH reconstruction is a type of local bone flap. The clavicle is detached medially and rotated downwards, keeping its feeding vessels intact. Thereafter, the rotated clavicle and osteotomized humerus are connected using plates and screws.

The most important aspect of this method is that the acromioclavicular joint is preserved to maintain continuation of the scapula and the clavicle. This feature contributed for postoperative shoulder stability after treatment without arthrodesis.

Several procedures exist for the reconstruction of the proximal humerus after wide resection of malignant tumors. Shoulder arthrodesis is a suitable choice for limb salvage reconstruction that uses vascularized fibular grafts. This procedure provides a stable shoulder girdle and enhances function [9]. Recently, a double-barrel vascularized fibular graft was used to decrease complications caused by the low stability of a single fibular autograft [12, 13]. However, Tsukushi et al. described problems with arthrodesis, stating that it was difficult to attach the reconstructed graft to the scapula and that prolonged postoperative immobilization was necessary to ensure bony union. They also described difficulties associated with performing thoracotomies, which are used to treat ipsilateral lung metastases, among individuals who underwent arthrodesis [9].

Replacement of the proximal humerus with a prosthesis may provide good results for patients when the deltoid muscle or rotator cuff is preserved. The use of prostheses was initially reported around 1970 [14–16]. Cannon et al. reported that proximal humeral endoprosthesis was a durable reconstruction method as it provided a stable platform for elbow and hand function [1]. In addition, it is generally the least time-consuming option for the administration of postoperative chemotherapy and radiotherapy [5]. However, infection is the most common and severe surgical complication associated with the procedure, occurring at a rate of greater than 10%. Superior subluxation of the implant has also been reported as a complication [4, 17].

Sling procedures that implement fibular grafts have been reported since early times [18]. A recent study described a procedure in which a free vascularized fibula was grafted to the proximal humerus after wide resection of a tumor, as nonvascularized grafts longer than 12 cm are more likely to cause stress fractures [19]. The tendons of the biceps femoris and the palmaris longus together were used to suspend the head of the fibula from the acromion. Although revascularization of the fibula requires skill in microscopy, the sling procedure is meritorious as it is easier to perform than an arthrodesis and there is no need for postoperative immobilization. However, some complications were reported; bony protrusion of the acromion sometimes caused pain and irritation of the skin [5] and flail shoulder without the continuity of bone triggered postoperative instability and loss of lifting ability [20].

Also, donor site morbidity after harvesting fibular graft, such as peroneal nerve palsy, toe clawing, ankle instability, and flexor halluces longus weakness has been reported [12]. To avoid this morbidity, using allograft could be considered. Some authors have reported the experience of reconstruction with allograft [6, 7], but it is not widespread in our country now.

Upon considering the aforementioned information and postoperative shoulder stability, we performed CPH

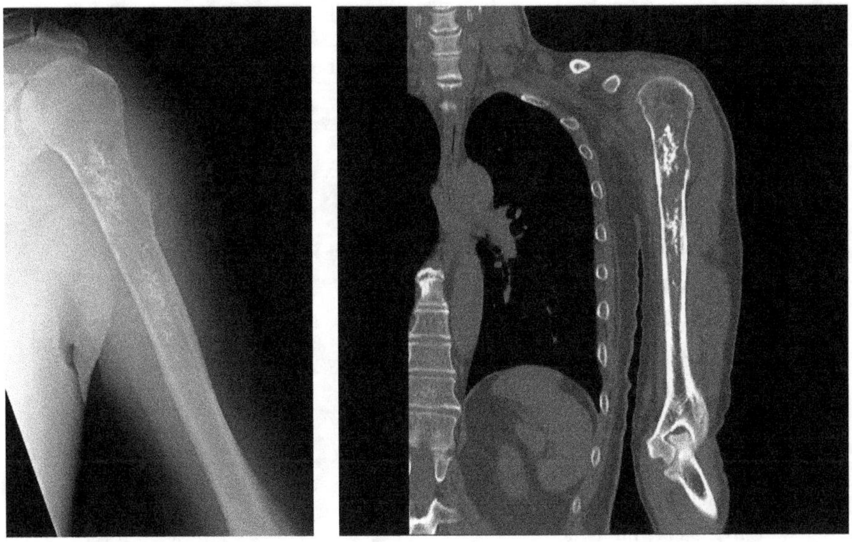

(a) (b)

FIGURE 4: (a) A plain radiography and (b) CT of the left humerus. Bone marrow calcification and cortical expansion of the proximal humerus are observed.

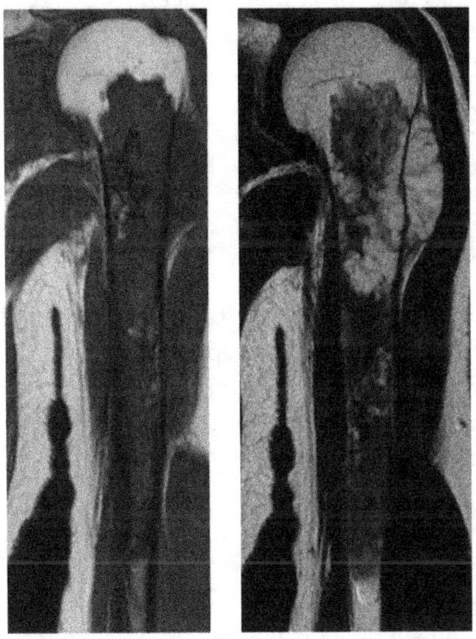

(a) (b)

FIGURE 5: MRI findings of the left humerus. (a) T1 weighted imaging of the coronal view shows isosignals extending from the metaphysis to the diaphysis. (b) T2-weighed imaging shows intramedullary heterogenous changes with extraosseous high signals in the proximal humerus.

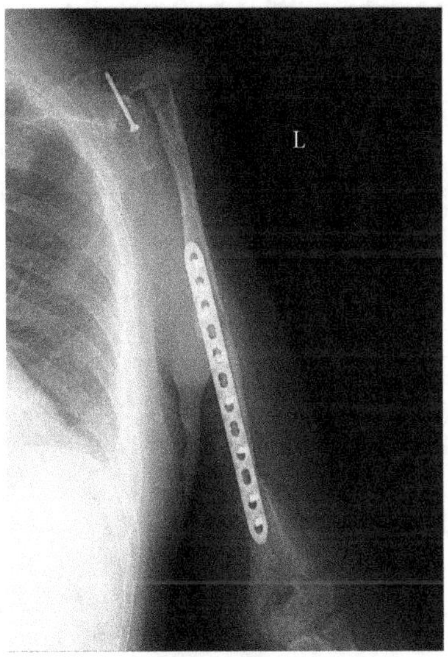

FIGURE 6: Postoperative XP. The rotated clavicle, the free fibula graft, and the distal humerus are fixed with a titanium plate, and bony union is observed among them.

reconstruction on our cases. We did not elect to perform shoulder arthrodesis since our patients had the possibilities of undergoing pulmonary metastasectomy in the future and since their physical activity was not expected to increase as they were elderly people over the age of 65. Reconstruction with a prosthesis was not appropriate because complication rates were relatively high and the procedure would not help them maintain shoulder function after resection of the deltoid muscle and rotator cuff [9, 17]. In addition, we did not adopt sling procedure to avoid donor site trouble or complex microsurgery.

Although studies of CPH reconstruction have been performed, they involved young patients, presumably because of the development of this method for limb deficiencies. Prior to this study, only one case of CPH reconstruction involving an elderly patient had been reported [8], but postoperative upper limb function was not discussed.

We did not observe postoperative complications in our patients. In previous reports, prominence of the acromioclavicular joint with skin perforations, recurrent fractures, infections, or ruptured acromioclavicular ligaments were

TABLE 1: Complication rate and MSTS score after reconstruction of proximal humerus.

Authors	Reconstruction method	Number of patients	Complication rate	MSTS score (%)
Cannon et al. [1]	Prosthesis	83	27%	63
Wafa et al. [4]	Prosthesis	34	38%	83
Sulamaa [3]	Arthrodesis	5	40%	58.3–85.0
Wada et al. [5]	Vascularized fibula graft	8	75%	79
Getty and Peabody [6]	Allograft	16	69%	70
Potter et al. [7]	Allograft	17	65%	71
	Prosthesis	16	44%	69
Kitagawa et al. [8]	Arthrodesis	4	25%	(87/1 case)
	Prosthesis	10	30%	(68/5 cases)
	Clavicula pro humero	7	14%	(71.5/2 cases)
Nishida et al. [2]	Clavicula pro humero	2	50%	80
Tsukushi et al. [9]	Clavicula pro humero	7	14%	69
Current authors	*Clavicula pro humero*	*2*	*0%*	*68.5*

observed after CPH reconstruction [2, 8, 21]. However, the postoperative complication rate was considered modest compared to that of other methods (Table 1).

In this study, the average postoperative upper limb function was 68.5%, which was evaluated using the MSTS scoring system. This was comparable to that of previous reports of CPH reconstruction that examined relatively younger subjects [2, 8, 9]. The upper limb function after CPH reconstruction was comparable to that of other reconstruction methods (Table 1). We particularly found CPH reconstruction to be appropriate after the excision of deltoid muscle.

In this study, the average period of bony union of the rotated clavicle to the humerus after CPH reconstruction was 8.5 months, which seemed approximately the same as previously described [9]. The literature looking into the factors affecting duration of bone union after CPH reconstruction is scarce. On the other hand, there was a report that bone union after vascularized fibular grafts was not markedly influenced by chemotherapy of radiotherapy [22]. Considering that CPH reconstruction was similar to vascularized fibular grafts at a point to preserve the blood supply of autologous bone graft, we thought that these additional therapies would not have much effect on bone union after CPH reconstruction although further studies would be needed.

In this study, the upper limb length after reconstruction was almost the same as that of the unaffected side. It is believed that shortening of reconstructed proximal humerus is beneficial for elbow and wrist function [2], but reconstruction without length discrepancy did not have any problem. Considering the cosmetic problem, reconstructions that enable the length of the upper limb to remain similar to that of its preoperative length are desirable.

In conclusion, we examined two cases of CPH reconstruction in elderly patients and the results were satisfactory. The clavicula pro humero method of reconstruction was useful not only for young patients but also for elderly patients for reconstruction after proximal humeral tumor resection.

Consent

Informed consent has been obtained from both patients in this manuscript.

Disclosure

The authors did not receive grants or external funding in support of our research or preparation of this manuscript. The authors did not receive payments or other benefits or a commitment or agreement to provide such benefits from any commercial entity.

References

[1] C. P. Cannon, G. U. Paraliticci, P. P. Lin, V. O. Lewis, and A. W. Yasko, "Functional outcome following endoprosthetic reconstruction of the proximal humerus," *Journal of Shoulder and Elbow Surgery*, vol. 18, no. 5, pp. 705–710, 2009.

[2] Y. Nishida, S. Tsukushi, Y. Yamada, Y. Kamei, K. Toriyama, and N. Ishiguro, "Reconstruction of the proximal humerus after extensive extraarticular resection for osteosarcoma: a report of two cases with clavicula pro humero reconstruction," *Oncology Reports*, vol. 20, no. 5, pp. 1105–1109, 2008.

[3] M. Sulamaa, "Upper extremity phocomelia: a contribution to its operative treatment," *Clinical Pediatrics*, vol. 2, pp. 251–257, 1963.

[4] H. Wafa, K. Reddy, R. Grimer et al., "Does total humeral endoprosthetic replacement provide reliable reconstruction with preservation of a useful extremity?" *Clinical Orthopaedics and Related Research*, vol. 473, no. 3, pp. 917–925, 2015.

[5] T. Wada, M. Usui, K. Isu, S. Yamawakii, and S. Ishii, "Reconstruction and limb salvage after resection for malignant bone tumour of the proximal humerus. A sling procedure using a free

vascularised fibular graft," *The Journal of Bone & Joint Surgery—British Volume*, vol. 81, no. 5, pp. 808–813, 1999.

[6] P. J. Getty and T. D. Peabody, "Complications and functional outcomes of reconstruction with an osteoarticular allograft after intra-articular resection of the proximal aspect of the humerus," *Journal of Bone and Joint Surgery—Series A*, vol. 81, no. 8, pp. 1138–1146, 1999.

[7] B. K. Potter, S. C. Adams, J. D. Pitcher Jr., T. I. Malinin, and H. T. Temple, "Proximal humerus reconstructions for tumors," *Clinical Orthopaedics and Related Research*, vol. 467, no. 4, pp. 1035–1041, 2009.

[8] Y. Kitagawa, D. M. Thai, and P. F. Choong, "Reconstructions of the shoulder following tumour resection," *Journal of Orthopaedic Surgery*, vol. 15, no. 2, pp. 201–206, 2007.

[9] S. Tsukushi, Y. Nishida, M. Takahashi, and N. Ishiguro, "Clavicula pro humero reconstruction after wide resection of the proximal humerus," *Clinical Orthopaedics and Related Research*, no. 447, pp. 132–137, 2006.

[10] Y. Mimata, J. Nishida, K. Sato, Y. Suzuki, and M. Doita, "Glenohumeral arthrodesis for malignant tumor of the shoulder girdle," *Journal of Shoulder and Elbow Surgery*, vol. 24, no. 2, pp. 174–178, 2015.

[11] W. Winkelmann, "Clavicula pro Humero—eine neue Operationsmethode für maligne Tumoren des proximalen Humerus," *Zeitschrift für Orthopädie und Unfallchirurgie*, vol. 130, no. 3, pp. 197–201, 1992.

[12] J. Nishida and T. Shimamura, "Vascularized bone reconstructive approaches after tumor resection," *Current Orthopaedic Practice*, vol. 22, no. 4, pp. 309–314, 2011.

[13] K. Wieser, K. Modaressi, F. Seeli, and B. Fuchs, "Autologous double-barrel vascularized fibula bone graft for arthrodesis of the shoulder after tumor resection," *Archives of Orthopaedic and Trauma Surgery*, vol. 133, no. 9, pp. 1219–1224, 2013.

[14] H. J. Burrows, J. N. Wilson, and J. T. Scales, "Excision of tumours of humerus and femur, with restoration by internal prostheses," *Journal of Bone and Joint Surgery—Series B*, vol. 57, no. 2, pp. 148–159, 1975.

[15] F. F. Parrish, "Allograft replacement of all or part of the end of a long bone following excision of a tumor," *The Journal of Bone & Joint Surgery—American Volume*, vol. 55, no. 1, pp. 1–22, 1973.

[16] G. Mollowitz, "Vitalium endprosthesis in sarcoma of the proximal humerus," *Chirurg*, vol. 37, no. 3, pp. 130–132, 1966.

[17] M. I. O'Connor, F. H. Sim, and E. Y. S. Chao, "Limb salvage for neoplasms of the shoulder girdle: intermediate reconstructive and functional results," *The Journal of Bone & Joint Surgery—American Volume*, vol. 78, no. 12, pp. 1872–1888, 1996.

[18] K. Clark, "A case of replacement of the upper end of the humerus by a fibular graft reviewed after twenty-nine years," *The Journal of Bone & Joint Surgery—British Volume*, vol. 41, no. 2, pp. 365–368, 1959.

[19] W. F. Enneking, J. L. Eady, and H. Burchardt, "Autogenous cortical bone grafts in the reconstruction of segmental skeletal defects," *Journal of Bone and Joint Surgery—Series A*, vol. 62, no. 7, pp. 1039–1058, 1980.

[20] Y. Nishida and S. Tsukushi, "Reconstruction modalities after resection for malignantbone tumor of the proximal humerus," *Kotsu Kansetsu Jintai*, vol. 19-12, pp. 1143–1150, 2006.

[21] R. W. Rödl, G. Gosheger, C. Gebert, N. Lindner, T. Ozaki, and W. Winkelmann, "Reconstruction of the proximal humerus after wide resection of tumours," *The Journal of Bone & Joint Surgery—British Volume*, vol. 84, no. 7, pp. 1004–1008, 2002.

[22] P. H. Hilven, L. Bayliss, T. Cosker et al., "The vascularised fibular graft for limb salvage after bone tumour surgery: A Multicentre Study," *Bone and Joint Journal*, vol. 97-B, no. 6, pp. 853–861, 2015.

26

Small Split Doses of CD34$^+$ Peripheral Blood Stem Cells to Support Repeated Cycles of Nonmyeloablative Chemotherapy

Maxim Yankelevich,[1] Sureyya Savasan,[1] Igor Dolgopolov,[2] Roland Chu,[1] and George Mentkevich[2]

[1]*Division of Hematology/Oncology, Department of Pediatrics, Children's Hospital of Michigan, Wayne State University, 3901 Beaubien Street, Detroit, MI 48201, USA*
[2]*Institute for Pediatric Oncology, N.N. Blokhin Russian Cancer Research Center, 24 Kashirskoye Shosse, Moscow 115478, Russia*

Correspondence should be addressed to Maxim Yankelevich; myankele@med.wayne.edu

Academic Editor: Josep M. Ribera

Cumulative myelosuppression is the main limiting factor for administration of repeated cycles of chemotherapy. We present a case series of five pediatric patients with high-risk solid malignancies who received small split peripheral blood stem cells (PBSC) doses of less than 1×10^6/kg CD34$^+$ cells obtained after a single leukapheresis procedure and given after repeated cycles of ICE (ifosfamide, carboplatin, and etoposide) chemotherapy. Mean duration to absolute neutrophil count (ANC) recovery to >1000/mm^3 and platelet recovery to $>50 \times 10^3$/mm^3 was 17.1 and 24.3 days. Using split doses of PBSC prevented prolonged neutropenia after repeated cycles of submyeloablative chemotherapy.

1. Introduction

Cumulative myelosuppression is the main limiting factor for administration of repeated cycles of intensive chemotherapy such as ICE when patients can tolerate only a limited number of full-dose chemotherapy cycles even with the use of growth factors [1].

One strategy to reduce hematological toxicity is the infusion of autologous PBSC after chemotherapy. The minimal recommended dose of hematopoietic progenitors for successful transplantation after myeloablative chemotherapy was described as 2 to 2.5×10^6/kg of CD34$^+$ cells [2].

Less is known about the minimal doses of CD34$^+$ cells that would still support enhanced hematopoietic reconstitution after nonmyeloablative conventional therapy regimens. PBSC support at doses exceeding 2×10^6/kg allowed maintaining dose intensity of nonmyeloablative conventional chemotherapy in patients with solid tumors [3–12]. Patients required multiple leukapheresis procedures to provide more than 2×10^6/kg of CD34$^+$ cells per cycle to support several chemotherapy cycles. Here, we report a retrospective analysis of our clinical experience where we used split doses of less than 1×10^6/kg CD34$^+$ cells obtained after one leukapheresis procedure to support repeated cycles of chemotherapy in pediatric patients with solid tumors.

2. The Case Series

Five patients were treated at the N.N. Blokhin Russian Cancer Research Center (Moscow, Russia) and the Children's Hospital of Michigan (Detroit, MI). We obtained informed consents for chemotherapy and PBSC collection from all patients included in this analysis. The patients received repeated cycles of ICE (ifosfamide 9000 mg/m^2, carboplatin 500 mg/m^2, and etoposide 500 mg/m^2) chemotherapy supported by autologous PBSC. Three patients had a single leukapheresis procedure following 2nd to 4th cycle of chemotherapy and G-CSF stimulation, and the product was split into four equal doses. In two patients (patients 2 and 4, Table 1), we used PBSCs obtained after leukapheresis procedures that did not collect required numbers of CD34$^+$ cells to support myeloablative chemotherapy and otherwise

TABLE 1: PBSC support and hematopoietic recovery after postinduction cycles of ICE; comparison of induction and postinduction cycles.

Pts. no.	Cycle no.	Chemotherapy	Number of $CD34^+$ cells $\times 10^6$/kg	Days to ANC > 1000/mm^3	Days to Plt > 50 $\times 10^9$/L	Fever
1	3	ICE + GM-CSF	0.35	18	20	ND
	4	ICE + GM-CSF	0.35	23	34	Yes
2	3	ICE	0.3	17	21	No
3	3	ICE + G-CSF	0.8	16	22	No
	4	ICE + G-CSF	0.8	16	22	No
	5	ICE + G-CSF	0.8	16	25	No
	6	ICE + G-CSF	0.8	16	25	Yes
4	3	ICE + GM-CSF	1.8	15	22	ND
5	5	ICE + G-CSF	0.82	17	26	No
	6	ICE + G-CSF	0.82	17	26	Yes
Mean	—	—	0.76	17.1	24.3	—

Hematopoietic toxicity	ICE cycles 1 and 2 ($n = 10$)	ICE cycle 3 and subsequent cycles with PBSC support ($n = 10$)	p
Mean days to ANC > 1000/mm^3	17.6	17.1	0.28
Mean days to Plt > 50 $\times 10^9$/L	21.8	24.3	0.053

ND, no data available.

would be discarded. The PBSCs were reinfused 24 hours after completion of consolidation chemotherapy cycles followed by G-CSF or GM-CSF stimulation. We used the number of days from the start of chemotherapy to ANC recovery to > 1000/mm^3 to evaluate hematopoietic toxicity. We compared these data to induction chemotherapy cycles administered without PBSC support in the same patients. We used the Student's t-test to determine the significance of differences.

The following is a short description of each patient's case:

Patient 1 was a 2-year-old male with stage 4 anaplastic Wilms' tumor whose metastatic lung disease was refractory to the first line of chemotherapy, and he was switched to ICE. He subsequently received 4 cycles of ICE chemotherapy with PBSC support after cycles 3 and 4. He had partial radiological response (PR) to chemotherapy and subsequently received high-dose melphalan with PBSC support; however, he developed a second disease recurrence 3 months after transplant.

Patient 2 was a 17-year-old female with stage 4 favorable histology Wilms' tumor who developed both pulmonary and abdominal recurrence 10 months after initial therapy. She was treated with abdominal tumor resection and 4 cycles of ICE chemotherapy with PBSC support after cycle 3 (an infusion of 0.3×10^6 $CD34^+$ cells/kg from apheresis that did not collect required dose for myeloablative therapy was given). She had PR to chemotherapy. She then received high-dose thiotepa and melphalan with autologous bone marrow transplant. She developed recurrent disease 4 months after transplant.

Patient 3 was a 9-year-old male with stage 3 favorable histology Wilms' tumor who had pulmonary recurrence 13 months after his initial therapy and was treated with 6 cycles of ICE chemotherapy with PBSC support after cycles 3 through 6. He had PR to chemotherapy and was alive without signs of disease more than 10 years off therapy at the time of this report.

Patient 4 was a 1.5-year-old male with stage 3 Wilms' tumor abdominal recurrence. He underwent complete abdominal tumor resection and then received ICE chemotherapy as a consolidation with PBSC support after cycle 3 (an infusion of 1.8×10^6 $CD34^+$ cells/kg from apheresis that did not collect required dose for myeloablative therapy was given). The patient was still under therapy at the time of this report.

Patient 5 was a 20-year-old female with metastatic PNET with primary abdominal tumor and multiple metastases to the lungs, lymph nodes, and vagina. She underwent abdominal surgeries and received ICE chemotherapy. She had very good partial response after the first two cycles but developed significant hematological toxicities after cycles 3 and 4 even with 30% chemotherapy dose reductions. She received her ICE cycles 5 and 6 at full dose followed by 0.82×10^6/kg $CD34^+$ cells support per cycle and tolerated them well with significant reduction of hematological toxicity. The ANC recovery to > 1000/mm^3 was on day 26 after cycle 4 and on day 17 after cycles 5 and 6. Platelet count recovery to > 50,000/mm^3 was on day 29 after cycle 4 and on day 26 after cycles 5 and 6. She subsequently remained in remission for 7 months but developed metastatic recurrence thereafter and died of disease.

Severe myelosuppression was the main toxicity observed in all patients receiving ICE chemotherapy. The doses of infused $CD34^+$ cells ranged 0.3 to 1.8×10^6/kg (mean 0.76×10^6/kg), and in 9 out of 10 PBSC infusions, the dose of $CD34^+$ cells was below 1×10^6/kg (Table 1). In patients who started to receive PBSC support after their 3rd and subsequent cycles, there were no significant differences in ANC recovery between the first 2 induction cycles and the subsequent cycles given with PBSC support (17.6 days after cycles 1 and 2 versus 17.1 days after cycle 3 and subsequent cycles, $p = 0.28$). All PBSC-supported cycles were given at the full planned doses.

3. Discussion

ICE chemotherapy is one of the effective regimens in pediatric solid tumors [13–16]. However, dose intensity of repeated cycles decreases due to hematological toxicity: multiple publications report the necessity to de-escalate chemotherapy dosing after the third and subsequent cycles of ICE regimen [1, 13, 15, 16], and while median days to ANC and platelet recovery after the first 2 cycles were reported around 18 and 22 days, respectively [1, 13, 14], recovery times significantly increase after subsequent cycles. Thus, Yankelevich et al. [14] reported 26 and 30 median days to ANC and platelet recovery following the second two cycles of ICE. In this report, we demonstrate that split PBSC doses obtained from one leukapheresis procedure and containing less than 1×10^6 $CD34^+$ cells per kg provide sufficient support for ANC recovery after repeat cycles of ICE chemotherapy. Several reports described PBSC support at a traditional dose range of $>2.5 \times 10^6$/kg. Hawkins et al. [6] and Bensimhon et al. [8] used at least $2–2.5 \times 10^6$/kg $CD34^+$ cells per cycle after several cycles of intensive chemotherapy similar to ICE in children with solid tumors. To collect these cell numbers, patients had to have multiple (up to 6) leukapheresis procedures. The average number of days to ANC recovery to $> 500/mm^3$ was 15–17 [6]. Bensimhon et al. showed that after giving 4.9 to 10×10^6/kg of stem cells after 3rd cycle of cyclophosphamide/carboplatin, the median time to ANC recovery to $> 750/mm^3$ ranged from 14 to 16 days [8]. These parameters of hematological recovery are similar to our data obtained with much smaller doses of $CD34^+$ cells (Table 1).

Leukapheresis is an expensive procedure commonly requiring central line placement and additional use of growth factors to mobilize stem cells. It takes multiple leukapheresis procedures over several days to collect the desired $CD34^+$ cell dose [6–8, 10]. Using small split doses of PBSC may provide effective support for multiple cycles of conventional chemotherapy. $CD34^+$ stem cell doses below 2×10^6/kg are safe and may be efficient after conventional cycles of chemotherapy providing protection from cumulative myelotoxicity.

References

[1] M. S. Cairo, V. Shen, M. D. Krailo et al., "Prospective randomized trial between two doses of granulocyte colony-stimulating factor after ifosfamide, carboplatin, and etoposide in children with recurrent or refractory solid tumors: a children's cancer group report," *Journal of Pediatric Hematology/Oncology*, vol. 23, no. 1, pp. 30–38, 2001.

[2] C. H. Weaver, B. Hazelton, R. Birch et al., "An analysis of engraftment kinetics as a function of the $CD34^+$ content of peripheral blood progenitor cell collections in 692 patients after the administration of myeloablative chemotherapy," *Blood*, vol. 86, no. 10, pp. 3961–3968, 1995.

[3] C. L. Shapiro, L. Ayash, L. J. Webb et al., "Repetitive cycles of cyclophosphamide, thiotepa, and carboplatin intensification with peripheral-blood progenitor cells and filgrastim in advanced breast cancer patients," *Journal of Clinical Oncology*, vol. 15, no. 2, pp. 674–683, 1997.

[4] G. D. Long, R. S. Negrin, C. F. Hoyle et al., "Multiple cycles of high dose chemotherapy supported by hematopoietic progenitor cells as treatment for patients with advanced malignancies," *Cancer*, vol. 76, no. 5, pp. 860–868, 1995.

[5] R. Pettengell, P. J. Woll, N. Thatcher, T. M. Dexter, and N. G. Testa, "Multicycle, dose-intensive chemotherapy supported by sequential reinfusion of hematopoietic progenitors in whole blood," *Journal of Clinical Oncology*, vol. 13, no. 1, pp. 148–156, 1995.

[6] D. S. Hawkins, J. Felgenhauer, J. Park et al., "Peripheral blood stem cell support reduces the toxicity of intensive chemotherapy for children and adolescents with metastatic sarcomas," *Cancer*, vol. 95, no. 6, pp. 1354–1365, 2002.

[7] K. R. Pradhan, C. S. Johnson, T. A. Vik, L. S. Sender, and S. G. Kreissman, "A novel intensive induction therapy for high-risk neuroblastoma utilizing sequential peripheral blood stem cell collection and infusion as hematopoietic support," *Pediatric Blood and Cancer*, vol. 46, no. 7, pp. 793–802, 2006.

[8] P. Bensimhon, J. G. Villablanca, L. S. Sender et al., "Peripheral blood stem cell support for multiple cycles of dose intensive induction therapy is feasible with little risk of tumor contamination in advanced neuroblastoma: a report from the Children's Oncology Group," *Pediatric Blood and Cancer*, vol. 54, no. 4, pp. 569–602, 2010.

[9] R. I. Jakacki, C. Jamison, S. A. Heifetz, K. Caldemeyer, M. Hanna, and L. Sender, "Feasibility of sequential high-dose chemotherapy and peripheral blood stem cell support for pediatric central nervous system malignancies," *Medical and Pediatric Oncology*, vol. 29, no. 6, pp. 553–559, 1997.

[10] S. Leyvraz, L. Perey, G. Rosti et al., "Multiple courses of high-dose ifosfamide, carboplatin, and etoposide with peripheral-blood progenitor cells and filgrastim for small-cell lung cancer: a feasibility study by the European Group for Blood and Marrow Transplantation," *Journal of Clinical Oncology*, vol. 17, no. 11, pp. 3531–3539, 1999.

[11] P. Lorigan, P. J. Woll, M. E. R. O'Brien, L. F. Ashcroft, M. R. Sampson, and N. Thatcher, "Randomized phase III trial of dose-dense chemotherapy supported by whole-blood hematopoietic progenitors in better-prognosis small-cell lung cancer," *Journal of the National Cancer Institute*, vol. 97, no. 9, pp. 666–674, 2005.

[12] S. Leyvraz, S. Pampallona, G. Martinelli et al., "A threefold dose intensity treatment with ifosfamide, carboplatin, and etoposide for patients with small cell lung cancer: a randomized trial," *Journal of the National Cancer Institute*, vol. 100, no. 8, pp. 533–541, 2008.

[13] P. Van Winkle, A. Angiolillo, M. Krailo et al., "Ifosfamide, carboplatin, and etoposide (ICE) reinduction chemotherapy in a large cohort of children and adolescents with recurrent/refractory sarcoma: the Children's Cancer Group (CCG) experience," *Pediatric Blood and Cancer*, vol. 44, no. 4, pp. 338–347, 2005.

[14] M. Yankelevich, I. Dolgopolov, R. Ravshanova et al., "Efficacy and toxicity of ICE/CCE chemotherapy with or without GM-CSF in relapsed or refractory Wilms' tumor. A single institution study," *International Journal of Pediatric Hematology/Oncology*, vol. 6, pp. 331–338, 2000.

[15] F. Bracho, M. D. Krailo, V. Shen et al., "A phase I clinical, pharmacological, and biological trial of interleukin 6 plus granulocyte-colony stimulating factor after ifosfamide, carboplatin, and etoposide in children with recurrent/refractory solid tumors: enhanced hematological responses but a high incidence of grade III/IV constitutional toxicities," *Clinical Cancer Research*, vol. 7, no. 1, pp. 58–67, 2001.

[16] M. S. Cairo, V. Davenport, O. Bessmertny et al., "Phase I/II dose escalation study of recombinant human interleukin-11 following ifosfamide, carboplatin and etoposide in children, adolescents and young adults with solid tumours or lymphoma: a clinical, haematological and biological study," *British Journal of Haematology*, vol. 128, no. 1, pp. 49–58, 2004.

27

Surgical Management of Pilocytic Astrocytoma of the Optic Nerve

Ifeoluwa Apanisile and Tamás Karosi

Department of Otolaryngology and Head and Neck Surgery, B-A-Z County Central Hospital and University Teaching Hospital, Miskolc, Hungary

Correspondence should be addressed to Tamás Karosi; karositamas@gmail.com

Academic Editor: Jeanine M. Buchanich

Optic nerve astrocytomas (ONAs) are frequent types of optic nerve gliomas (ONGs), which can affect the visual pathway. An 18-year-old male patient was admitted to our department with right-sided intraorbital/retrobulbar swelling, which progressively grew over several months. Clinical examination showed right-sided diplopia, mydriasis, low visual acuity (0.4), exophthalmus (3 cm), epiphora, and severe retrobulbar pain. There was a family history of high-grade (IV) astrocytomas in which two of the family members died due to the disease. Preoperative MRI scan revealed a soft tissue mass around the retrobulbar area of the right eye with intact orbital bony walls. Surgery was performed whereby it was dissected freely from the muscles and was separated from the optic nerve and the globe. Histopathologic analysis confirmed a benign astrocytoma. The follow-up examination revealed no recurrent or residual tumor. A systemic review of the literature indicates that early diagnosis and experienced multidisciplinary management are required in case of unilateral, resectable forms of ONAs with no distant metastasis, in order to provide a long-time survival of patients. Surgical intervention of unilateral ONAs is a relatively safe procedure, allowing complete or partial tumor removal with minimal morbidity and low recurrence rate.

1. Introduction

Optic nerve astrocytomas (ONAs) usually affect the visual pathway, mainly in the pediatric age group. In the orbit, ONAs might arise from the optic nerve and tend to be a dura-bound fusiform swelling with distinct imaging and histologic characteristics. These tumors often extend into the optic chiasm and into the frontal brain lobe and may be associated with neurofibromatosis (type I), respectively [1].

Pilocytic astrocytoma (PA) form of ONA is a rare, slow-growing glioma, classified as grade-I tumor by the World Health Organization (WHO) [2] (Table 1). It typically occurs in children and young adults [2]. Only one-third of patients are older than 18 years of age, and only 17% are older than 30 years. There are no clinical features that are unique to these tumors. Signs and symptoms are usually of several months' duration and are directly related to the size, location, and presence of tumor-associated hydrocephalus [2].

The macroscopic appearance of ONAs is typically well-circumscribed, cyst-like mass with a discrete mural nodule. Microscopically, the tumor often reveals a biphasic pattern in which more compact areas composed of bipolar areas and brightly eosinophilic Rosenthal-fibers that alternate with looser, spongier areas with prominent microcysts. Eosinophilic granular bodies are found in both compact and loose areas [2, 3].

The present study reports a case of a young male patient with unilateral ONA in association with no distant metastasis. The neuroradiological and histopathologic findings and multidisciplinary management are discussed in detail.

2. Case Report

An eighteen-year-old male patient was referred to the outpatient ward of our department on November 2016. He was diagnosed with a right-sided retrobulbar tumor at the ophthalmology department of another medical institution

Table 1: Selected CNS gliomas. Comparison of basic histopathologic findings and immunostaining characteristics*.

Selected CNS tumor	WHO grade	Histopathology	MIB-1/Ki-67 LI	p53
Pilocytic astrocytoma	I	Biphasic piloid and spongy glial cell regions	<10%	<5%
Diffuse astrocytoma	II	+ Diffuse infiltration and cytoplasmic atypia	<10%	<5%
Anaplastic astrocytoma	III	+ Anaplasia and high mitotic activity	>10%	>5%
Glioblastoma	IV	+ Microvascular proliferation and/or necrosis	>10%	>5%
Ganglioglioma	I	Uniform, monomorphic glial cell and ganglion cell components, diffuse infiltration, and rare mitosises	<5%	<5%
Anaplastic ganglioglioma	III	+ Anaplasia, increased mitotic activity, vascular proliferation, and necrosis	>5%	>5%

*Immunostaining characteristics are general guidelines and must be utilised in conjunction with histopathologic features.

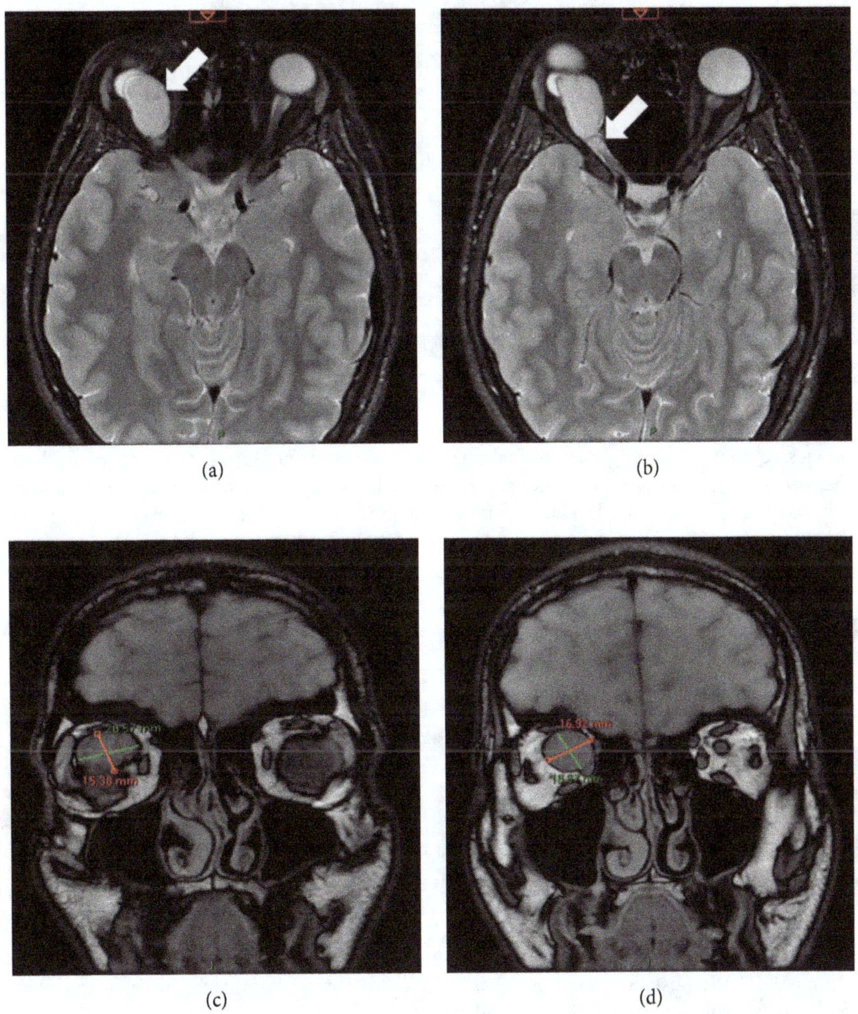

Figure 1: Preoperative MRI scans. (a) A well-defined tumor (white arrow) with vivid signal intensity in the right orbit. (b) The tumor cannot be separated from the optic nerve, followed by the foramen optic (white arrow). (c) The T2-weighted image shows the exact position and size of the tumor. (d) The dorsal edge of the previous shot.

(ophthalmological examination and orbital MRI were performed); however, the ophthalmological team declined to perform the surgical procedure (Figures 1 and 2).

Since our department functions as a tertiary orbital surgery center, after thorough preoperative investigations, we agreed to proceed with the surgery. The symptoms of the patient started about half a year before he was examined at our department. There was no significant information from his past medical history. However, from the family history, it should be noted that his brother died two years earlier due to high-grade (IV) astrocytoma (glioblastoma multiforme), affecting the left side of temporal lobe.

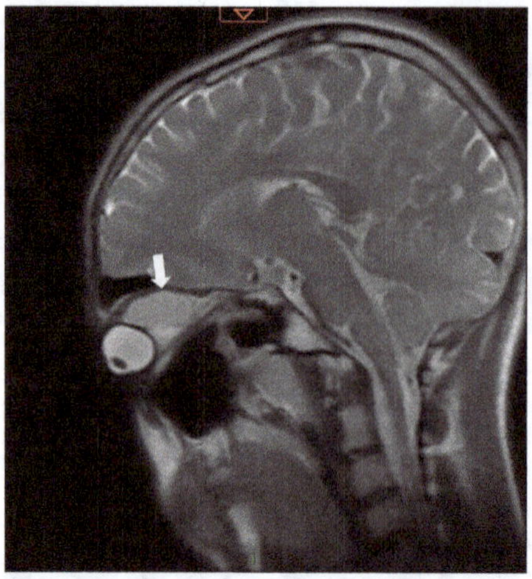

Figure 2: Sagittal T1-weighted MRI. The exact position and extent of the tumor and its relation to the optic nerve are clearly visible. There is a noticeable ocular bulb dislocation (white arrow).

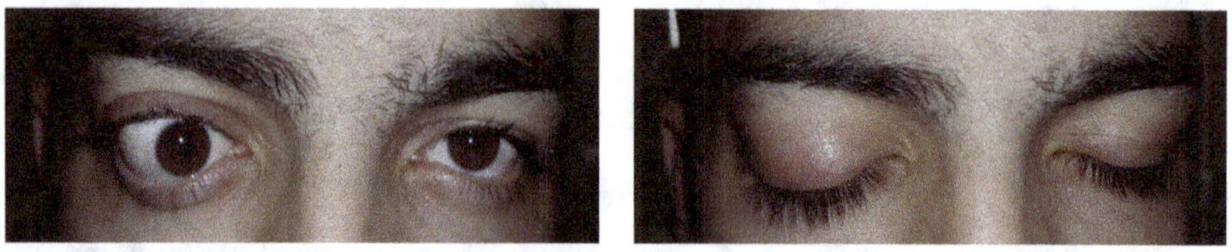

(a) (b)

Figure 3: Preoperative images. (a) Observe the right exophthalmus, the downward and outward dislocation of the ocular bulb, which places the pupil's axis toward the medial. Hypoglobus and anisocoria (right-sided mydriasis) are clearly visible symptoms. The movements of the ocular bulb are completely blocked cranially and laterally. (b) The previous images with closed eyes. On the right side, the upper eyelid closure is incomplete.

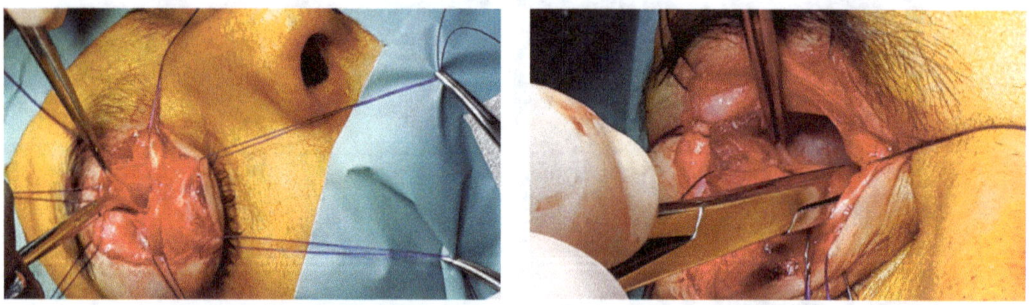

(a) (b)

Figure 4: Intraoperative images. (a) We raise the split Tenon-case with clips. The ocular muscles are elevated by several suture threads. (b) Retrobulbar area filled with the bluish-gray color, encapsulated tumor.

Ophthalmological and clinical examination revealed right-sided diplopia, mydriasis, low visual acuity (0.4), right-sided exophthalmus (3 cm), epiphora, significant eye movement disorders, and severe retrobulbar pain. Exophthalmus was not only evident, but also it clearly dislocates the ocular bulb caudally and laterally. The symptoms started slowly and progressed gradually until eye vision was severely impaired. On the other hand, exophthalmus progressed rapidly.

Preoperative orbital MRI scan revealed the size and exact position of the soft tissue mass around the retrobulbar area of the right eye, its relation to the optic nerve, and the ocular bulb with intact orbital bony walls (Figures 1 and 2).

Figure 3 illustrates the ophthalmological status of opened eyelid and closed eyelid immediately before surgery. After application of preoperative medications, we successfully performed superolateral orbitotomy under general anesthesia. The total duration of the surgery was 69 minutes (see Video

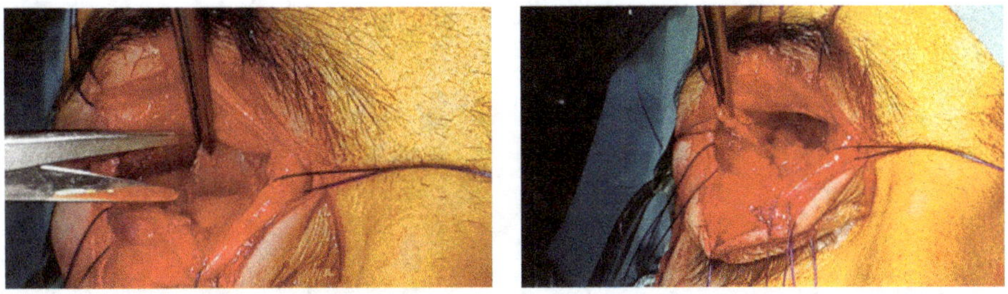

(a) (b)

FIGURE 5: Intraoperative images. (a) By elevating the tumor, we bluntly dissect it carefully from the dorsal surface of the ocular bulb and from the optic nerve. (b) Demonstration of the surgical cavity after successful removal of the tumor.

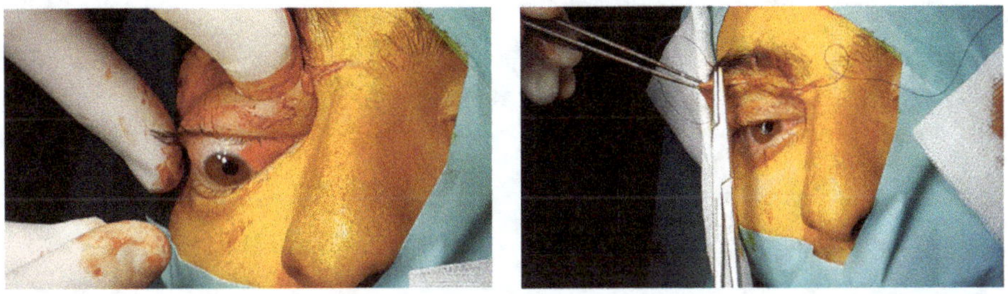

(a) (b)

FIGURE 6: Intraoperative images. (a) Checking ocular bulb movements and relieving any movement constrictions. (b) End stage of the surgery: wound closure with intracutaneous sutures. We could observe the disappearance of the exophthalmus. The mydriasis appeared to increase, and pupil decentralized.

files in Supplementary Material available online at https://doi.org/10.1155/2017/4283570). When performing the surgery, we made infraciliary incision to expose the surgical field; thereafter, we bluntly dissected the orbital fat tissue and mobilized the superior rectus muscle, medial rectus muscle, and superior oblique muscle, respectively. Thereafter, we carefully and bluntly separated soft tissues from the muscular structures. Firstly, we applied pressure gauzes, hot saline-soaked gauzes, and sometimes careful and limited usage of electrocoagulation to control bleeding without damaging the surrounding structures. We could observe the tumor infiltrating the dorsal surface of the ocular bulb, closely related to the optic nerve (Supplementary Material).

The tumor had a definite encapsulated and cystic character; however, it clearly showed inhomogeneous gelatinous fragments of solid tumor (Figures 4–6). The tumor was carefully removed from the optic nerve, which was followed up to orbital apex. The mobilized tissue was pulled in a ventral direction and then separated from the dorsal surface of the ocular bulb. The surgical cavity was disinfected with polyvidone-iodide solution, and then a tiny rubber drain was placed into the orbit (Supplementary Material).

Prior to wound closure, we checked the eye globe mobility and tension, and we observed that no distension was detectable. The eye muscles were placed in their original anatomical position. The individual soft tissue sections were reconstructed with 4.0 PDS sutures. We reconstructed the orbicularis oculi muscle and the superior levator palpebral muscle with 4.0 Monosyn, using simple sutures. The skin edges were intracutaneously closed with 4.0 Dafilon stitches (Figures 4–6) (Supplementary Material). It should be noted that we did not require ophthalmology consultation during the surgical procedure. Perioperatively, Tobradex eye drops, local ice pack cooling, and systemic antibiotic treatment (Rocephin 2×2 g iv.) were used for 3 days.

The eye was covered with photosensitivity pads. During the early postoperative monitoring, chemosis and eyelid swelling were observed; however, it resolved after 1 week of treatment (methyl-prednisolone: 2×40 mg iv., and calcium gluconate: 2×10 ml iv.). The 8th day after the surgery, the patient was discharged. Histopathologic examination confirmed the diagnosis of benign glial cell tumor based on the expression of neuron-specific enolase (NSE) and synaptophysin (S-100), while cytokeratin AE1/3 reaction and Mib1 markers were negative (Figure 7). Clinical follow-up examination 3 weeks later revealed persistent mydriasis, but exophthalmus, diplopia, and eye movement abnormalities were eliminated. No visual acuity impairment was observed. Postoperative follow-up MRI examination revealed no residual tumor (Figure 8). Informed consent was obtained from the patient for this study and publication of accompanying images and videos. Our study was performed according to the Declaration of Helsinki.

3. Discussion

Optic nerve astrocytomas (ONAs) are usually low-grade tumors although their presentation and clinical course are highly variable and unpredictable (Table 1). Gliomas

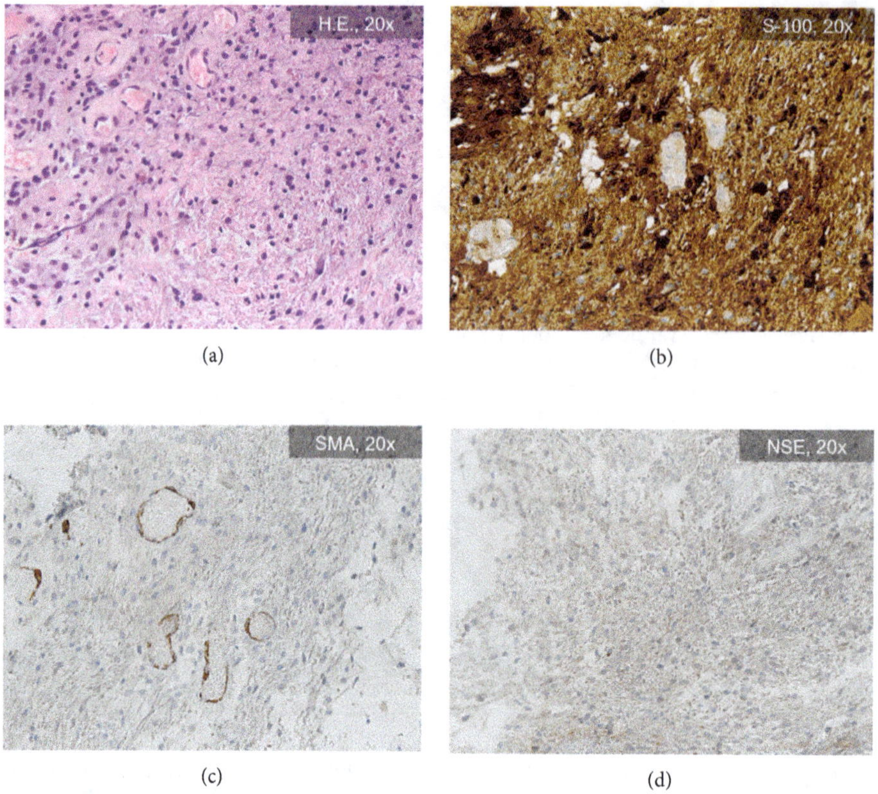

FIGURE 7: Images of histopathologic examination of the surgical specimen. (a) Hematoxylin-eosin staining represents a solid tumor with several cells showing a vortical pattern. (b) Tumor cells show intense S-100-specific immunoreaction. (c) The smooth muscular actin- (SMA-) specific immunoreaction is practically negative. (d) The neuron-specific enolase- (NSE-) specific immunoreaction represents a strong granular cytoplasmic positivity.

presenting in adulthood are generally very aggressive with rapid decline in vision leading to spread throughout the central nervous system and death [4, 5].

ONGs are extraordinarily rare and seldom seen in routine clinical practice. The pilocytic variant of glioma (astrocytoma) usually affects childhood or early adolescents and is benign and noninvasive in nature [6–8]. These tumors, in most instances, affect the anterior optic pathway and clinically manifest as uniocular visual loss and proptosis [4, 9–11].

There are two possible explanations for the origin of the tumor. One possibility is that brain heterotopia occurred during development, with subsequent sequestration and anatomic discontinuity. This would have been followed by tumor development with effacement of all heterotopic brain tissue. A second possibility is mesenchymal stem cells giving rise to the tumor. The presence of a complete layer of meninges and a cystic cavity would favor a developmental outpouching of embryonic brain rather than a mesenchymal stem cell derivation. It is interesting to note that the glioma was "invading" the surrounding orbital fat through a dural defect. It is worth speculating whether this defect may have represented the point at which the heterotopic tissue was tethered to the rest of the brain before losing its anatomic connection [12]. In general, gliomas of the posterior optic pathways rarely present with proptosis. However, the absence of proptosis does not necessarily preclude sparing of the intraorbital segments of the optic nerve. Optic pathway gliomas are known to be associated with neurofibromatosis type 1; however, our patient did not seem to have this condition [13].

When imaged in cross section, two thirds of all ONAs demonstrate a classic appearance: a cystic mass with an enhancing mural nodule. However, less common appearances are quite nonspecific [14]. A feature specific of this benign neoplasm is that in many cases it displays histologic and imaging features that are commonly seen in higher grade neoplasms and appear incongruous for a slow-growing brain tumor with fairly bland histologic characteristics, such as microvascular proliferation, infiltration of surrounding tissues and structures, intratumoral hemorrhage, intense enhancement on postcontrast images, and leptomeningeal dissemination [15].

Understanding the natural history of these tumors is essential if patients are to receive optimal treatment. For WHO grade I gliomas, the surgical outcome is usually good (Table 1). Poor prognosis is observed for gliomas invading the optic pathways from adjacent parts of the brain, such as the hypothalamus, or suprasellar region [16].

Good quality MRI has almost negated the need for surgical biopsy and is invaluable in the accurate planning of treatment [17]. Surgical excision is only very rarely indicated and is usually limited to those patients with a tumor confined to a single optic nerve and documented radiological evidence of tumor progression toward, but not involving, the optic

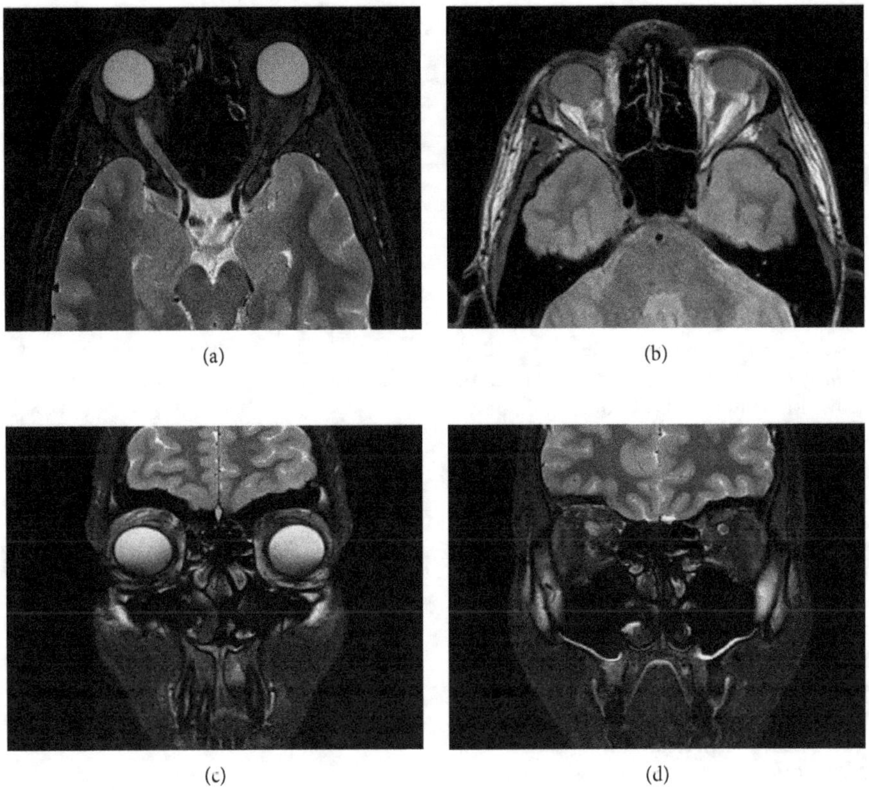

FIGURE 8: Postoperative MRI scans (3 months). Axial and coronal T1 (a, c) and T2-weighted (b, d) MRI images show normal anatomical conditions with no residual tumor mass.

chiasm. For aggressive tumors, biopsy may be indicated to confirm diagnosis prior to commencing adjuvant therapy [18, 19]. The treatment of ONA is highly individualized, and clinicians should be aware of the benefits and disadvantages of the various treatment options [20].

Although gross total resection of the tumor is often curative, location in critical or deep areas (such as the brainstem and hypothalamus) can render it unresectable and require additional management approaches [21]. Strategies for treating ONA in critical or deep areas, such as chiasmatic and brainstem ONAs, include observation and combinations of surgery, chemotherapy, and radiotherapy. Recent studies have demonstrated that chemotherapy should be the first-line treatment strategy for all patients who have radiological and/or clinical progression, although the best choice of agent(s) remains unclear. Radiotherapy is proven to be effective in combating recurrent and progressive disease, but the side effects of such treatment must always be considered. At present, multifractionated conformal radiotherapy remains the most widely used treatment, but newer techniques of delivering focused radiation continue to advance and may be more beneficial [22]. Although pathological diagnosis remains the gold standard, preoperative diagnosis of tumor behavior and extent is of utmost importance in selecting the appropriate therapeutic management in every single case. Quite often, the diagnosis of ONA is initially made or suggested on the basis of an imaging study. Therefore, it is important for all radiologists to be aware of the many clinical and radiological manifestations of this tumor type.

4. Conclusion

Prompt clinical suspicion aided by imaging and histopathologic studies can aid in early diagnosis and subsequent management to improve outcome and reduce morbidity. In this case, surgical excision was done with clinical improvement seen. As mentioned earlier, follow-up MRI examination is planned few months later, and depending on the result, appropriate next management plan will be adequately applied.

Disclosure

All authors have read the final version of the manuscript with full agreement of submission. This paper has not been submitted elsewhere simultaneously, and it is not under consideration in other journals or books. We declare that it is an original report.

References

[1] H. S. Mudhar, M. Nuruddin, and S. Roy, "Primary orbital cystic pilocytic astrocytoma," *Ocular Oncology and Pathology*, vol. 2, pp. 280–284, 2016.

[2] J. Shapey, H. V. Danesh-Meyer, and A. H. Kaye, "Diagnosis and management of optic nerve glioma," *Journal of Clinical Neuroscience*, vol. 18, no. 12, pp. 1585–1591, 2011.

[3] T. J. Cummings, J. M. Provenzale, S. B. Hunter et al., "Gliomas of the optic nerve: histological, immunohistochemical (MIB-1 and p53) and MRI analysis," *Acta Neuropathologica*, vol. 99, no. 5, pp. 563–570, 2000.

[4] E. C. Alvord Jr. and S. Lofton, "Gliomas of the optic nerve or chiasm. Outcome by patients' age, tumour site and treatment," *Journal of Neurosurgery*, vol. 68, no. 1, pp. 85–98, 1988.

[5] M. Eghtedari, S. F. Fattahi, N. Owji, M. J. Ashraf, M. R. Khalili, and B. Geramizadeh, "Optic nerve glioma with complete intraocular extension," *Journal of Current Ophthalmology*, vol. 28, no. 4, pp. 228–231, 2016.

[6] E. Czyzyk, S. Jóźwiak, M. Roszkowski et al., "Optic pathway gliomas in children with and without neurofibromatosis 1," *Journal of Child Neurology*, vol. 18, no. 7, pp. 471–478, 2003.

[7] J. L. Zeid, J. Charrow, M. Sandu et al., "Orbital optic nerve gliomas in children with neurofibromatosis type 1," *Journal of AAPOS*, vol. 10, no. 6, pp. 534–539, 2006.

[8] A. M. Chutorian, J. F. Schwartz, R. A. Evans, and S. Carter, "Optic gliomas in children," *Neurology*, vol. 14, pp. 83–95, 1964.

[9] R. J. Packer, P. J. Savino, L. T. Bilaniuk et al., "Carboplatin and vincristine for recurrent and newly diagnosed low-grade gliomas of childhood," *Journal of Clinical Oncology*, vol. 11, no. 5, pp. 850–856, 1993.

[10] M. Ulutas, S. Boyacı, A. Akakın, T. Kılıç, and K. Aksoy, "Surgical anatomy of the cavernous sinus, superior orbital fissure, and orbital apex via a lateral orbitotomy approach: a cadaveric anatomical study," *Acta Neurochirurgica*, vol. 158, no. 11, pp. 2135–2148, 2016.

[11] N. Lamba, D. P. Dworak, S. A. Patel, and R. Chennuri, "A case report of primary orbital non-Hodgkin's lymphoma causing complete vision loss," *GMS Ophthalmology Cases*, vol. 6, 2016.

[12] A. J. Scheiner, W. C. Frayer, L. B. Rorke, and K. Heher, "Ectopic brain tissue in the orbit," *Eye*, vol. 13, no. 2, pp. 251–254, 1999.

[13] S. Thiagalingam, M. Flaherty, F. Billson et al., "Neurofibromatosis type 1 and optic pathway gliomas: follow up of 54 patients," *Ophthalmology*, vol. 111, no. 3, pp. 568–577, 2004.

[14] E. D. Feijó, A. C. Nery, F. R. Caiado, A. M. Prehis, and R. M. Limongi, "Extraconal cystic schwannoma mimicking an orbital dermoid cyst," *Arquivos Brasileiros de Oftalmologia*, vol. 79, no. 4, pp. 258–260, 2016.

[15] A. Ducasse, J. C. Merol, F. Bonnet, F. Litré, C. Arndt, and I. Larré, "Adult orbital tumors," *Journal Français d'Ophtalmologie*, vol. 39, no. 4, pp. 387–399, 2016.

[16] N. M. Miller, "Primary tumors of the optic nerve and its sheath," *Eye*, vol. 18, no. 11, pp. 1026–1037, 2004.

[17] T. T. Shen, O. Sakai, H. D. Curtin et al., "Magnetic resonance imaging of primaryanterior visual pathway tumours," *International Ophthalmology Clinics*, vol. 41, no. 1, pp. 171–180, 2001.

[18] B. Gorkem, A. Majed, B. Laura, J. G. Ben et al., "Aggressive low-grade optic nerve glioma in adults," *Neuro-Opthalmology*, vol. 38, no. 6, pp. 297–309, 2014.

[19] A. A. Campbell, S. R. Grob, and M. K. Yoon, "Novel surgical approaches to the orbit," *Middle East African Journal of Ophthalmology*, vol. 22, no. 4, pp. 435–441, 2015.

[20] I. Dallan, P. Castelnuovo, M. Turri-Zanoni et al., "Transorbital endoscopic assisted management of intraorbital lesions: lessons learned from our first 9 cases," *Rhinology*, vol. 54, no. 3, pp. 247–253, 2016.

[21] M. Seiichiro, H. Yoshinori, H. Kentaro, and S. Naokatu, "Superolateral orbitotomy for intraorbital tumors: comparison with the conventional approach," *Journal of Neurological Surgery Part B: Skull Base*, vol. 77, no. 6, pp. 473–478, 2016.

[22] M. Alireza, A. Amelot, D. Chauvet, L. M. Terrier, G. Lot, and O. Bekaert, "Poor prognosis and challenging treatment of optic nerve malignant gliomas: literature review and case report series," *World Neurosurgery*, vol. 97, pp. 751.e1–751.e6, 2016.

28

Tracheal Chondrosarcoma: Systematic Review of Tumor Characteristics, Diagnosis, and Treatment Outcomes with Case Report

Emily A. Kutzner,[1] Joshua S. Park,[2] Salman Zaheer,[3] and Jared C. Inman[2]

[1]*School of Medicine, Loma Linda University, 11175 Campus St., Loma Linda, CA 92350, USA*
[2]*Department of Otolaryngology-Head and Neck Surgery, Loma Linda University Medical Center, 11234 Anderson St., Suite 2586A, Loma Linda, CA 92354, USA*
[3]*Department of Cardiothoracic Surgery, Loma Linda University Medical Center, 11234 Anderson St., Suite 1637, Loma Linda, CA 92354, USA*

Correspondence should be addressed to Emily A. Kutzner; ekutzner@llu.edu

Academic Editor: Ossama W. Tawfik

To our knowledge this is the first systematic review of tracheal chondrosarcoma treatment outcomes. Management insights are thoroughly discussed. Men constitute 93.8% of cases, and most of these occur in the distal trachea. The most common symptom, dyspnea, occurs in virtually all patients. Extratracheal extension had occurred in 78.6% of patients. Definitive treatment with tracheal resection showed no recurrences in 10 patients with mean follow-up of 3.1 years. Adjuvant radiotherapy may be utilized for improving local control when open complete resection cannot be performed, but only after endoscopic excision of gross tumor.

1. Introduction

Tracheal chondrosarcomas are exceptionally rare, with only 17 cases having been reported in the English literature, to date. Moreover, the whole body of literature for different subsites of chondrosarcoma is also underwhelming in its discussion of advanced treatment decisions in high risk or surgically difficult areas to address, specifically multimodality treatment options. A systematic review of the current English-language literature was performed in an effort to further characterize these rare tumors and to determine treatment outcomes with different management techniques—namely, surgical excision with negative margins. Additionally, we include our own case of a 61-year-old male patient with tracheal chondrosarcoma treated with open tracheal resection and end-to-end anastomosis, without adjuvant therapy.

2. Materials and Methods

A systematic literature review of all cases of tracheal chondrosarcoma reported in English literature was performed independently by two authors (E.K., J.I.). The PubMed database, Cochrane Library, Web of Science, and Google Scholar were searched, using the medical subject heading terms of "tracheal chondrosarcoma," "trachea chondrosarcoma", "chondrosarcoma", "cartilaginous tumor trachea", "trachea", and "tracheal" to accumulate cases reported during the time period of 1966 (when PubMed was officially started) to January 4, 2016. We limited the search to include only cases published in the English-language literature. Inclusion criteria required a diagnosis of primary tracheal chondrosarcoma. The references included in these cases as well as those included in additional relevant articles were incorporated as references in this review. Two additional cases, one with an English abstract listed on PubMed and one referenced in several other case reports, were published in Japanese and were excluded from this study [1, 2]. Another two case reports published in English in 1954 and 1959 (prior to our the start of our inclusion period) were referenced in several of the case reports in this study; however the tumors in these reports were poorly described and relatively uncharacterized

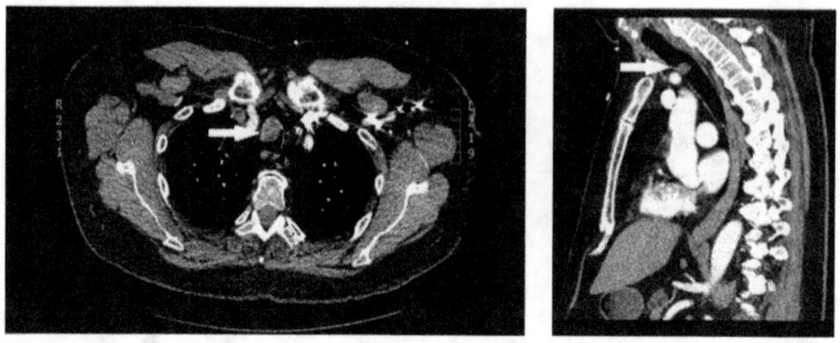

(a)

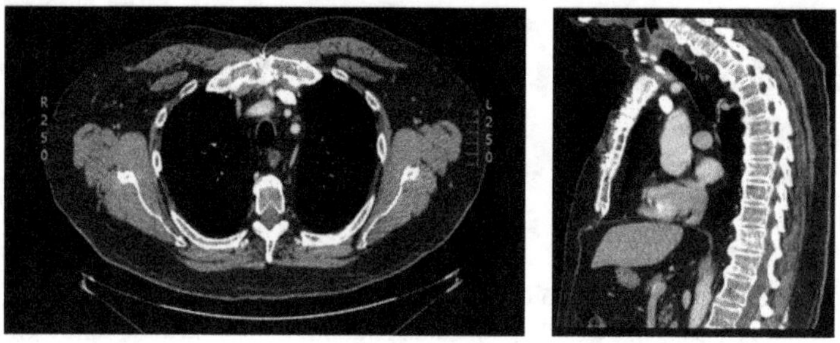

(b)

FIGURE 1: CT scan preoperative axial and sagittal views of the tumor (white arrows, (a)); postoperative views of resected trachea (b).

[3, 4]. Two authors independently performed the literature search and data extraction, combined their findings, and removed duplicates (E.K., J.I.). Details of the literature selection strategy are diagramed in Figure 2 following the PRISMA statement format from 2009 [5]. Patient data from the case reports were recorded in Excel ©2013 and pertinent, or predominately present, data were analyzed and used for cohort analysis. Each discrepancy or uncertainty was explored and resolved by author consensus. Institutional review board was applied for and granted exemption.

3. Results

The description of our experience with a unique case of tracheal chondrosarcoma is detailed below, and our specific patient details are outlined in Table 1, along with the data extracted from the previously reported cases of tracheal chondrosarcoma [6–20]. Our review yielded 15 previously reported cases of tracheal chondrosarcoma in the English literature, the majority of which involved elderly men, with most lesions occurring in the lower trachea. Further data extraction is compiled in Tables 2 and 3 [6–20].

A 61-year-old morbidly obese male patient with a 4-year history of stable obstructive sleep apnea (OSA) presented to Loma Linda University Medical Center Emergency Department with a 2-day history of acute dyspnea. The patient had been experiencing progressively worsening dyspnea over the course of approximately 2 months.

A neck computed tomography (CT) scan demonstrated an intraluminal tracheal mass, 2.2 × 2.1 × 1.3 cm in size, obstructing approximately 75% of the tracheal lumen (Figure 1). The tumor origin was 6 cm caudal to the true vocal folds, at the level of the innominate artery. There was a suspicion of extraluminal extension but no calcification appreciated on CT (Figure 1).

Initially, the patient underwent endoscopic debulking of tumor to restore the airway and obtain pathology specimens. Approximately 75% of the gross tumor was removed at that time. Based on the final pathology report from these specimens, the patient was diagnosed with grade 1 chondrosarcoma of the trachea.

Definitive treatment for this patient was open tracheal resection. Transcervical exposure with mini-sternotomy was performed and endotracheal endoscopic video-assisted methylene blue was injected transtracheally to identify the margins of the tracheal resection. Once the tracheal margins were marked and visualized externally, the innominate artery was retracted while a 4 cm tracheal sleeve, including the tumor, was resected. On gross appearance, the tumor was firm, mucosalized, and cartilaginous. Margins were clear by 1.2 cm superiorly and 1.4 cm inferiorly. The free ends of the trachea were approximated by primary anastomosis, using 2-0 and 4-0 polydioxanone sutures, placed externally submucosally in standard fashion. Grillo stitches were placed to remove tension from the trachea in case of excessive patient movement.

The postoperative course was uneventful. The patient remained on a ventilator with the endotracheal tube balloon positioned distal to the tracheal anastomosis for 48 hours. He then underwent flexible bronchoscopy, which confirmed that the mucosa of the anastomosis appeared "sealed." The patient was then weaned off the ventilator, extubated, and placed on prophylactic proton-pump inhibitor and Valsalva/anticoughing precautions with head of bed elevation. A swallow study the following day was normal, a diet was begun, and the patient was discharged on postoperative day four. The

Table 1: Selected characteristics of 18 cases of tracheal chondrosarcoma.

Year	First author	Sex	Age	Symptoms	Symptom duration (months)	Location	Grade (1–3)	Extratracheal extension	Size (cm)	Calcification	Treatment	Number of recurrences	Follow-up (years)
1967	Daniels	M	73	D, C, W	7	Lower	2	NR	2.5	NR	(1) ER[‡] (2) ER	5 (local)	AWD, 3.0
1973	Fallahnejad	F	48	D, C, W	16	Upper	NR	Present	4.0	None	R	0	NED, 5.0
1978	Weber	M	71	D, C, Ho	4	Middle	NR	Present	3.0	Present	R	0	NED, 5.0
1985	Slasky	M	58	D	24	Lower	2	Present	2.0	Present	R	0	NED, 2.5
1986	Arévalo	M	74	D, P	0.25	Upper	1	Present	2.0	Present	R	0	NED, 1.0
1988	Matsuo	M	72	D, He	7	Middle	1	Present	5.0	None	(1) IR[‡] (2) LaR (3) R	1	NED, 0.5
1990	Salminen	M	57	D, C	3	Lower	3	Present	2.3	None	IR	5 (local & distant)	DOD, 14
1994	Leach	M	72	D	36	Lower	3	Present	6.5	Present	R	NR	NR
1998	Farrell	M	87	D	12	Middle	2	Present	3.0	NR	(1) ER[*,‡] (2) ER (3) Rad	2 (local)	AWD, 1.0
1997	Kiriyama	M	54	D, W	1	Lower	1	NR	2.0	Present	LaDeb/R[§]	0	NED, 3.5
2003	Maish	M	78	D	3	Lower	1	Present	NR	None	LaDeb/R[§]	0	NED, 0.5
2008	Umezu	M	34	D, He, W	8	Upper	1	Present	2.5	Present	R	0	NED, 6.3
2009[†]	Wagnetz	M	34	D, C, W	18	Upper	2	None	2.0	Present	ER/R[§]	NR	NR
2010	Mendonça	M	72	D, W, O	12	Upper	1	Present	NR	Present	LaDeb/Rad[§]	0	NED, 7.0
2010[†]	de Almeida	M	35	D	NR	Upper	2	None	NR	Present	R	NR	NR
2016	Kutzner	M	61	D	2	Lower	1	None	2.2	Present	ER/R[§]	0	NED, 1.0

M, male; F, female; NR, not recorded; C, cough; D, dyspnea; W, wheeze; Ho, hoarse; P, pneumonia; He, hemoptysis; O, odynophagia; R, resection; ER, endoscopic resection; IR, incomplete resection; LaR, laser resection; LaDeb/R, laser debulking/resection; UNK, unknown; Rad, radiotherapy; NED, no evidence of disease; AWD, alive with disease; DOD, died of disease. [*]Refused resection. [†]Patient with Maffucci Syndrome. [‡]Patient with recurrences treated in numerical order. [§]Patient symptomatically treated with laser debulking or with endoscopic resection prior to definitive treatment of resection or radiotherapy.

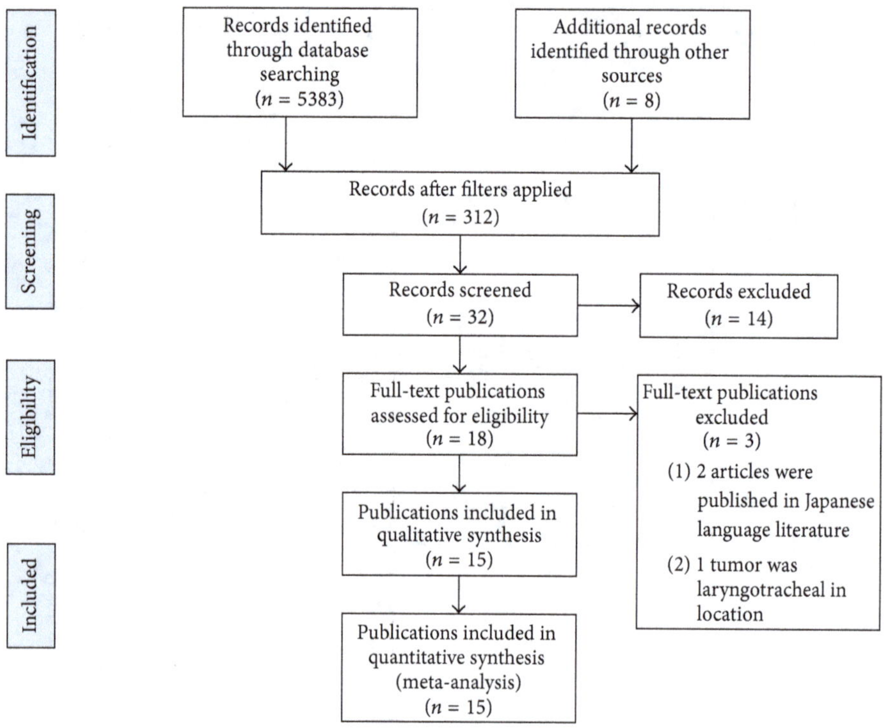

FIGURE 2: PRISMA diagram of the literature selection process.

TABLE 2: Analysis of selected characteristics of tracheal chondrosarcoma [6–20].

Characteristic		Mean	Median	Mode	Range
Age (years)		61.3	66	72	34–87
Size (cm)		3.0	2.5	2.0	2.0–6.5
Symptom duration (months)		10.2	7	7	0.25–36
	Number of cases/number reported	Percentage			
Male	15/16	93.8%			
Symptoms					
Dyspnea	16/16	100.0%			
Wheeze	6/16	37.5%			
Cough	5/16	31.3%			
Hemoptysis	2/16	12.5%			
Hoarseness	1/16	6.3%			
Odynophagia	1/16	6.3%			
Grade					
1	7/14	50.0%			
2	5/14	35.7%			
3	2/14	14.3%			
Tracheal location					
Lower	7/16	43.8%			
Upper	6/16	37.5%			
Middle	3/16	18.8%			
Calcification	10/14	71.4%			
Extratracheal	11/14	78.6%			

TABLE 3: Patient recurrence rates with regard to treatment modality [6–20].

Definitive treatment modality	Follow-up reported	Number of cases				Length of follow-up (years)			Recurrence rate
		REC	NED	AWD	DOD	Mean	Median	Range	
Open resection ([7–10, 13, 15–18, 20], present case)	11	0	10	0	0	3.1	3	0.5–6.3	0%
Endoscopic resection only [6, 14]	2	7	0	2	0	2	2	1–3	100%
Incomplete resection [11, 12]	2	5	1	0	1	7.3	7.3	0.5–14.0	100%
Endoscopic resection + XRT [19]	1	0	1	0	0	7	7	7	0%
Overall	16	12*	13	2	1	4.8	5	0.5–14.0	75%

XRT: external beam radiation therapy; REC, recurrence; NED, no evidence of disease; AWD, alive with disease; DOD, died of disease. *Multiple recurrences in small number of patients.

patient was alive without disease recurrence 1 year after surgery, based on follow-up CT (Figure 1) and in office bronchoscopy. In this case, the patient was elected by clinical judgment to be kept intubated for 48 hours, pending future bronchoscopy for mucosal healing before extubation due to the degree of tension placed on the 4 cm sleeve anastomosis intraoperatively and the proximity of the tracheal anastomosis to the innominate artery—clinically anastomotic failure was deemed to be highly morbid in this diabetic, morbidly obese man.

4. Discussion

Chondrosarcomas are rare, accounting for only 0.2% of malignancies of the head and neck [21]. These cartilaginous tumors most frequently originate in the pelvis, femur, humerus, and ribs. Only 10–12% of all chondrosarcomas occur in the head and neck area, where the most common sites of origin include the larynx and maxillonasal regions [22, 23]. Our analysis of 16 cases, including the present one, revealed that these tumors occur most often in the elderly, with an average age of 61.3 years at the time of diagnosis and a range of 34–87 years. Two cases occurred in younger males, aged 34 and 35, with Maffucci Syndrome, a rare disease in which diffuse enchondromatosis and cutaneous hemangiomas occur throughout the body [18, 20]. There is a considerable propensity for males, as only one of the recorded patients was female. These tumors occur most frequently in the lower third of the trachea (43.8%), followed by the upper third (37.5%) and the middle third (18.8%). The average tumor size is 3.0 cm, with a range of 2.0–6.5 cm.

Patients with tracheal chondrosarcoma are often asymptomatic until the tumor occludes greater than 75% of the tracheal lumen [14, 17]. The most commonly reported symptoms include dyspnea (the most common symptom, occurring in 100% of these patients), nonproductive cough, and wheeze. As the "alarm sign" of hemoptysis is present only in 12.5% of these cases, the above combination of symptoms can often lead to misdiagnosis of this condition as an acute exacerbation of asthma or chronic obstructive pulmonary disease (COPD) [12, 14, 16, 17].

Computed tomography (CT) is the imaging method of choice for tracheal chondrosarcomas [16]. CT allows for the determination of tumor size, location, presence/absence of calcification, degree of luminal obstruction, and the presence/absence of extratracheal extension [16, 17]. Calcification is present in 71.4% of these tumors and extratracheal extension is observed in 78.6%.

Bronchoscopy is the gold standard for diagnosis, as it allows for collection of pathology specimens as well as for symptomatic treatment of airway compromise via endoscopic resection or laser debulking of the tumor [16].

Unlike chondrosarcomas of the bone and lung, chondrosarcomas of the head and neck tend to be low-grade and slow-growing, with low risk of metastasis [14, 24]. Lymph node involvement occurs in only 5% of cases, and distant metastases occur in only 7–18% [24, 25]. Thus, the lethality of these tumors stems not from distant metastasis but from local aggression, intra-axial invasion, and a high local recurrence rate if not adequately resected [24–27]. Of note, 71% of high-grade (grade 3) chondrosarcomas of the head and neck present with distant metastases [24, 28, 29].

There is one reported case of tracheal chondrosarcoma, which developed distant metastases following malignant transformation of an incompletely resected tracheal chondroma into a grade 3 chondrosarcoma—a case which proved fatal even after multiple resections, 14 years following diagnosis and initial therapy [12].

Definitive treatment for the majority of the patients in this review (11/16) was open surgical resection, with negative margins, of the involved portion of the trachea. No recurrences have been reported in this group of patients, to date. Contrastingly, recurrent disease has been reported in both of the patients (100%) who underwent endoscopic resection as definitive treatment of the tumor [6, 14]. External beam radiotherapy was utilized as adjunctive treatment following laser resection of the tumor in one patient with grade 1 chondrosarcoma in whom open resection was absolutely contraindicated, and the patient remained disease-free 7 years later [19]. Adjuvant radiotherapy has also been used alongside repeat endoscopic resection to treat disease recurrence in a patient who initially underwent endoscopic resection as definitive treatment, after he had refused open resection of the tumor. This patient was alive with the disease at 1-year follow-up [14]. Table 3 shows the extracted, combined patient surveillance status at follow-up and the disease recurrence rate with regard to treatment modality [6–20].

As chondrosarcomas of the trachea are exceedingly rare, a review of other head and neck chondrosarcoma subsites and whole body sites with treatment analysis should also be considered when discussing treatment options. In the head and neck, one of the most common subsites for chondrosarcomas to originate is the larynx. Achieving adequate resection of these tumors while sparing laryngeal function is ideal. Endoscopic removal, thyrotomy, laryngofissure, are partial laryngectomy are laryngeal function-sparing techniques that can achieve wide excision of the tumor along with a sufficient margin of uninvolved cartilage [30]. Unfortunately, however, up to 75% of these tumors involve the cricoid cartilage, which is considered crucial for laryngeal function [30–32]. Traditionally, total laryngectomy has been recommended for tumors involved in greater than 50% of the cricoid cartilage. However, CO2 lasering and reconstructive techniques such as thyrotracheal anastomosis over a stent and rib graphs suggest that laryngeal function can still be preserved in these patients [30, 33]. Importantly, recurrence rates of laryngeal chondrosarcomas have been reported at 35–40%, with a tendency for late recurrence [30]. Thus, patients with head and neck chondrosarcomas should be followed continuously, with a high level of suspicion for recurrence [22]. The prognosis of low-grade laryngeal chondrosarcoma, when treated adequately, shows an overall survival rate of 95% at 10 years. Tumor grade, composition, and type of surgical procedure performed should be considered when determining individual prognoses [30, 33–35].

As there are no evidence-based recommendations for margin control in head and neck chondrosarcomas, broadening our discussion to include the optimal treatment for whole body chondrosarcomas warrants consideration. Recent studies of low-grade chondrosarcomas in the extremities have found that aggressive intralesional curettage, with or without cryosurgery at the margin, may be an acceptable alternative to wide excision of these lesions [36, 37]. These initial studies demonstrate that recurrence rates after aggressive intralesional excision are relatively low and that they do not differ, significantly, from those of wide excision (3.8% recurred in intralesional excision and 1.8% recurred in wide excision). Postsurgical functionality is greater in patients treated conservatively with intralesional curettage than in those treated aggressively with wide excision [22, 35]. These findings may suggest that the aggressiveness of treatment modality of low-grade chondrosarcomas of the extremities may be tailored for each individual based on tumor characteristics that may help predict tumor behavior, such as location and degree of differentiation. For tumors originating in the trachea, recurrences may be more difficult to treat and aggressive intralesional treatment is not a likely viable option, as the integrity of the tracheal wall must be maintained in order to keep the air filled luminal space separate from the negative pressure mediastinal cavity. Of note, this particular long bone surgical concept difficultly reconciles with the data collected from the tracheal patients examined in this review because, in this study, the mean tumor size was 3.0 cm (range, 2.0–6.5 cm) and extratracheal extension was present in 78.6% of these patients. Partial excision, or complete gross tumor endoscopic resection with adjunctive treatment to the margin, is likely not feasible in most cases of tracheal chondrosarcoma, due to their size at diagnosis and/or the presence of extratracheal extension compromising the integrity of the tracheal wall. What this evolving long bone treatment paradigm may help show is that low-grade chondrosarcomas likely do not require the same degree of margin control as do other sarcomas in minimizing local recurrence rates. From this literature and the laryngeal chondrosarcoma literature, it seems evident that less aggressive margin clearance into normal tissue applies in low-grade chondrosarcomas, achieving acceptably low recurrence rates—unlike most other sarcomas. However, observation and recurrence in the trachea are not the same as an extremity, as the trachea must retain its patency for air-flow and tumors of any appreciable size would become symptomatic. Further research is needed on the overall recurrence rates of chondrosarcomas of varying histologic grades with regard to the precise degree of margin control.

Traditionally, chondrosarcomas have been thought to be relatively radioresistant, due, in part, to their low-grade nature [16, 24]. However, in recent studies, head and neck chondrosarcomas have shown a response to radiotherapy in certain circumstances [19, 24, 38–40]. As such, radiotherapy is now utilized as adjuvant therapy in high-grade tumors to combat local recurrence after surgical excision, inoperable tumors for palliation, recurrent tumors, patients with incomplete resection or positive margins, patients who are poor surgical candidates, and patients who refuse margin-clearing surgery [16, 24, 30].

Currently, no evidence exists to support the use of chemotherapy in the treatment of chondrosarcomas, although it is used by some in the treatment of high-grade tumors with a greater risk for metastases and should be considered in those with lymph node metastasis [22, 41].

References

[1] Y. Mine, K. Hirose, N. Itou et al., "A case of chondrosarcoma of the trachea," *The Journal of the Japan Society for Respiratory Endoscopy*, vol. 12, pp. 413–418, 1990.

[2] Y. Kaneda, S. Nawata, K. Sugi, T. Hirayama, and K. Esato, "Chondrosarcoma of the trachea—report of a case," *Nippon Kyobu Geka Gakkai Zasshi*, vol. 41, no. 9, pp. 1535–1540, 1993.

[3] H. J. Moersch, O. T. Clagett, and F. H. Ellis, "Tumors of the trachea," *Medical Clinics of North America*, vol. 38, no. 4, pp. 1091–1096, 1954.

[4] C. Jackson and C. L. Jackson, *Disease of the Nose, Throat and Ear*, W.B. Saunders Company, Philadelphia, Pa, USA, 1959.

[5] D. Moher, A. Liberati, J. Tetzlaff, and D. G. Altman, "Preferred reporting items for systematic reviews and meta-analyses: the PRISMA statement," *Annals of Internal Medicine*, vol. 151, no. 4, pp. 264–269, 2009.

[6] A. C. Daniels, G. H. Conner, and F. H. Straus, "Primary chondrosarcoma of the tracheobronchial tree," *Archives of Pathology & Laboratory Medicine*, vol. 84, pp. 615–624, 1967.

[7] M. Fallahnejad, D. Harrell, J. Tucker, J. Forest, and W. S. Blakemore, "Chondrosarcoma of the trachea," *The Journal of Thoracic and Cardiovascular Surgery*, vol. 65, pp. 210–213, 1973.

[8] A. L. Weber, M. Shortsleeve, M. Goodman, E. Montgomery, and H. C. Grillo, "Cartilaginous tumors of the larynx and trachea," *Radiologic Clinics of North America*, vol. 16, pp. 261–271, 1978.

[9] B. S. Slasky, R. L. Hardesty, and S. Wilson, "Tracheal chondrosarcoma with an overview of other tumors of the trachea," *Journal of Computed Tomography*, vol. 9, no. 3, pp. 225–231, 1985.

[10] M. Arévalo, J. Ordi, G. Renedo, R. Rami, and H. Oliva, "Chondrosarcoma of the trachea: Report of a case," *Respiration*, vol. 49, no. 2, pp. 147–151, 1986.

[11] T. Matsuo, S. Kinoshita, K. Iwasaki et al., "Chondrosarcoma of the trachea: a case report and literature review," *Acta Cytologica*, vol. 32, pp. 908–912, 1988.

[12] U.-S. Salminen, P. Halttunen, E. Taskinen, and S. Mattila, "Recurrence and malignant transformation of endotracheal chondroma," *The Annals of Thoracic Surgery*, vol. 49, no. 5, pp. 830–832, 1990.

[13] K. R. Leach, F. J. Martinez, J. W. Morelock, M. T. Korobkin, and M. B. Orringer, "Dyspnea and tracheal mass in an elderly man," *Chest*, vol. 105, no. 5, pp. 1555-1556, 1994.

[14] M. L. Farrell, J. L. Gluckman, and P. Biddinger, "Tracheal chondrosarcoma: a case report," *Head and Neck*, vol. 20, no. 6, pp. 568–572, 1998.

[15] M. Kiriyama, A. Masaoka, Y. Yamakawa, H. Niwa, I. Fukai, and T. Yamada, "Chondrosarcoma originating from the trachea," *Annals of Thoracic Surgery*, vol. 63, no. 6, pp. 1772-1773, 1997.

[16] M. Maish and A. A. Vaporciyan, "Chondrosarcoma arising in the trachea: a case report and review of the literature," *Journal of Thoracic and Cardiovascular Surgery*, vol. 126, no. 6, pp. 2077–2080, 2003.

[17] H. Umezu, M. Tamura, S. Kobayashi, N. Sawabata, K. Honma, and S. Miyoshi, "Tracheal chondrosarcoma," *General Thoracic and Cardiovascular Surgery*, vol. 56, no. 4, pp. 199–202, 2008.

[18] U. Wagnetz, D. Patsios, G. Darling, F. Las Heras, and D. Hwang, "Tracheal chondrosarcoma—a rare complication in Maffucci syndrome," *British Journal of Radiology*, vol. 82, no. 981, pp. e178-e181, 2009.

[19] V. Mendonça, M. Jorge, I. Monteiro-Grillo, M. J. Palhano, and S. Feijó, "Tracheal chondrosarcoma," *Clinical and Translational Oncology*, vol. 12, no. 8, pp. 576–580, 2010.

[20] J. R. de Almeida, N. A. Pagedar, S. Keshavjee, and R. Gilbert, "Chondrosarcoma of the trachea in a patient with Maffucci syndrome," *Journal of Otolaryngology—Head and Neck Surgery*, vol. 39, no. 2, pp. E12-E15, 2010.

[21] M. de Vincentiis, A. Greco, M. Fusconi, G. Pagliuca, S. Martellucci, and A. Gallo, "Total cricoidectomy in the treatment of laryngeal chondrosarcomas," *The Laryngoscope*, vol. 121, no. 11, pp. 2375–2380, 2011.

[22] P. Hong, S. M. Taylor, J. R. Trites, M. Bullock, J. G. Nasser, and R. D. Hart, "Chondrosarcoma of the head and neck: report of 11 cases and literature review," *Journal of Otolaryngology—Head and Neck Surgery*, vol. 38, no. 2, pp. 279–285, 2009.

[23] L. Gallego, L. Junquera, M. F. Fresno, and J. C. de Vicente, "Chondrosarcoma of the temporomandibular joint. A case report and review of the literature," *Medicina Oral, Patologia Oral y Cirugia Bucal*, vol. 14, no. 1, pp. E39-E43, 2009.

[24] S. Obeso, J. L. Llorente, J. P. Díaz-Molina, R. Sánchez-Fernández, J. Pablo Rodrigo, and C. Suárez, "Surgical treatment of head and neck chondrosarcomas," *Acta Otorrinolaringologica (English Edition)*, vol. 61, no. 4, pp. 262–271, 2010.

[25] D. S. Ruark, U. K. Schlehaider, and J. P. Shah, "Chondrosarcomas of the head and neck," *World Journal of Surgery*, vol. 16, no. 5, pp. 1010–1015, 1992.

[26] J. S. Oghalai, J. L. Buxbaum, R. K. Jackler, and M. W. McDermott, "Skull base chondrosarcoma originating from the petroclival junction," *Otology and Neurotology*, vol. 26, no. 5, pp. 1052–1060, 2005.

[27] J. E. Wanebo, R. E. Bristol, R. R. Porter, S. W. Coons, and R. F. Spetzler, "Management of cranial base chondrosarcomas," *Neurosurgery*, vol. 58, no. 2, pp. 249–254, 2006.

[28] A. G. Korten, H. J. ter Berg, G. H. Spincemaille, R. T. Van der Laan, and A. M. Van de Wel, "Intracranial chondrosarcoma: review of the literature and report of 15 cases," *Journal of Neurology, Neurosurgery & Psychiatry*, vol. 65, no. 1, pp. 88–92, 1998.

[29] P. Förander, T. Rähn, L. Kihlström, E. Ulfarsson, and T. Mathiesen, "Combination of microsurgery and Gamma Knife surgery for the treatment of intracranial chondrosarcomas," *Journal of Neurosurgery*, vol. 105, supplement, pp. 18–25, 2006.

[30] L. D. R. Thompson and F. H. Gannon, "Chondrosarcoma of the larynx: a clinicopathologic study of 111 cases with a review of the literature," *The American Journal of Surgical Pathology*, vol. 26, no. 7, pp. 836–851, 2002.

[31] M. Policarpo, F. Taranto, E. Aina, P. Valletti, and F. Pia, "Chondrosarcoma of the larynx: a case report," *Acta Otorhinolaryngological Italica*, vol. 28, pp. 38–41, 2008.

[32] Q. Wang, H. Chen, and S. Zhou, "Chondrosarcoma of the larynx: report of two cases and review of the literature," *International Journal of Clinical and Experimental Pathology*, vol. 8, no. 2, pp. 2068–2073, 2015.

[33] O. Y. Chin, P. M. Dubal, A. B. Sheikh et al., "Laryngeal chondrosarcoma: a systematic review of 592 cases," *The Laryngoscope*, vol. 127, no. 2, pp. 430–439, 2016.

[34] J. F. D. S. Oliveira, F. A. P. L. Branquinho, A. R. R. T. N. Monteiro, M. E. C. C. Portugal, and A. M. F. S. Guimarães, "Laryngeal chondrosarcoma—ten years of experience," *Brazilian Journal of Otorhinolaryngology*, vol. 80, no. 4, pp. 354–358, 2014.

[35] I. Buda, R. Hod, R. Feinmesser, and J. Shvero, "Chondrosarcoma of the larynx," *Israel Medical Association Journal*, vol. 14, pp. 681–684, 2012.

[36] M. Hickey, F. Farrokhyar, B. Deheshi, R. Turcotte, and M. Ghert, "A systematic review and meta-analysis of intralesional versus wide resection for intramedullary grade I chondrosarcoma of the extremities," *Annals of Surgical Oncology*, vol. 18, no. 6, pp. 1705–1709, 2011.

[37] D. Donati, S. Colangeli, M. Colangeli, C. Di Bella, and F. Bertoni, "Surgical treatment of grade I central chondrosarcoma," *Clinical Orthopaedics and Related Research*, vol. 468, no. 2, pp. 581–589, 2010.

[38] B. B. Burkey, H. T. Hoffman, S. R. Baker, A. F. Thornton, and K. D. McClatchey, "Chondrosarcoma of the head and neck," *Laryngoscope*, vol. 100, no. 12, pp. 1301–1305, 1990.

[39] A. R. Harwood, B. J. Cummings, and P. J. Fitzpatrick, "Radiotherapy for unusual tumors of the head and neck," *Journal of Otolaryngology*, vol. 13, no. 6, pp. 391–394, 1984.

[40] S. Gripp, H. Pape, and G. Schmitt, "Chondrosarcoma of the larynx: the role of radiotherapy revisited—a case report and review of the literature," *Cancer*, vol. 82, no. 1, pp. 108–115, 1998.

[41] B. B. Koch, L. H. Karnell, H. T. Huffman et al., "National cancer database report on chondrosarcoma of the head and neck," *Head & Neck*, vol. 22, no. 4, pp. 408–425, 2000.

29

Primary Angiosarcoma of the Spleen: Rare Diagnosis with Atypical Clinical Course

Filip Kohutek,[1] Ladislav Badik,[2] and Branislav Bystricky[1]

[1]*Department of Oncology, Faculty Hospital Trencin, Trencin, Slovakia*
[2]*Department of Radiology, Faculty Hospital Trencin, Trencin, Slovakia*

Correspondence should be addressed to Filip Kohutek; filip.kohutek@gmail.com

Academic Editor: Jose I. Mayordomo

Primary angiosarcoma of the spleen is a rare diagnosis with poor prognosis. Morphologically, it demonstrates conventional blood vessel differentiation. We present a case of 65-year-old female who underwent radical splenectomy for primary angiosarcoma of the spleen. After three-year disease-free interval, she was diagnosed with bone-only metastatic disease. Palliative radiotherapy and bisphosphonates kept her disease reasonably stable for another four years. After development of lung metastases, six cycles of single agent doxorubicin kept her progression-free for six years. Upon further progression in lungs, thirteen years after original diagnosis, lung biopsy confirmed metastatic splenic angiosarcoma in the lungs. She started weekly paclitaxel chemotherapy. Although splenic angiosarcoma generally carries grave prognosis, some patients may enjoy prolonged periods of disease stabilization. Durable benefit can be achieved in some patients with multimodality management. We review the literature focusing on systemic treatment for this rare tumor.

1. Introduction

Soft tissue sarcomas (STS) represent heterogeneous group of malignant tumors originating in mesenchymal tissue. These malignancies are rare and their treatment is usually centralized into large treatment centers. In the United States, estimated number of new cases of STS for 2016 is 12,310 and estimated number of deaths is 4,900 [1]. In Europe, average incidence of this group of malignancies is 4-5 patients/100,000 person-years [2]. According to WHO, STS can be classified into 40 morphological entities. There is a clear need for grouping of those numerous entities into larger groups in clinical practice as was done in non-Hodgkin's lymphomas.

Angiosarcomas contribute by less than 1% to all cases of STS. Malignant cells of angiosarcoma are derived from endothelial cells. Skin and visceral organs are mostly affected. On the contrary, only few cases of heart or large vessels involvement have been described. According to study of 98 cases by Shon et al. [3], there was no difference in prognosis between skin and visceral angiosarcoma.

However, the results of retrospective study of Fury et al. [4] showed that primary site of angiosarcoma actually had impact on its prognosis; better median survival (43.1 m versus 27.6 m) was observed in superficial (skin) angiosarcomas.

Herein we present a case of female patient with primary splenic angiosarcoma. Despite development of stage IV disease, long-time survival and good quality of life could be observed.

2. Case Report

65-year-old female patient was admitted to Faculty Hospital Trencin, Department of Surgery, in January 2003 with palpable abdominal mass in left hypochondrium. The patient was only complaining about mild abdominal pain. Her past medical history was unremarkable, and she did not have any known risk factors for angiosarcoma. Abdominal mass was detected by patient's general practitioner during regular health exam. CT was performed and large hypervascularised splenic tumor at size of 5 × 4 cm was detected. No metastases were present at the CT scan. Mild anaemia (haemoglobin 11 g/dL), leucocytosis (13.10 × 10^9/L), and thrombocytosis (507 × 10^9/L) could be observed in complete blood count. Biochemistry showed no abnormalities. Due to increased

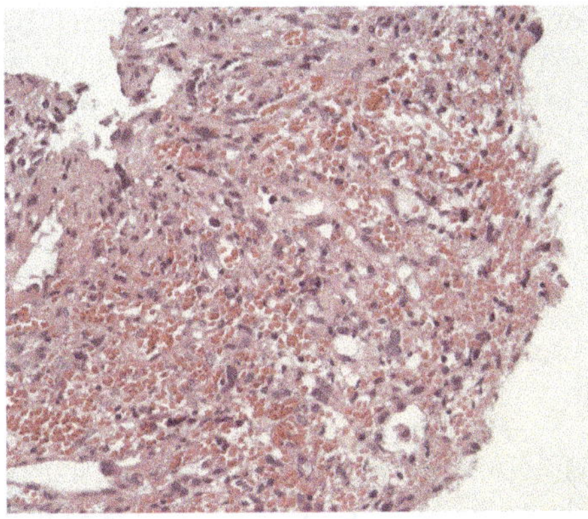

FIGURE 1: Primary splenic angiosarcoma. Staining with hematoxylin and eosin. 20-fold magnification.

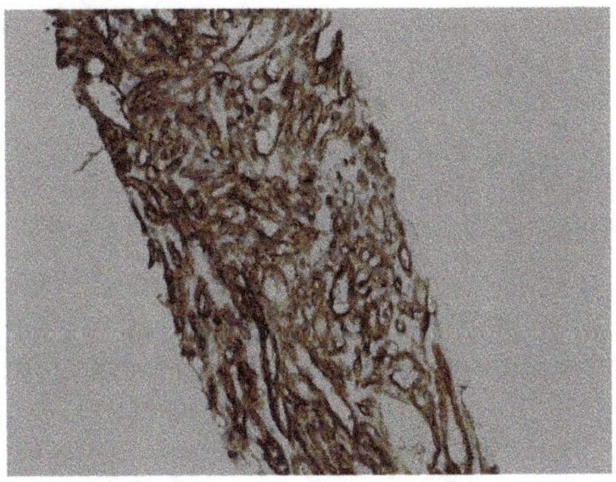

FIGURE 2: Primary splenic angiosarcoma. Immunohistochemical CD34 staining. 20-fold magnification.

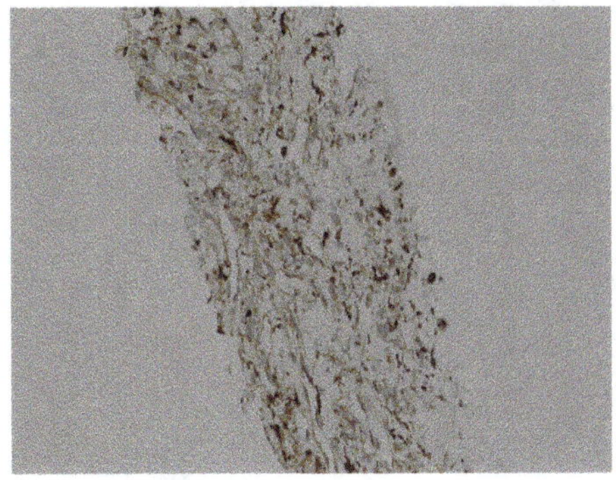

FIGURE 3: Primary splenic angiosarcoma. Immunohistochemical CD68 staining. 20-fold magnification.

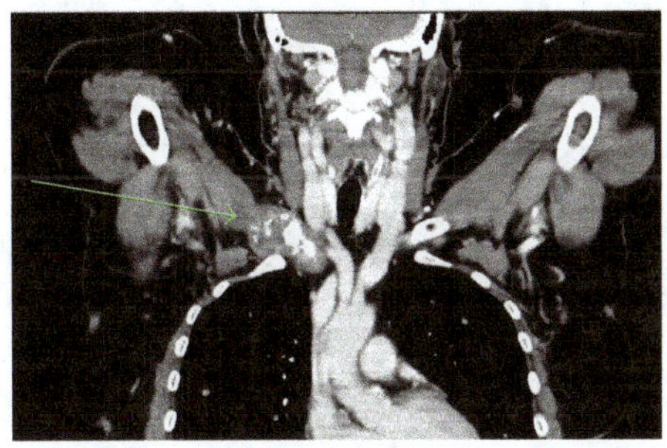

FIGURE 4: CT scan of thorax (multiplanar reconstruction). The green arrow points to osteolytic metastasis of right clavicle.

vascularity of tumor and possibility of seeding in localized malignancy, no CT-guided biopsy was performed. Subsequently, radical splenectomy was performed and definitive diagnosis of low-grade primary splenic angiosarcoma was made (Figures 1, 2, and 3). No adjuvant treatment was indicated due to low-grade disease and complete resection; routine follow-up was initiated. Three years later, the patient was complaining about 1-month lasting pain localized to upper thoracic spine and irradiating to neck and head. CT and bone scan was performed and multiple bone metastases (sacrum, left 11th rib, right scapula, right humerus, and right clavicle) were detected (Figure 4). Laboratory results showed no significant abnormalities in hematological or biochemical parameters. Palliative radiotherapy at dose of 20 Gy to right arm and clavicle was administered due to painful nature of these metastatic sites. Bisphosphonates were introduced into treatment as well. Palliative chemotherapy was proposed, but it was refused by patient. After 12 months, new metastatic deposit appeared at right sternoclavicular joint. Another course of palliative radiotherapy (20 Gy) was administered to affected site. Patient's attitude towards palliative chemotherapy did not change. However, during subsequent three years, no progression was detected on imaging.

Unfortunately, in 2010 new metastases in liver and axial skeleton were detected. With patient's approval, 6 cycles of palliative chemotherapy (doxorubicin 60 mg/m^2 triweekly) were given. During subsequent follow-up, no progression of disease was detected until 2016, when progression of metastatic lung lesions was noted. CT directed lung biopsy was performed (Figure 5). The result confirmed angiosarcoma metastasis. Vascular spaces were lined by atypical, highly pleomorphic cells with high nuclear to cytoplasm ratio. Intraluminally, occasional erythrocytes were seen. These cells were immunohistochemically positive for CD31, confirming vascular tumor arising from endothelial cells. MIB1 proliferation was 15% (Figure 6). At present, second-line chemotherapy (paclitaxel weekly) is ongoing.

3. Discussion

Exposure to radiation and lymphedema [5] and exposure to chemicals such as thorium, arsenic, and vinyl chloride are mostly recognized risk factors of angiosarcoma [6]. Retrospective study of Fayette et al. [5] showed that breast angiosarcoma contributes by 35% to all angiosarcomas. Whereas postoperative radiation following quadrantectomy or lumpectomy increases relative risk (RR) of angiosarcoma development more than 1,000 times, it can be concluded that breast angiosarcoma development is late adverse effect of adjuvant radiotherapy.

Splenic vascular tumors are currently classified into three broad categories: tumors arising from endothelial

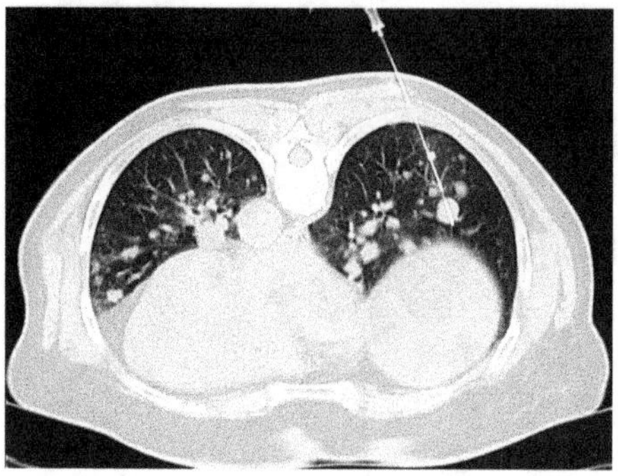

FIGURE 5: CT-guided needle biopsy of pulmonary metastasis of splenic angiosarcoma (20 G Trucut needle).

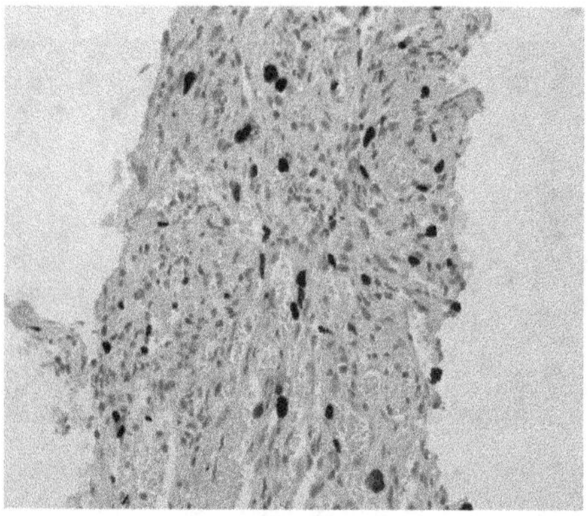

FIGURE 6: Pulmonary metastasis of splenic angiosarcoma. Immunohistochemical MIB1 staining. 20-fold magnification.

lining of blood vessels, lymphatic endothelium, and specialized endothelium (littoral/sinusoidal cells) with morphologic overlap between them [7].

It is presumed that splenic angiosarcoma originates from vascular endothelium of splenic sinuses [8]. It was described for the first time in 1879 by Langhans. Until now, only 300 cases of splenic angiosarcoma have been reported. Still, it is the most frequent nonlymphoid primary cancer of the spleen. Worldwide incidence of this disease reaches 0.14–0.25/million persons.

Natural course of this disease is usually characterized by rapid progression and unfavorable outcome for the patient. The most common symptom is abdominal pain and fullness with splenomegaly, anemia, and thrombocytopenia. Fatigue, weight loss, and fever are common systemic complaints of patients. Life threatening rupture of spleen is the first manifestation of this malignancy in numerous cases. Early appearance of metastases is typical; liver, lung, lymph nodes, and gastrointestinal system are preferred sites of metastases [9]. Median survival is only 5 months [10].

Considering rarity of this disease, no international guidelines are available for diagnosis and treatment of splenic angiosarcoma. If neoadjuvant treatment of intraabdominal sarcoma is intended, biopsy is indicated [11]. However, biopsy of highly vascularized spleen is considerably risk-bearing and is not usually performed. On CT scan, splenic angiosarcoma can present as heterogeneous mass with central hypoattenuation, except in acute bleeding, where high attenuation is observed. MRI shows hypointensive masses on T1 and high signal on T2 if necrosis or bleeding is present. Both imaging modalities can reveal splenomegaly and occasional splenic rupture with hemoperitoneum.

Radical surgical treatment (splenectomy) remains the only curative modality in the treatment of splenic angiosarcoma. Patients should undergo vaccination prior to or immediately after splenectomy in order to prevent severe bacterial infections. Splenectomy also provides tissue for histological examination. Although postoperative radiotherapy is associated with decreased local recurrence rate, it has not improved overall survival in intraabdominal sarcomas [12].

In unresectable stages, downstaging preceding surgery by neoadjuvant chemotherapy, radiotherapy, or chemoradiation can be attempted. If neoadjuvant therapy does not achieve sufficient down staging, treatment is palliative. Taxanes with or without gemcitabine are regarded as most effective in treatment of angiosarcoma.

In general, taxanes are considered to be effective in angiosarcoma but not in other soft tissue sarcomas. However, only limited data are available to support this statement.

Efficacy of weekly paclitaxel in advanced angiosarcoma was studied in phase II trial of French Sarcoma Group [13]. 30 patients with metastatic or locally advanced unresectable angiosarcoma were included into prospective study. Paclitaxel was administered at dose of $80\,mg/m^2$ on days 1, 8, and 15 of 4-week-long cycle. Taxane-based therapy achieved impressing results. Two-month-PFS was 74% and 4-month-PFS was 45%. Median time to progression (TTP) was 4 months and median overall survival (OS) was 8 months. Survival rates did not differ significantly in pretreated and chemotherapy-naive patients. Seven patients suffered from grade 3 or 4 toxicity and 1 patient died due to severe thrombocytopenia. Authors stated that paclitaxel-based chemotherapy of advanced angiosarcoma brought significant clinical benefit with acceptable toxicity.

Hirata et al. [14] published retrospective study of 41 patients with metastatic angiosarcoma. Patients were divided into 3 groups according to given treatment: taxane, nontaxane, and best-supportive care. Taxane-based chemotherapy achieved significant prolongation of PFS and OS compared to non-taxane-based chemotherapy and best-supportive care. Authors suggest that taxane-based chemotherapy may be more effective than nontaxane therapy in this setting.

The search for predictive factors of taxane chemotherapy brought first results. Expression of transducin-like enhancer of split 3 (TLE3) has been associated with better outcomes of taxane therapy [3].

As mentioned above, angiosarcoma is a malignancy originating from vascular endothelium and proangiogenic factors, such as vascular endothelial growth factor (VEGF), playing an important role in its pathogenesis. Sunitinib has been approved for imatinib-refractory GIST and in advanced renal-cell carcinoma utilizing its antiangiogenic effect. So far, no randomized controlled trials are available with sunitinib in treatment of advanced angiosarcoma. Several case reports have been published. Yoo et al. [15] published a case report of older woman with chemotherapy-refractory advanced angiosarcoma of retroperitoneum. Whereas patient's worsening performance status did not allow the use of another chemotherapy regimen, sunitinib was used as a last resort. Treatment with sunitinib was associated with impressing tumor control. Volume doubling time (VDT) of tumor based on serial CT scans was calculated. Compared to previous chemotherapy, VDT value on sunitinib was significantly longer (145 days on sunitinib versus 16 days on paclitaxel and 66 days on doxorubicin).

Sorafenib is a tyrosine-kinase inhibitor targeting several tyrosine-kinases such as BRAF, vascular endothelial growth factor receptor (VEGFR), and others [16]. Efficacy of sorafenib in angiosarcoma was studied in phase II trial [17] of French Sarcoma Group. In this trial, patients were divided into two groups: those with superficial angiosarcoma and those with visceral angiosarcoma. Sorafenib showed insufficient antitumor activity in both groups. Nine-month PFS was 3.8% in patients with superficial angiosarcoma and 0% in patients with visceral sarcomas. The trial was halted prematurely due to unsatisfying results. Another multicenter phase II trial of Maki et al. [18] studied activity of sorafenib against various histological subtypes of sarcomas. In this trial, sorafenib was administered to patients with advanced sarcoma at the dose of 400 mg twice a day. 14% of patients treated with sorafenib had a partial response (response rate 14%). Median PFS was 3.2 months and median OS was 14.3 months. However, in the angiosarcoma subgroup, PFS was 3.8 months and OS was 14.9 months. Contrary to previous French phase II trial, sorafenib proved to be efficient in treatment of angiosarcoma in this US trial. However, sorafenib showed no antitumor activity in other histological subtypes of sarcoma although it had minor activity against leiomyosarcoma.

Several case reports suggest that pazopanib may be effective in angiosarcoma treatment [19–21]. Phase III trial PALETTE by van der Graaf et al. [22] confirmed efficacy of pazopanib in advanced STS treatment in pretreated patients. Patients were divided into 2 arms: pazopanib monotherapy arm and placebo arm. Pazopanib treatment brought significant improvement of survival rates (PFS benefit of 3 months and OS benefit of 1.8 months). However, no relevant subanalysis for angiosarcoma is available in this trial.

Addition of bevacizumab to taxane-based chemotherapy was studied in randomized phase II trial of Ray-Coquard et al. [23]. Patients were treated with paclitaxel weekly (90 mg/m^2) or combination of paclitaxel (90 mg/m^2) weekly and bevacizumab (10 mg/kg biweekly). In the combination arm, six courses of bevacizumab were given and followed by maintenance therapy with bevacizumab (15 mg/kg triweekly) until progression. Primary endpoint was 6-month PFS. Six-month PFS rate was 54% in paclitaxel only arm and 57% in paclitaxel and bevacizumab arm. Median overall survival reached 19.5 months in paclitaxel only arm and 15.9 months in the combination arm. Authors concluded that addition of bevacizumab to paclitaxel failed to improve survival rates and recommended no further clinical investigation on this combination in advanced angiosarcoma treatment.

According to ESMO clinical practice guidelines, gemcitabine and docetaxel are an alternative to taxane-only chemotherapy of angiosarcoma. Efficacy of combination therapy consisting of gemcitabine, docetaxel, and bevacizumab (GDB) in treatment of soft tissue sarcomas was studied in phase II trial of Dickson et al. [24]. In the angiosarcoma subgroup, treatment with GDB combination resulted in at least partial responses in 60% of patients. Authors concluded that GDB combination represents a viable option in treatment of angiosarcomas.

Thalidomide is a drug well known for decades. It is presumed that thalidomide may play role in inhibition of angiogenesis, tumor necrosis factor inhibition, and immune system stimulation. However, exact effect of thalidomide on particular malignancies remains unclear [25]. Unfortunately, no RCTs but only few case reports are available on efficacy of thalidomide in advanced angiosarcoma treatment. Raina et al. [26] reported complete response in patient with secondary angiosarcoma of breast treated with thalidomide. In this case, thalidomide was chosen due to patient's advanced age (75 years) and questionable efficacy of chemotherapy. Complete response was achieved at the dose of 200 mg daily within 4 weeks. Adverse effects of thalidomide led to dose reduction (50 mg/daily) which resulted in disease recurrence after 8 weeks of dose reduction. Reestablishment of initial dose of 200 mg/daily led to disease stabilization.

Alvarado-Miranda et al. [27] published a case of 41-year-old woman with no history of malignancy with primary locally advanced angiosarcoma of left breast with axillary lymph node involvement. After neoadjuvant chemotherapy (four cycles of doxorubicin 50 mg/m^2/cisplatin 75 mg/m^2 in combination with thalidomide at dose of 200 mg daily followed by combined chemotherapy of paclitaxel 80 mg/m^2/ cisplatin 30 mg/m^2 with thalidomide at the dose of 200 mg/ daily), complete pathological response was observed. Subsequently, mastectomy and axillary lymph node dissection were performed and 6-month-long disease-free survival was observed.

These case reports suggest efficacy of thalidomide in angiosarcoma treatment. However, further investigation, preferably RCTs, is required to confirm these results.

In 2015, Banavali et al. [28] reported a case of 69-year-old woman with relapsing metastatic skin angiosarcoma treated with a combination of metronomic chemotherapy and non-selective beta-blocker propranolol. The patient was treated with low doses of cyclophosphamide and etoposide along with nonsteroid anti-inflammatory drug (NSAID) celecoxib and propranolol. The treatment was delivered according to particular schedule. Propranolol at the dose of 20 mg twice a day was delivered since the malignancy was positive for beta-adrenergic receptor. The treatment was associated with complete response after 2 cycles of treatment. Progression occurred 20 months after initiation of metronomic treatment. Patient died 7 months later. Authors underlined the fact that metronomic treatment proved to be innovative yet inexpensive therapy, the outcomes of which can be compared to more conventional regimens and modern and expensive targeted therapies.

Although angiosarcoma is generally considered to be rapidly progressive, our patient is surviving 13 years after being diagnosed with this malignancy. To our knowledge, this is one of the longest survivals of adult splenic angiosarcoma reported in literature, in addition to one patient reported by Hsu et al. [29]. Notably, metastatic spread occurred only 3 years (2006) after initial diagnosis (2003). It is unusual that systemic treatment had not been administered until 4 years (2010) later. No progression was detected during this 4-year-long interval in metastatic disease. Finally, first-line chemotherapy resulted in 6-year-long progression-free survival.

Several cases of long-term survival of patients with metastatic angiosarcoma have been reported. In 1988, Rosner [30] published case report of two patients with angiosarcoma of breast surviving more than 10 years after mastectomy and vinblastine-based adjuvant chemotherapy.

Hara et al. [31] presented a case of 48-year-old woman with localized splenic angiosarcoma. Splenectomy was performed and 3 courses of adjuvant chemotherapy were administered. CHOP regimen (cyclophosphamide, doxorubicin, vincristine, and prednisolone) was chosen in this setting. Moreover, due to poor prognosis, high-dose chemotherapy and autologous peripheral blood stem-cell transplantation (auto-PBSCT) were performed. This radical treatment brought 6-year-long complete remission. Afterwards, rapid course of recurring disease with massive metastatic spread and worsening of performance status led to patient's death within several months.

Finally, retrospective study of Fayette et al. [5] showed that survival rates in angiosarcoma are influenced by primary site of angiosarcoma. If angiosarcoma originates in visceral organs such as liver, spleen, bone, or heart, worse survival rates can be observed. On the other side, authors reported that significant proportion of patients with initially metastatic disease survived beyond 8 years after being diagnosed with angiosarcoma.

It is obvious that significant proportion of patients with advanced angiosarcoma may experience long-term survivorship. This long-term survivorship might be determined by unrecognized prognostic factors. However, it is unclear whether selection of systemic treatment contributes to this long-term survivorship. Without identifying these prognostic factors, this question remains unanswered.

4. Conclusion

Optimal treatment for primary splenic angiosarcoma remains unknown. ESMO and NCCN provide guidelines based on limited data and treatment outcomes for primary splenic angiosarcoma are poor in most patients. However, as suggested above, strict selection of patients based on prognostic and predictive factors and subsequent tailored therapy might bring impressive results. The research should focus on identifying those prognostic and predictive factors. However due to rarity of this disease, this task may be a question of long-term research.

Consent

Written informed consent was obtained from the patient for publication of this case report and accompanying images.

Acknowledgments

The authors would like to express their gratitude to Medicyt Laboratories, Ltd., for providing photographic material used in this article.

References

[1] American Cancer Society, *Cancer Facts and Figures 2016*, 2016, http://www.cancer.org/acs/groups/content/@research/document/acspc-047079.pdf.

[2] The ESMO/European Sarcoma Network Working Group, "Soft tissue and visceral sarcomas: ESMO Clinical Practice Guidelines for diagnosis, treatment and follow-up," *Annals of Oncology*, vol. 25, supplement 3, pp. iii102–iii112, 2014.

[3] W. Shon, S. M. Jenkins, D. T. Ross et al., "Angiosarcoma: a study of 98 cases with immunohistochemical evaluation of TLE3, a recently described marker of potential taxane responsiveness," *Journal of Cutaneous Pathology*, vol. 38, no. 12, pp. 961–966, 2011.

[4] M. G. Fury, C. R. Antonescu, K. J. Van Zee, M. F. Brennan, and R. G. Maki, "A 14-year retrospective review of angiosarcoma: clinical characteristics, prognostic factors, and treatment outcomes with surgery and chemotherapy," *Cancer Journal*, vol. 11, no. 3, pp. 241–247, 2005.

[5] J. Fayette, E. Martin, S. Piperno-Neumann et al., "Angiosarcomas, a heterogeneous group of sarcomas with specific behavior depending on primary site: a retrospective study of 161 cases," *Annals of Oncology*, vol. 18, no. 12, pp. 2030–2036, 2007.

[6] A. Gupta, M. M. Patnaik, and H. V. Naina, "Angiosarcoma of the prostate gland following brachytherapy for prostatic adenocarcinoma," *Current Urology*, vol. 8, no. 2, pp. 109–112, 2014.

[7] J. L. Kutok and C. D. M. Fletcher, "Splenic vascular tumors," *Seminars in Diagnostic Pathology*, vol. 20, no. 2, pp. 128–139, 2003.

[8] M. Despoina, D. Dionysios, A. Georgios, S. Konstantinos, K. Efstratios, and Z.-S. Adamantia, "Primary angiosarcoma of the spleen: an oncological enigma," *Case Reports in Oncological Medicine*, vol. 2014, Article ID 193036, 4 pages, 2014.

[9] B. Xu, X. Xie, X. Zhou, M. Zhai, and W. Yang, "Spontaneous rupture of primary splenic angiosarcoma: a case report," *Oncology Letters*, vol. 10, no. 5, pp. 3271–3273, 2015.

[10] Y.-F. Duan, Y. Jiang, C.-X. Wu, and F. Zhu, "Spontaneous rupture of primary splenic angiosarcoma: a case report and literature review," *World Journal of Surgical Oncology*, vol. 11, article 53, 2013.

[11] National Comprehensive Cancer Network, NCCN Clinical Practice Guidelines in Oncology, Soft Tissue Sarcoma v. 2.2016, National Comprehensive Cancer Network, https://www.nccn.org/professionals/physician_gls/pdf/sarcoma.pdf.

[12] J. J. Jones, C. N. Catton, B. O'Sullivan et al., "Initial results of a trial of preoperative external-beam radiation therapy

and postoperative brachytherapy for retroperitoneal sarcoma," *Annals of Surgical Oncology*, vol. 9, no. 4, pp. 346–354, 2002.

[13] N. Penel, B. N. Bui, J.-O. Bay et al., "Phase II trial of weekly paclitaxel for unresectable angiosarcoma: the ANGIOTAX Study," *Journal of Clinical Oncology*, vol. 26, no. 32, pp. 5269–5274, 2008.

[14] T. Hirata, K. Yonemori, M. Ando et al., "Efficacy of taxane regimens in patients with metastatic angiosarcoma," *European Journal of Dermatology*, vol. 21, no. 4, pp. 539–545, 2011.

[15] C. Yoo, J.-E. Kim, S.-K. Yoon et al., "Angiosarcoma of the retroperitoneum: report on a patient treated with sunitinib," *Sarcoma*, vol. 2009, Article ID 360875, 4 pages, 2009.

[16] S. Sleijfer, "Phase II studies in soft tissue sarcoma: time for reappraisal," *The Oncologist*, vol. 17, no. 2, pp. 154–156, 2012.

[17] I. Ray-Coquard, A. Italiano, E. Bompas et al., "Sorafenib for patients with advanced angiosarcoma: a phase II trial from the french sarcoma group (GSF/GETO)," *Oncologist*, vol. 17, no. 2, pp. 260–266, 2012.

[18] R. G. Maki, D. R. D'Adamo, M. L. Keohan et al., "Phase II study of sorafenib in patients with metastatic or recurrent sarcomas," *Journal of Clinical Oncology*, vol. 27, no. 19, pp. 3133–3140, 2009.

[19] H. Tomita, Y. Koike, M. Asai et al., "Angiosarcoma of the scalp successfully treated with pazopanib," *Journal of the American Academy of Dermatology*, vol. 70, no. 1, pp. e19–e21, 2014.

[20] H. Miura and H. Shirai, "Low-dose administration of oral pazopanib for the treatment of recurrent angiosarcoma," *Clinical and Experimental Dermatology*, vol. 40, no. 5, pp. 575–577, 2015.

[21] S. Kitamura, H. Hata, K. Imafuku, N. Haga, E. Homma, and H. Shimizu, "Pazopanib can preserve cosmetic quality of life even in end-stage angiosarcoma," *Clinical and Experimental Dermatology*, vol. 40, no. 8, pp. 931–933, 2015.

[22] W. T. A. van der Graaf, J.-Y. Blay, S. P. Chawla et al., "Pazopanib for metastatic soft-tissue sarcoma (PALETTE): a randomised, double-blind, placebo-controlled phase 3 trial," *The Lancet*, vol. 379, no. 9829, pp. 1879–1886, 2012.

[23] I. L. Ray-Coquard, J. Domont, E. Tresch-Bruneel et al., "Paclitaxel given once per week with or without bevacizumab in patients with advanced angiosarcoma: a randomized phase II trial," *Journal of Clinical Oncology*, vol. 33, no. 25, pp. 2797–2802, 2015.

[24] M. A. Dickson, D. R. D'Adamo, M. L. Keohan et al., "Phase II trial of gemcitabine and docetaxel with bevacizumab in soft tissue sarcoma," *Sarcoma*, vol. 2015, Article ID 532478, 7 pages, 2015.

[25] G. Fraiman, A. K. Ganti, A. Potti, and S. Mehdi, "Angiosarcoma of the small intestine: a possible role for thalidomide?" *Medical Oncology*, vol. 20, no. 4, pp. 397–401, 2003.

[26] V. Raina, M. Sengar, N. K. Shukla et al., "Complete response from thalidomide in angiosarcoma after treatment of breast cancer," *Journal of Clinical Oncology*, vol. 25, no. 7, pp. 900–901, 2007.

[27] A. Alvarado-Miranda, L. Bacon-Fonseca, U. Lara-Medina Fernando, H. Maldonado-Martínez, and C. Arce-Salinas, "Thalidomide combined with neoadjuvant chemotherapy in angiosarcoma of the breast with complete pathologic response: case report and review of literature," *Breast Care*, vol. 8, no. 1, pp. 74–76, 2013.

[28] S. Banavali, E. Pasquier, and N. Andre, "Targeted therapy with propranolol and metronomic chemotherapy combination: sustained complete response of a relapsing metastatic angiosarcoma," *ecancermedicalscience*, vol. 9, article 499, 2015.

[29] J.-T. Hsu, H.-M. Chen, C.-Y. Lin et al., "Primary angiosarcoma of the spleen," *Journal of Surgical Oncology*, vol. 92, no. 4, pp. 312–316, 2005.

[30] D. Rosner, "Angiosarcoma of the breast: long-term survival following adjuvant chemotherapy," *Journal of Surgical Oncology*, vol. 39, no. 2, pp. 90–95, 1988.

[31] T. Hara, H. Tsurumi, S. Kasahara et al., "Long-term survival of a patient with splenic angiosarcoma after resection, high-dose chemotherapy, and autologous peripheral blood stem cell transplantation," *Internal Medicine*, vol. 49, no. 20, pp. 2253–2257, 2010.

30

Hypokalemic Paralysis Secondary to Immune Checkpoint Inhibitor Therapy

Pragathi Balakrishna[1] **and Augusto Villegas**[2]

[1] *PGY3 Internal Medicine, Orange Park Medical Center, Orange Park, FL, USA*
[2] *Department of Hematology and Oncology, Orange Park Medical Center, Orange Park, FL, USA*

Correspondence should be addressed to Pragathi Balakrishna; pragathibalakrishna@gmail.com

Academic Editor: Constantine Gennatas

Introduction of immune checkpoint inhibitors (ICIs) has led to significant improvements in the treatment of multiple malignancies. Anti-programmed cell death protein 1 (PD-1) and anti-cytotoxic T-lymphocyte antigen 4 (CTLA-4) are two essential ICIs that have been FDA approved since 2011. As the use of immunotherapy in melanoma and other malignancies increases, the potential of adverse events also increases. Overall, anti-PD-1 agents are well tolerated. In rare instances, colitis, endocrinopathies, skin, and renal toxicities have been observed. A 58-year-old male with a history of stage 4 cutaneous melanoma presented with quadriplegia while on nivolumab. Routine blood test revealed low potassium, low bicarbonate, and high serum creatinine. Admission diagnosis included hypokalemia, acute kidney injury, and renal tubal acidosis. The offending drug was discontinued, and the patient was started on high-dose corticosteroids. On discharge, paralysis was resolved. Renal function and potassium were normalized. Nivolumab was discontinued, and he was started on pembrolizumab. Literature suggests that, although rare, patients receiving ICE may develop immune-mediated nephritis and renal dysfunction. The mainstay of immune-related adverse event (irAE) management is immune suppression. Hence, given the increasing frequency of immunotherapy use, awareness should be raised in regard to irAEs and their appropriate management.

1. Introduction

Immune checkpoint inhibitors (ICIs) are emerging as revolutionary drugs targeting a variety of malignancies such as melanoma, non-small-cell lung carcinoma (NSCLC), and renal cell carcinoma (RCC) [1]. Three checkpoint protein inhibitory antibodies have been FDA approved for melanoma since 2011. These are nivolumab and pembrolizumab, which block programmed death 1 receptor (PD-1), and ipilimumab, which blocks cytotoxic T-lymphocyte-associated antigen 4 (CTLA-4) receptor [2]. PD-1 transmits inhibitory signals to immune cells, leading to decreased proliferation and apoptosis. Cancer cells express PD-L1, the ligand of PD-1, allowing the tumor to escape attack by effector T cells. Immune checkpoint inhibitors encompass blocking antibodies to the PD-1/PD-L1 and CTLA-4 checkpoint molecules. These drugs block the PD-1/PD-L1 interaction, enhancing the cellular response against the tumor (Figure 1) [3].

Nivolumab and pembrolizumab are anti-PD-1 antibodies which are indicated for metastatic melanoma. They have shown superior progression-free survival (PFS) among patients with advanced melanoma [4, 5]. A trial comparing nivolumab to dacarbazine in previously untreated patients showed a 12-month survival rate of 73% versus 42%, respectively [6]. Another phase 1 clinical trial studied the progression-free survival amongst patients with advanced melanoma treated with pembrolizumab. This trial showed a 12-month progression-free survival rate of 35% in patients regardless of previous ipilimumab treatment and a 12-month progression-free survival rate of 52% in treatment-naïve patients [5].

On the one hand, ICIs have dramatically improved the outcome of metastatic melanoma and other cancers such as

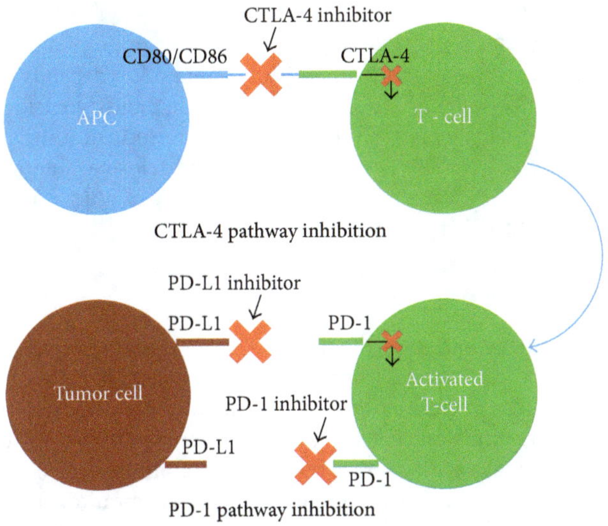

FIGURE 1: Mechanism of action of immune checkpoint inhibitors. CTLA-4 = cytotoxic T-lymphocyte antigen 4, PD-1 = programmed cell death protein 1, PD-L1 = programmed death-ligand 1.

NCSLC and RCC [7]. However, the therapy is associated with immune-related adverse events (irAEs), which were observed in 5% of patients [4]. The basis for the majority of these adverse events is a hyperactivated T-cell response with reactivity directed against normal tissue, resulting in the generation of high levels of CD4 T-helper cell cytokines or increased migration of cytolytic CD8 T cells within normal tissues [2]. Overall, anti-PD-1 agents are well tolerated with low-grade fatigue, diarrhea, pruritus, nausea, and decreased appetite occurring as the most common adverse events. Sometimes colitis, endocrinopathies, skin toxicity, and renal toxicities have been observed [8]. Acute renal failure has been reported in < 1% of the patients treated with nivolumab monotherapy or in combination studies for melanoma or NSCLC. Patients with renal injury typically present with elevations in serum creatinine and are treated with steroids which lead to clinical improvement and resolution in most cases [9]. Here, we present a patient with advanced melanoma who developed metabolic acidosis, hypokalemic paralysis, and acute renal failure during treatment with anti-PD1 antibodies.

2. Case Report

A 58-year-old Caucasian male with a history of metastatic melanoma presented with severe weakness. The patient was initially diagnosed with cutaneous melanoma of the back in May 2008 (American Joint Committee of Cancer (AJCC) Stage 1b; T2a, N0, M0; BRAF V600 mutation not detected) and underwent wide local excision with clear margins. In April 2014, he presented with progressive shortness of breath and significant weight loss over the past 3–4 weeks. CT angiography of the chest showed mediastinal and hilar lymphadenopathy, along with numerous pulmonary nodules throughout both lungs ranging between 6 mm and 3.5 cm. CT abdomen and MRI brain were done which ruled out any liver lesion or brain metastasis. Biopsy of the lung nodules confirmed metastatic melanoma (BRAF V600 mutation not detected), and treatment with anti-CTLA-4 antibody, ipilimumab (3 mg/kg), was initiated. The patient received this treatment regimen for 3 months but then was lost to follow-up. In November 2014, he agreed to start therapy with nivolumab, an anti-PD- L1 antibody. Ten months later, he presented with progressive quadriplegia, lower extremity weakness worse than upper extremity weakness, developing over a few days. He reported that, due to the weakness, he fell and was unable to get up on his own. His home medication list included only nivolumab. Routine blood test in ED revealed potassium of 1.7 mEq/L, bicarbonate of 9 mEq/L, chloride of 116 mEq/L, sodium of 139 mEq/L (anion gap 14, delta ratio of 2), serum creatinine of 2.64 mg/dL (baseline of 0.91 mg/dL 3 weeks prior), and elevated eosinophils of 6%. Admission diagnosis included hypokalemia, hyperchloremic normal anion gap metabolic acidosis, acute kidney injury (AKI), and eosinophilia. Urinalysis revealed 1+ protein (urine protein/creatinine ratio of 1.42), fractional excretion of sodium of 1.9%, amorphous urine sediment, and 24-hour urine potassium of 159 mEq/L, hence indicating intrinsic kidney injury such as acute interstitial nephritis, acute tubular necrosis, or glomerulonephritis. Pertinent negatives in his blood work included normal thyroid-stimulating hormone levels. Retroperitoneal ultrasound showed normal kidneys with no solid mass, stone, or obstruction. Urinary bladder also appeared normal. There was no history suggestive of previous kidney disease; autoimmune diseases such as sjögrens, lupus nephritis, or rheumatoid arthritis (RA); thyroid disorders; diabetes; vomiting; excessive alcohol use; dehydration; or exposure to nephrotoxic agents such as antibiotics, contrast, or analgesics. Based on these findings, progressive quadriplegia was secondary to hypokalemia which was due to type 1 RTA, most likely irAE secondary to anti-PD-1 antibody therapy. The offending drug was discontinued, and the patient was started on intravenous hydrocortisone 100 mg every 6 hours for 2 days, followed by a tapering dose lasting 4 weeks. IV replacement therapy with potassium and bicarbonate was also initiated. Renal biopsy was considered but was not done as the patient responded well to steroids with return of renal function to normal. Quadriplegia gradually improved which correlated to improvement in serum potassium levels. By day 3 of hospitalization, the quadriplegia had resolved. Serum creatinine, hypokalemia, and other electrolyte imbalance improved. On discharge, renal function, potassium, and bicarbonate were normal. Subsequently, he was started on pembrolizumab, another anti-PD-1 antibody, which the patient has tolerated well.

3. Discussion

As the use of immunotherapy in melanoma and other malignancies increases, the potential of adverse events (AEs) also increases. Safety reports for anti-PD-1's are available for > 2,000 patients participating in ongoing studies. Some side effects may be caused by an inflammatory mechanism [10]. Manufacturer information for nivolumab suggests that patients receiving nivolumab may develop immune-mediated nephritis and renal dysfunction (1.2% (23/1994) of patients). The median time to onset was 4.6 months (range: 23 days to 12.3 months) [11]. Immune-mediated nephritis and renal dysfunction led to permanent discontinuation of the medication in 0.3% and withholding of it in 0.8% of patients. All patients received high-dose corticosteroids (at least 40 mg prednisone equivalents per day) for a median duration of 21 days (range: 1 day to 15.4 months). Complete resolution occurred in 48% of patients [11]. Patients with immune-mediated nephritis present with some combination of the following laboratory findings: increased plasma creatinine, eosinophilia/eosinophiluria, characteristic urine sediment, and variable degree of proteinuria and rarely with evidence of tubulointerstitial damage such as Fanconi syndrome and renal tubular acidosis (RTA) [12]. A meta-analysis demonstrated that the use of immune checkpoint inhibitors was associated with an increased risk of immune-related renal toxicity [13]. As per common toxicity criteria (CTC), renal toxicity grade for urinary electrolyte wasting (e.g., RTA) is categorized from grade 0 to grade 4: grade 0 being none; grade 1 being asymptomatic, not requiring treatment; grade 2 being mild, reversible, and manageable with oral replacement; grade 3 being reversible but requiring IV replacement; and grade 4 being irreversible, requiring continued replacement. Grade 3 and 4 are considered as high-grade toxicity [14]. Three studies compared nivolumab with other chemotherapeutic agents in advanced melanoma. The incidence of all-grade renal toxicities in the nivolumab treatment arm ranged from 0.7 to 1.9% versus high-grade toxicities which ranged from 0 to 0.5% [13]. In our patient, based on the clinical presentation, the renal toxicity was grade 3. To our knowledge, this is the first case report of type 1 RTA associated with severe hypokalemia, caused by an immune checkpoint inhibitor. The patient had a basal metabolic profile studies prior to administering the medication, which was within normal range. Initial severe hypokalemia prompted further workup which led to identifying and characterizing his dysfunction. The differential diagnosis for RTA in a patient with no prior history of kidney disease includes medications, autoimmune disease particularly Sjögren syndrome or RA, kidney transplantation, nephrocalcinosis, medullary sponge kidney, chronic obstructive uropathy, cirrhosis, and sickle cell anemia [15]. A complete workup done ruled out most of these causes. Timing of his symptoms and the associated use of nivolumab, in the absence of any other precipitating factors (other medications and infection), pointed to immunotherapy being the most likely cause. The mainstay of immune-related adverse event (irAE) management is immune suppression, including high-dose steroids, immunosuppressants, and potentially TNF-α inhibitors [16]. Several specific algorithms are being developed for the management of the anti-PD-1 AEs. For most grade 1 toxicities, treatment can be continued with careful monitoring and supportive measures. Grade 2 toxicities usually resolve by withholding the drug and with administration of steroids. For grade 3 and 4 toxicities, discontinuation of the offending agent, use of high-dose corticosteroids, and a renal consultation and consideration for imaging or renal biopsy as appropriate are indicated [10]. Restarting of anti-PD-1 antibodies depends on the severity of the AEs. For majority of grade 1 and 2 toxicities, the drug can be safely but carefully restarted. In patients with grade 3 toxicity, retreatment requires close evaluation of the risks. Patients with grade 4 toxicity should not be rechallenged [3].

4. Conclusion

In summary, our case highlights a rare yet serious irAE of anti-PD-1 antibodies. Immune checkpoint inhibitors are an important advancement in the treatment of various cancers; however, this comes at the expense of a unique pattern of irAEs. Renal toxicity is rare but could be an important cause of morbidity in these patients [10]. Close monitoring of patients and a high degree of clinical suspicion is recommended when treating patients with immune checkpoint inhibitors. Early intervention with either careful monitoring of the patient or discontinuing the offending agent is the key to the management of these complications.

References

[1] R. J. Motzer, B. Escudier, D. F. McDermott et al., "Nivolumab versus everolimus in advanced renal-cell carcinoma," *New England Journal of Medicine*, vol. 373, no. 19, pp. 1803–1813, 2015.

[2] J. S. Weber, J. C. Yang, M. B. Atkins, and M. L. Disis, "Toxicities of immunotherapy for the practitioner," *Journal of Clinical Oncology*, vol. 33, no. 18, pp. 2092–2099, 2015.

[3] J. Escandon, S. Peacock, A. Trabolsi, D. B. Thomas, A. Layka, and J. Lutzky, "Interstitial nephritis in melanoma patients secondary to PD-1 checkpoint inhibitor," *Journal for ImmunoTherapy of Cancer*, vol. 5, no. 1, p. 3, 2017.

[4] S. L. Topalian, M. Sznol, D. F. McDermott et al., "Survival, durable tumor remission, and long-term safety in patients with advanced melanoma receiving nivolumab," *Journal of Clinical Oncology*, vol. 32, no. 10, pp. 1020–1030, 2014.

[5] A. Ribas, O. Hamid, A. Daud et al., "Association of pembrolizumab with tumor response and survival among patients with advanced melanoma," *JAMA*, vol. 315, no. 15, pp. 1600–1609, 2016.

[6] C. Robert, G. V. Long, B. Brady et al., "Nivolumab in previously untreated melanoma without BRAF mutation," *New England Journal of Medicine*, vol. 372, no. 4, pp. 320–330, 2015.

[7] J. Larkin, V. Chiarion-Sileni, R. Gonzalez et al., "Combined nivolumab and ipilimumab or monotherapy in untreated melanoma," *New England Journal of Medicine*, vol. 373, no. 1, pp. 23–34, 2015.

[8] S. L. Topalian, F. S. Hodi, J. R. Brahmer et al., "Safety, activity, and immune correlates of anti-PD-1 antibody in cancer," *New England Journal of Medicine*, vol. 366, no. 26, pp. 2443–2454, 2012.

[9] L. Hofmann, A. Forschner, C. Loquai et al., "Cutaneous, gastrointestinal, hepatic, endocrine, and renal side-effects of anti-PD-1 therapy," *European Journal of Cancer*, vol. 60, pp. 190–209, 2016.

[10] H. Linardou and H. Gogas, "Toxicity management of immunotherapy for patients with metastatic melanoma," *Annals of Translational Medicine*, vol. 4, no. 14, p. 272, 2016.

[11] Highlights of prescribing information, "Opdivo (nivolumab) injection, for intravenous use, Initial U.S. approval: 2014," 2017, http://packageinserts.bms.com/pi/pi_opdivo.pdf.

[12] K. Neelakantappa, G. R. Gallo, and J. Lowenstein, "Ranitidine-associated interstitial nephritis and Fanconi syndrome," *American Journal of Kidney Diseases*, vol. 22, no. 2, pp. 333–336, 1993.

[13] O. Abdel-Rahman and M. Fouad, "A network meta-analysis of the risk of immune-related renal toxicity in cancer patients treated with immune checkpoint inhibitors," *Immunotherapy*, vol. 8, no. 5, pp. 665–674, 2016.

[14] Cancer Therapy Evaluation Program, "Common Toxicity Criteria, Version 2.0 DCTD, NCI, NIH, DHHS March 1998," 1998, https://ctep.cancer.gov/protocoldevelopment/electronic_applications/docs/ctcv20_4-30-992.pdf.

[15] L. A. Hechanova, *Renal Tubular Acidosis*, Merck Manual Professional Version, Merck Sharp & Dohme Corp, Kenilworth, NJ, USA, 2017.

[16] J. S. Weber, K. C. Kahler, and A. Hauschild, "Management of immune-related adverse events and kinetics of response with ipilimumab," *Journal of Clinical Oncology*, vol. 30, no. 21, pp. 2691–2697, 2012.

31

Cardiac Relapse of Acute Myeloid Leukemia after Allogeneic Hematopoietic Stem Cell Transplantation

María Facenda-Lorenzo,[1] Ana Sánchez-Quintana,[2] Alejandro Quijada-Fumero,[1] Ana Laynez-Carnicero,[1] Joaquín Breña-Atienza,[2] Francisco J. Poncela-Mireles,[1] Juan M. Llanos-Gómez,[3] Ana I. Cabello-Rodríguez,[2] and María Ramos-López[1]

[1]*Servicio de Cardiología, Hospital Universitario de La Candelaria, Carretera del Rosario No. 145, 38010 Santa Cruz de Tenerife, Spain*
[2]*Hematology Service, University Hospital Nuestra Señora de La Candelaria, Santa Cruz de Tenerife, Tenerife, Canarias, Spain*
[3]*Radiology Service, University Hospital Nuestra Señora de La Candelaria, Santa Cruz de Tenerife, Tenerife, Canarias, Spain*

Correspondence should be addressed to María Facenda-Lorenzo; mariacarax@hotmail.com

Academic Editor: Yoshihito Yokoyama

Secondary or metastatic cardiac tumors are much more common than primary benign or malignant cardiac tumors. Any tumor can cause myocardial or pericardial metastasis, although isolated or combined tumor invasion of the pericardium is more common. Types of neoplasia with the highest rates of cardiac or pericardial involvement are melanoma, lung cancer, and breast and mediastinal carcinomas. Acute myeloid leukemia (AML) is the most common type of acute leukemia in adults. Initial treatment involves chemotherapy followed by consolidation treatment to reduce the risk of relapse. In high-risk patients, the treatment of choice for consolidation is hematopoietic stem cell transplantation (HSCT). Relapse of AML is the most common cause of HSCT failure. Extramedullary relapse is rare. The organs most frequently affected, called "sanctuaries," are the testes, ovaries, and central nervous system. We present a case with extramedullary relapse in the form of a solid cardiac mass.

1. Introduction

Secondary or metastatic cardiac tumors are much more common than primary benign or malignant cardiac tumors. They usually appear after the age of 50 years in patients of either sex [1]. Metastasis to the heart can occur by direct invasion (mediastinal tumors), hematogenous spread, lymphatic spread, and intracavitary extension through the inferior vena cava [2]. Any tumor can cause myocardial or pericardial metastasis, although isolated or combined tumor invasion of the pericardium is more common. Types of neoplasia with the highest rates of heart or pericardial involvement are melanoma, lung cancer, breast carcinoma, and mediastinal carcinomas [3]. Clinical presentation depends primarily on the size of the tumor and its anatomical location rather than histological type. Thus, the symptoms can be grouped into three main categories: pericardial involvement can produce pericardial effusion or, less frequently, pericarditis, and myocardial involvement is associated with atrial or ventricular arrhythmias, with varying degrees of blockages and angina due to compression or tumor embolization, while right intracavitary tumors can cause right heart occupation [4]. Transthoracic echocardiography (TTE) is the primary diagnostic procedure, followed by computed tomography (CT) and cardiac magnetic resonance imaging (MRI) to verify positive findings and to analyze other structures of the mediastinum and chest [1]. The final diagnosis requires histologic confirmation. Treatment of such tumors is generally associated with poor results and unfavorable prognosis [1].

Acute myeloid leukemia (AML) is a hematologic malignancy caused by the clonal transformation of a cell of myeloid lineage which proliferates abnormally, leading to the accumulation of immature myeloid cells in bone marrow (BM) and blood. AML is the most common type of acute leukemia in adults and its incidence increases with age [5]. In young patients, AML is a potentially curable disease. Initial treatment involves chemotherapy, aimed at inducing remission of cancer cells, followed by consolidation treatment

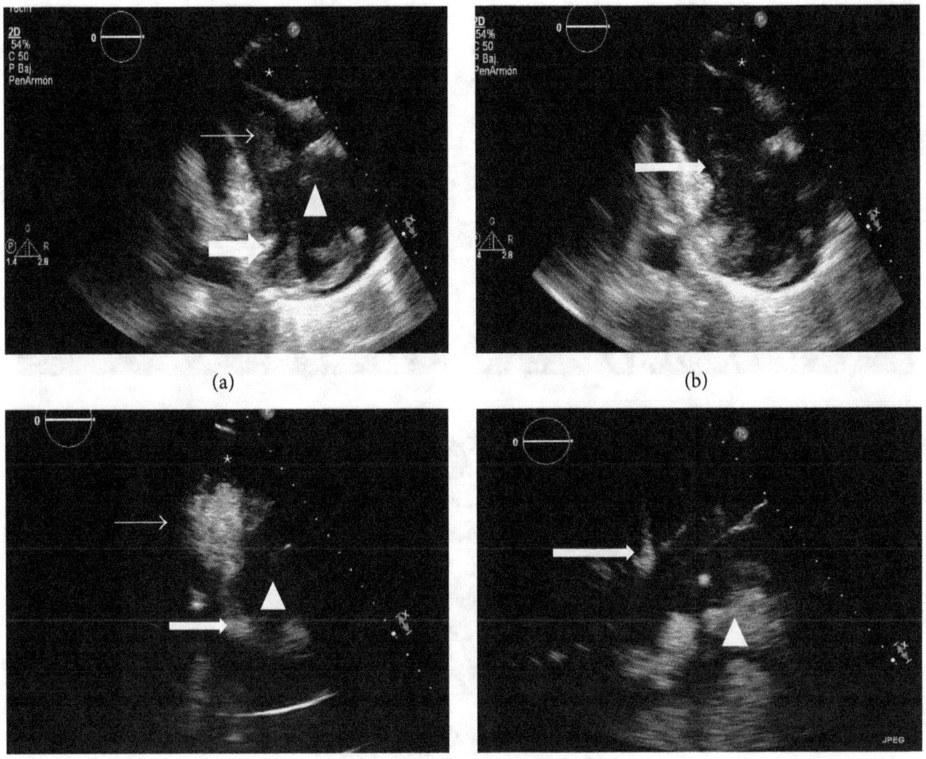

(a) (b) (c) (d)

FIGURE 1: Transthoracic echocardiography with SonoVue® contrast enhancement: (a) shows a homogeneous mass (arrowhead) in the right atrium (RA, thick arrow) which hindered blood flow to the right ventricle (RV, thin arrow), containing contrast medium. Pericardial effusion (star). (b) Same plane image showing stenosis at the tricuspid valve (arrow), with some contrast passing to the RV, as well as tricuspid stenosis. Pericardial effusion (star). (d) Echocardiogram showing contrast in most of the RV (thin arrow) and RA (thick arrow). The arrowhead refers to the homogeneous atrial mass. Pericardial effusion (star). (e) Subcostal plane, showing the contrast (arrowhead) and reflux into the suprahepatic veins (arrow).

to reduce the risk of relapse. In high-risk patients the treatment of choice for consolidation is hematopoietic stem cell transplantation (HSCT) from a compatible donor [5].

Recurrence of AML is the most common cause of HSCT treatment failure, occurring in up to 40% of patients who are refractory to first-line treatment. Extramedullary relapse is considered rare although its reported incidence varies from 0.65% to more than 20% [6]. AML may be located at a single site or manifest diffusely with multiorgan involvement. The organs most often affected, called "sanctuaries," are the testes, ovaries, and central nervous system, but bones, paranasal sinuses, breast tissue, skin, gastrointestinal tract, and the kidneys can also be affected [6, 7].

2. Case Presentation

We report the case of a 61-year-old woman diagnosed with AML without maturation in September 2013. Conventional cytogenetic analysis revealed 46,XX. PCR analyses did not reveal NPM1 or FLT3/ITD mutation. She received induction chemotherapy with daunorubicin and cytarabine with primary refractoriness and reinduction chemotherapy with fludarabine, cytarabine, and idarubicin (FLAG-IDA) with which complete remission was achieved. Consolidation was performed with allogeneic matched-sibling HSCT in January 2014, with thiotepa, fludarabine, and busulfan conditioning. Posttransplant complications presented as cytomegalovirus infection and acute gastric graft versus host disease (GVHD). One year after HSCT, immunosuppression (IS) was withdrawn, after which the patient presented chronic GVHD of the liver and eyes, which required the reintroduction of IS with sirolimus and corticosteroids. As part of follow-up, TTE performed in October 2014 showed no evidence of structural or valvular heart disease.

In August 2015 the patient was admitted to the emergency department with symptoms of malaise, fever, and pain characteristic of pericarditis. Physical examination revealed a blood pressure of 120/60 mmHg and mild 45-degree jugular venous distension. Cardiopulmonary auscultation showed decreased vesicular murmur in bases with symptoms of pleural effusion, no added noise and arrhythmic low-pitched heart sounds, and slight lower limb edemas. The electrocardiogram showed atrial fibrillation with controlled ventricular voltages and low generalized response. TTE showed left cavities of normal size and function and a dilated right ventricle (RV) with a mass of maximum diameter of 30 mm in the right atrium (RA) that hindered blood flow from the RA to the RV (mean tricuspid gradient of 8 mmHg). TTE with contrast (SonoVue) showed thickened, rigid RA walls and an anchored mass measuring 30 × 33 mm, seemingly dependent

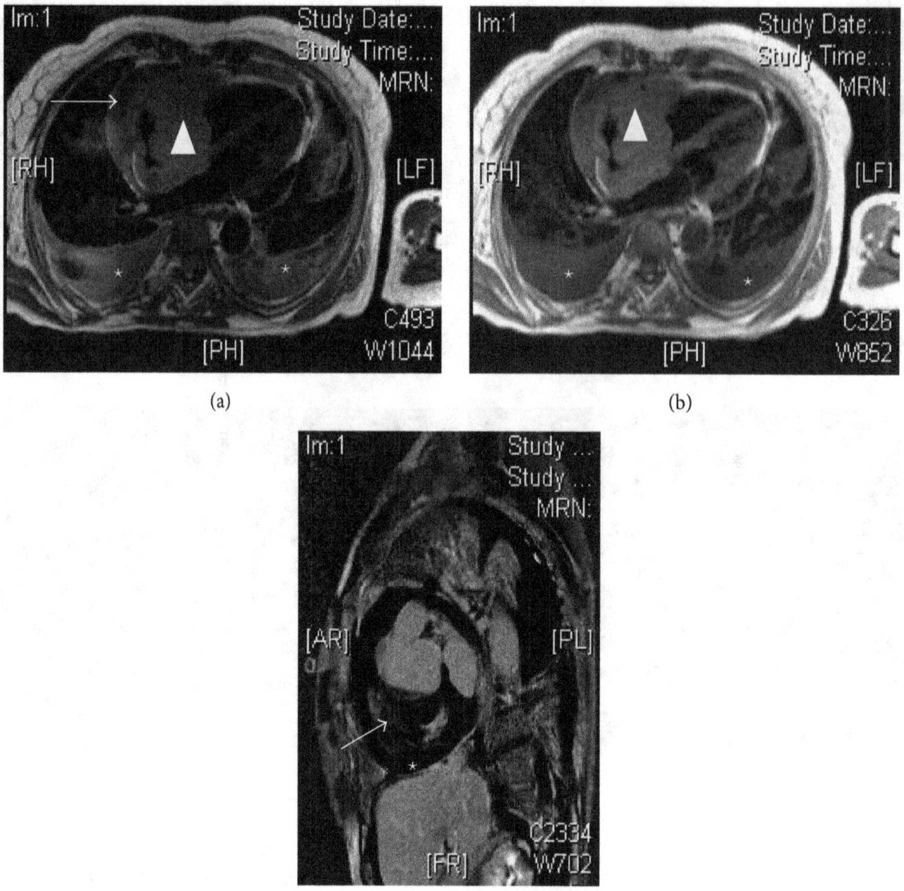

(a) (b) (c)

Figure 2: Cardiac magnetic resonance imaging (MRI). (a) Axial T2 cardiac section, showing an isointense homogeneous mass with respect to the RA myocardium (arrowhead), with pericardial effusion (arrow) and bilateral pleural effusion (star). (b) Axial T1 section, similar to the previous image, showing an isointense homogeneous mass with respect to the myocardium that occupies almost all of the RA, without fat infiltration (arrowhead) and bilateral pleural effusion (star). (c) shows the short-axis RV with delayed gadolinium enhancement and a pattern of diffuse and ill-defined enhancement (arrow). Pericardial effusion (star).

on the interatrial septum, extending to the lateral side of the RV, and moderate pericardial effusion (anterior 10 mm, posterior 8 mm, and RV free wall 13 mm) without evidence of hemodynamic compromise (Figures 1(a)–1(d)). Cardiac MRI (Figures 2(a)–2(c)) showed a mass with irregular edges occupying almost the whole RA, with concentric wall involvement and extension to basal segments of the RV free wall, encompassing the right coronary artery without causing stenosis, measuring 53 × 62 mm on the 4-chamber axis. The mass was homogeneous, isointensewith respect to the myocardium, without presenting fatty infiltration or hypervascularization on perfusion sequence, with a diffuse and delayed enhancement pattern, ill-defined, and non-specific, as well as moderate-severe pericardial effusion and bilateral pleural effusion. Thoracic-abdominal-pelvic CT scan showed a RA mass extending to the RV, as well as pleural and pericardial effusion.

Atrial mass biopsy (Figures 3(a)–3(d)) showed fragments of necrotic tissue with groups of viable blast-like cells, compatible with morphologic and immunophenotypic leukemic infiltration. In addition, BM aspirate confirmed the presence of relapse. After reinduction with FLAG-IDA, infectious and cardiologic complications appeared in the form of slow atrial fibrillation, which was treated with isoproterenol. Finally the patient died 10 days after reinitiating chemotherapy.

3. Discussion

Previous publications have reported that leukemia can metastasize to the heart [1, 8], usually presenting as diffuse infiltration of the pericardium and myocardium [9]. Also, extramedullary relapse after HSCT is known to occur in some patients, but usually later than isolated bone marrow relapses (mean 13 versus 6 months after HSCT). Most of these patients have a history of chronic GVHD and only a minority have extramedullary disease at diagnosis. The novelty of the present case is that the relapse manifested as a solid heart mass, which is exceptional in AML. On reviewing the literature we found very few cases of cardiac relapse after HSCT and mainly in acute lymphoblastic leukemia [10–13]. However, we did find one case of pericardial involvement after BM transplantation for AML [14].

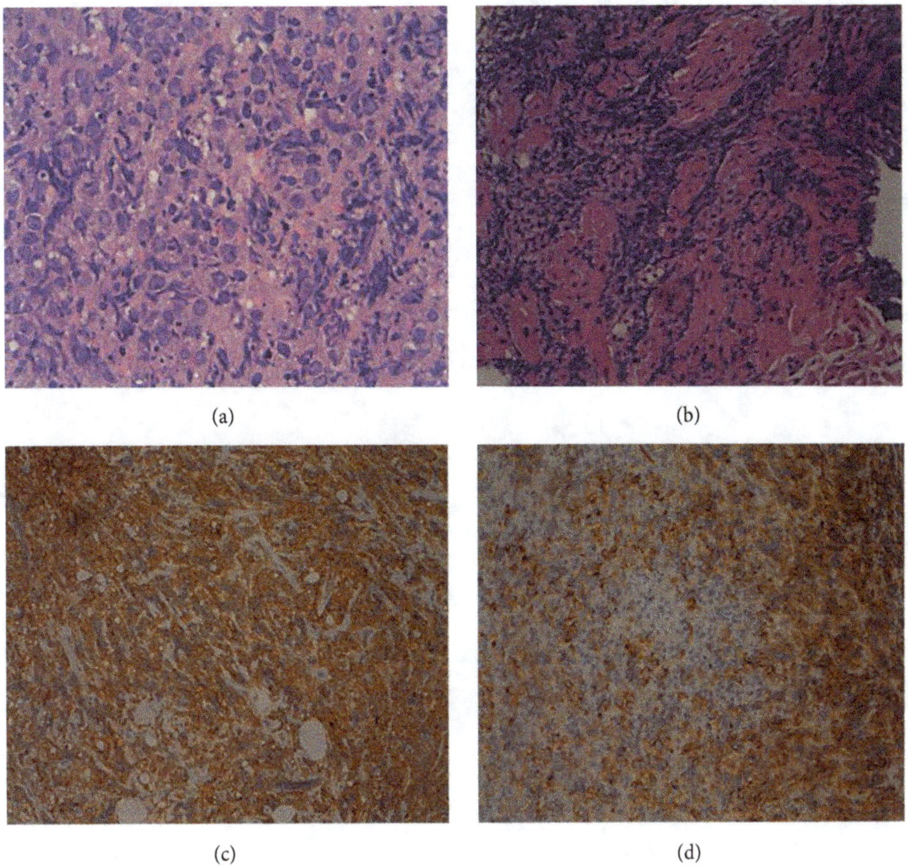

FIGURE 3: Histological findings. ((a) and (b)) The endomyocardial biopsy showed blastic infiltrate associated with myocardial necrosis (hematoxylin and eosin stain). ((c) and (d)) Infiltrating cells were strongly positive for CD45 (c) and CD34 (d).

The present case once again illustrates the importance of imaging techniques and biopsy to confirm the diagnosis of any cardiac mass, taking into account neoplasms in the differential diagnosis. It also illustrates that extramedullary relapse after BM transplant for AML can, exceptionally, take the form of a solid cardiac tumor. To our knowledge, this has not been previously reported.

References

[1] B. Hudzik, K. Miszalski-Jamka, J. Glowacki et al., "Malignant tumors of the heart," *Cancer Epidemiology*, vol. 39, no. 5, pp. 665–672, 2015.

[2] J. Butany, V. Nair, A. Naseemuddin, G. M. Nair, C. Catton, and T. Yau, "Cardiac tumours: diagnosis and management," *Lancet Oncology*, vol. 6, no. 4, pp. 219–228, 2005.

[3] A. D. Goldberg, R. Blankstein, and R. F. Padera, "Tumors metastatic to the heart," *Circulation*, vol. 128, no. 16, pp. 1790–1794, 2013.

[4] I. A. Paraskevaidis, C. A. Michalakeas, C. H. Papadopoulos, and M. Anastasiou-Nana, "Cardiac tumors," *ISRN Oncology*, vol. 2011, Article ID 208929, 5 pages, 2011.

[5] L. Finn, L. Sproat, M. G. Heckman et al., "Epidemiology of adult acute myeloid leukemia: impact of exposures on clinical phenotypes and outcomes after therapy," *Cancer Epidemiology*, vol. 39, no. 6, pp. 1084–1092, 2015.

[6] W. B. Clark, S. A. Strickland, A. J. Barrett, and B. N. Savani, "Extramedullary relapses after allogeneic stem cell transplantation for acute myeloid leukemia and myelodysplastic syndrome," *Haematologica*, vol. 95, no. 6, pp. 860–863, 2010.

[7] G. Chong, G. Byrnes, J. Szer, and A. Grigg, "Extramedullary relapse after allogeneic bone marrow transplantation for haematological malignancy," *Bone Marrow Transplantation*, vol. 26, no. 9, pp. 1011–1015, 2000.

[8] M. De Lazzari, M. Fedrigo, M. Perazzolo Marra et al., "Relapsing leukemia infiltrating the heart," *Circulation: Heart Failure*, vol. 8, no. 6, pp. 1133–1134, 2015.

[9] K. Reynen, U. Köckeritz, and R. H. Strasser, "Metastases to the heart," *Annals of Oncology*, vol. 15, no. 3, pp. 375–381, 2004.

[10] T. Hori, N. Suzuki, N. Mizue, N. Hatakeyama, M. Takamuro, and H. Tsutsumi, "Relapse of T-cell all after stem cell transplant presenting as hypertrophic cardiomyopathy: the value of non-invasive diagnostic imaging in detecting cardiac leukemia," *Pediatric Blood and Cancer*, vol. 46, no. 1, pp. 108–111, 2006.

[11] T. Facon, J. P. Jouet, P. Fenaux et al., "Isolated pericardial and mediastinal relapse following allogeneic bone marrow transplantation for acute lymphoblastic leukemia," *Transplantation*, vol. 51, no. 5, pp. 1125–1126, 1991.

[12] T. L. Wright, P. G. Bardy, P. Disney, S. Moore, and N. Horvath, "Isolated cardiac recurrence of acute lymphoblastic leukemia characterized by t(11;19) two years after unrelated allogeneic bone marrow transplantation," *Cancer Genetics and Cytogenetics*, vol. 137, no. 2, pp. 146–149, 2002.

[13] K. Chang, D.-Y. Kim, K.-H. Lee et al., "An isolated cardiac relapse after allogeneic hematopoietic stem cell transplantation for acute lymphoblastic leukemia," *The Korean Journal of Internal Medicine*, 2016.

[14] H. Einsele, G. Ehninger, A. Vallbracht et al., "Isolated pericardial relapse following allogeneic bone marrow transplantation for acute myelogenous leukemia," *Bone Marrow Transplantation*, vol. 4, no. 3, pp. 323–325, 1989.

32

Spontaneous Tumor Lysis Syndrome in a Patient with a Dedifferentiated Endometrial Adenocarcinoma

Shinichi Harada,[1] Keiki Nagaharu,[1,2] Youichirou Baba,[3] Tetsuya Murata,[3] Toshiro Mizuno,[2] and Keiki Kawakami[1]

[1]*Department of Hematology and Oncology, Suzuka General Hospital, Yamanohana 1275-53, Suzuka, Mie Prefecture 513-8630, Japan*
[2]*Department of Hematology and Oncology, Mie University Hospital, Edobashi 2-174, Tsu, Mie Prefecture 514-0001, Japan*
[3]*Department of Pathology, Suzuka General Hospital, Yamanohana 1275-53, Suzuka, Mie Prefecture 513-8630, Japan*

Correspondence should be addressed to Keiki Nagaharu; keiki.nagaharu@gmail.com

Academic Editor: Gerassimos P. Vandoros

Tumor lysis syndrome (TLS) is an oncological emergency caused by massive cytolysis of malignant cells. This syndrome eventually induces metabolic abnormalities. TLS is observed mainly among tumors with rapid cell proliferation or high sensitivity to antineoplastic treatment. In rare cases, TLS occurs without any cytotoxic treatment. Previous reports have shown that alternative stress including proceeding infection or an operation might play a role in TLS. However, exact mechanism of spontaneous TLS remains unknown. Here, we describe a case of a 59-year-old woman who presented with dedifferentiated endometrial adenocarcinoma and developed TLS without any cytotoxic chemotherapy. Although spontaneous TLS in solid malignancies are extremely rare, clinicians should consider the possibilities of TLS especially in aggressive solid tumors.

1. Background

Tumor lysis syndrome (TLS) is a life-threatening oncological emergency. Rapid cell death releases a large amount of nucleic acids, proteins, and electrolytes, leading to metabolic abnormalities such as hyperuricemia, hyperphosphatemia, hyperkalemia, and hypocalcemia [1]. This syndrome was first reported in 1929 [2] and has been commonly recognized as one of the comorbidities after chemotherapy. The key factors of TLS include a short doubling time, rapid proliferation, large tumor burden, disseminated tumor, and high sensitivity to antineoplastic drugs. However, it has been reported that some cases without therapeutic intervention would develop the TLS. Particularly, in hematological malignancies, there have been some cases of TLS. Spontaneous TLS cases in solid malignancy is extremely rare. Here, we present a rare case of dedifferentiated endometrial adenocarcinoma with spontaneous TLS.

2. Case Presentation

A 59-year-old woman was admitted to our hospital because of an 8-day history of fever and malaise. Her medical history included hypertension without medication. Upon admission, her vital parameters were blood pressure of 107/73 mmHg, pulse rate of 111 bpm, and body temperature of 37.0°C. She was alert (Glasgow coma scale; E4V5M6). She had a distended abdomen without tenderness. Pitting edema of the dorsum of the feet was seen. Other physical examinations were unremarkable. Laboratory tests (Table 1) showed an elevated white blood cell (WBC) count of 19300/μL (normal range: 3200–9800/μL), lactate dehydrogenase (LDH) activity of 444 IU/L (normal range: 100–250 IU/L), and C-reactive protein level of 14.48 mg/dL (normal range: 0.00–0.30 mg/dL). Human T-lymphotropic virus type 1 (HTLV-1) antibodies were positive without abnormal lymphocytes. Obtained blood and urinary culture revealed no pathogens.

She was treated with hydration and ceftriaxone for the suspicion of urinary tract infection. Fever continued and urinary output declined gradually. Investigation by computed tomography revealed multiple masses in the uterus, ascites, disseminated small nodules, and right hydronephrosis because of the tumor. No atrophy was seen in either kidney. Cytomorphological evaluation of ascites revealed large atypical cells. These cells were scattered with loose adhesion

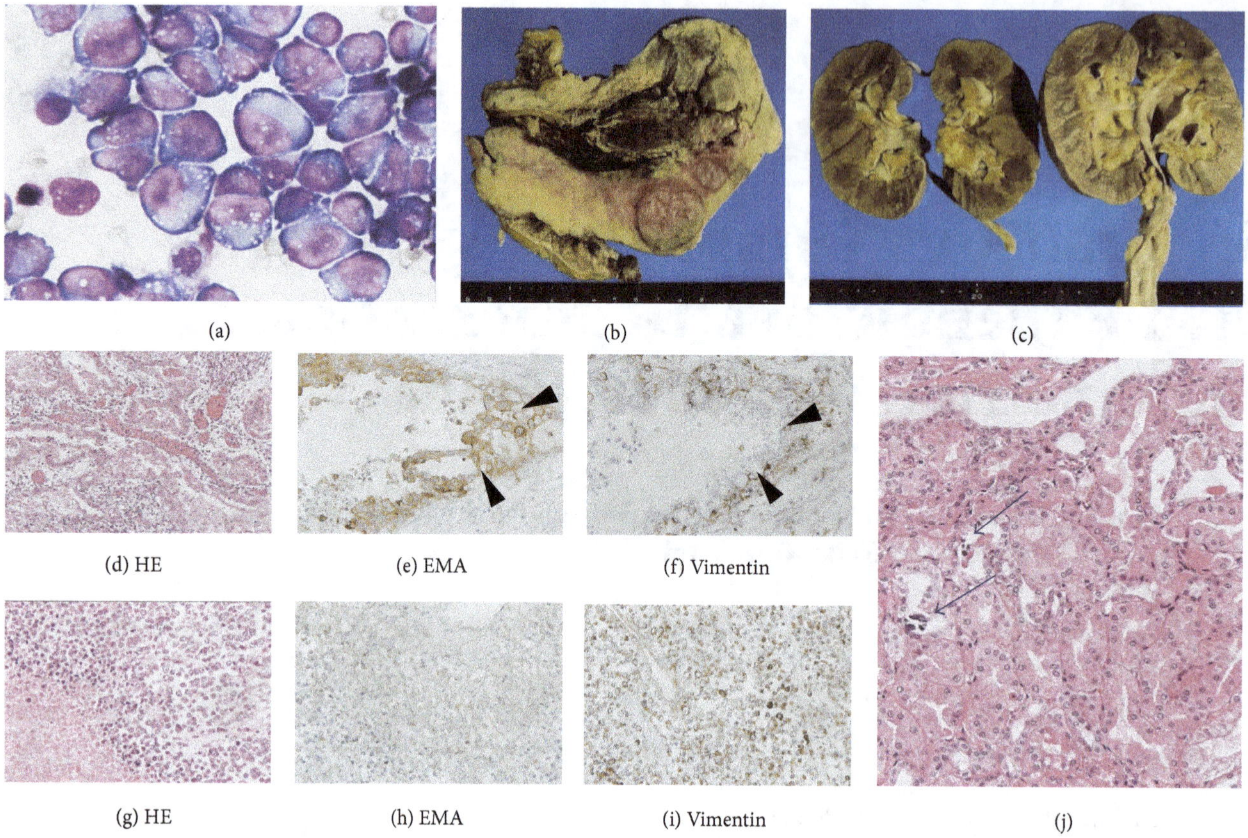

FIGURE 1: Histopathological findings of ascites and autopsy. (a) Cytomorphological evaluation of ascites revealed large abnormal cells mimicking lymphoma. (b, c) Autopsy showed an enlarged uterus. There was no apparent invasion in both kidneys. Small nodules were scattered throughout omentum. (d–i) Hematoxylin and eosin (HE) staining of the uterus showed two types of malignant cells (d, g) characterized by coexisting endometrial carcinoma and undifferentiated immature malignant cells. These endometrial malignant cells were positive for epithelial membrane antigen (EMA) (e) and negative for vimentin (f). Undifferentiated immature malignant cells were negative for EMA (h) and positive for vimentin (i). (j) HE staining of the kidney showed no malignant invasion and many small stones were seen in microtubules.

mimicking malignant lymphoma (Figure 1(a)). Based on the cytological evaluation and positivity for HTLV-1 antibodies, she was suspected to have malignant lymphoma. Then, she was referred to hematology department.

On day 5 in hospital (the first day in the hematology department), her performance status was 3 (Eastern Cooperative Oncology Group). Her malaise and fever were sustained, and she developed anuria. Reevaluation of the laboratory tests showed elevated uric acid 18.8 mg/dL (normal range: <6.8 mg/dL), creatinine of 5.18 (normal range: <0.80 mg/dL), and LDH activity of 622 IU/L. Disseminated intravascular coagulopathy was also diagnosed (Table 1). We diagnosed the tumor lysis syndrome and she was treated with furosemide and rasburicase. Anuria did not improve despite these treatments, and continuous hemodialysis was induced.

On day 6 in hospital, she experienced a sudden cardiopulmonary arrest. Although cardiopulmonary resuscitation was performed, she expired. Autopsy indicated pulmonary embolism without intravascular invasion of tumor cells. Pathological evaluation for uterus showed differentiated endometrioid adenocarcinoma component with squamous differentiation (Figures 1(d), 1(e), and 1(f)) and undifferentiated carcinoma component (Figures 1(g), 1(h), and 1(i)). Epithelial membrane antigen (EMA) expression was diffusely positive in differentiated endometrioid adenocarcinoma lesion (Figure 1(e), arrowhead) but negative for undifferentiated carcinoma lesion (Figure 1(h)). On the other hand, vimentin staining was negative in differentiated adenocarcinoma lesion (Figure 1(f), arrowhead) and positive in undifferentiated carcinoma lesion (Figure 1(i)). Neuroendocrine tumor constitution was not observed. Diagnosis of the uterine tumor indicated dedifferentiated endometrial adenocarcinoma (DEAC). Disseminated malignant cells were also observed in her lungs, liver, greater omentum, and mesentery. These lesions showed invasion of round cells like those seen in ascites. The MIB-1 (proliferative) index was approximately 60%. Microcalcification was seen in proximal tubules to collecting ducts of bilateral kidneys (Figure 1(j)). Final diagnosis was spontaneous TLS caused by DEAC of the uterus.

TABLE 1: Laboratory tests upon admission.

On admission		Fifth day		Reference range
Alb	3.3 g/dL	Alb	2.7 g/dL	3.5–4.5 g/dL
AST	16 IU/L	AST	35 IU/L	10–35 IU/L
ALT	7 IU/L	ALT	12 IU/L	10–35 IU/L
LDH	444 IU/L	LDH	662 IU/L	100–250 IU/L
BUN	17.8 mg/dL	BUN	66.4 mg/dL	<20 mg/dL
Cre	1.52 mg/dL	Cre	5.18 mg/dL	<0.80 mg/dL
Na	126 mEq/L	Na	126 mEq/L	135–145 mEq/L
K	4.9 mEq/L	K	5.7 mEq/L	3.5–4.5 mEq/L
Cl	89 mEq/L	Cl	83 mEq/L	95–108 mEq/L
UA	9.0 mg/dL	UA	18.8 mEq/L	<6.8 mEq/L
CRP	14.48 mg/dL	CRP	27.6 mg/dL	<0.30 mEq/L
		Ca	10.0 mg/dL	8.5–10.5 mg/dL
		P	9.3 mg/dL	2.7–4.6 mg/dL
CEA	5.7 ng/mL			0–5 ng/mL
CA19-9	2294 IU/mL			0–37 IU/mL
CA125	506 IU/mL			0–35 IU/mL
HTLV-1 antibody	Positive			Negative

TABLE 2: Review of spontaneous TLS in patients with solid tumors.

Tumor	Age	Sex	UA (mg/dL)	K (mEq/L)	Ca (mg/dL)	P (mg/dL)	Ref
Adenocarcinoma unknown origin	50	M	37	6.5	8.3	9.2	[3]
Adenocarcinoma unknown origin	59	F	26.5	ND	6.5	8.8	[4]
Adenocarcinoma unknown origin	71	F	10.3	5.78	9.6	6	[5]
Breast lobular carcinoma	62	F	10.1	ND	10.1	6	[6]
Cholangiocarcinoma	66	M	9.9	4.8	8.7	3.8	[7]
Colon cancer	82	F	20.4	ND	5.7	5.5	[8]
Gastric adenocarcinoma	36	M	16.9	5.6	7	6.9	[9]
Gastric adenocarcinoma	51	M	27.9	5.3	8.9	15.2	[10]
Germ cell tumor	13	F	28	5.6	7.2	7.3	[11]
Germ cell tumor	22	M	18	7.2	9.6	7.2	[12]
Germ cell tumor	52	M	21.8	7.9	5	7.1	[13]
Germ cell tumor	24	M	24	8.5	7.6	10	[13]
Hepatocellular carcinoma	72	M	20.1	4.5	7.2	5.4	[8]
Hepatocellular carcinoma	76	M	16.3	6.9	7.7	8.9	[14]
Hepatocellular carcinoma	70	M	22.9	6	11	6.9	[15]
Lung adenocarcinoma	72	M	12.6	7	8.2	8.3	[16]
Lung SCC	74	M	15.4	5.2	ND	4.7	[17]
Lung small cell lung cancer	53	M	8.3	6.1	ND	5.3	[18]
Maxillary SCC	53	M	20.9	7.6	6.2	11.8	[19]
Melanoma	69	M	24.6	6.3	8.4	3.8	[20]
Merkel cell cancer	87	F	13.9	5.6	7.3	7.2	[21]
Ovarian carcinoma	71	F	10.3	5.78	9.7	5.8	[22]
Pancreatic adenocarcinoma	56	F	14.3	7.5	4	6.3	[23]
Pheochromocytoma	80	M	16.5	6.6	8.4	5.8	[8]
Prostate cancer	72	M	28.1	4.9	8	8.3	[24]
Prostate cancer	56	M	16.4	5.7	10	11.7	[25]
Renal cell carcinoma	56	M	24.6	5	9.4	10.5	[26]
Sarcoma	49	F	14.3	5.1	7.7	6.9	[27]

3. Discussion

TLS usually refers to the constellation of metabolic disturbances that may follow the initiation of cancer treatment. The incidence of TLS has been reported as 4%–42% [28]. The variation of incidence depends on the types of malignancy. The TLS consensus panel recommended the risk-stratified prevention of TLS. In view of pathogenesis, the risk factors of TLS include tumor-related intrinsic and host-related extrinsic factors. Tumor-related intrinsic factors include a high proliferation rate, and host-related extrinsic factors are age, volume depletion, WBC count, and renal function [1]. Based on a PubMed search, at least 28 cases of spontaneous TLS have been reported in patients with solid tumors (Table 2). The literature search was using PubMed with the following medical keywords: {spontaneous} and {tumor lysis syndrome} OR {TLS}. These previous cases showed that several types of tumors have been reported to date. Contrary to the case of aggressive hematological tumors, not all cases have exhibited high proliferation. Although pathological findings of our case revealed high MIB-1 index, this value is not so high compared to that of hematological malignancies. These cases might have the host-related extrinsic factors. Some cases have been reported to be caused by host-related factors such as proceeding infection [29], the contrast dye iohexol [30], operations [31], and even anesthesia [32]. Our case has no apparent coexisting risks and we finally diagnosed her as having spontaneous TLS.

DEAC of the uterus is defined as containing both a low-grade endometrioid adenocarcinoma and undifferentiated carcinoma population. It has been reported as a rare but highly aggressive uterine cancer [33]. The undifferentiated component of DEAC sometimes can be confused with other tumors including lymphoma [34]. Taraif et al. reported that 80% of patients with DEAC die within 12 months of diagnosis [35]. Our case exhibited highly aggressive clinical course, as was suggested in several previous reports.

In conclusion, we experienced the extremely rare case of spontaneous TLS with DEAC. In the cases with DEAC, clinicians should pay attention to spontaneous TLS. Further investigations for new strategy to treat DEAC patients are needed.

References

[1] J. Hochberg and M. S. Cairo, "Tumor lysis syndrome: Current perspective," *Haematologica*, vol. 93, no. 1, pp. 9–13, 2008.

[2] J. Bedrna and J. Polcák, "Akuter harnleiterverschluss nach bestrahlung chronischer leukämien mit röntgenstrahlen," *Medizinische Klinik*, vol. 25, pp. 1700-1701, 1929.

[3] D. R. Crittenden and G. L. Ackerman, "Hyperuricemic Acute Renal Failure in Disseminated Carcinoma," *Archives of Internal Medicine*, vol. 137, no. 1, pp. 97–99, 1977.

[4] N. Saini, K. Pyo Lee, S. Jha et al., "Hyperuricemic Renal Failure in Nonhematologic Solid Tumors: A Case Report and Review of the Literature," *Case Reports in Medicine*, vol. 2012, pp. 1–5, 2012.

[5] Y. Wang, C. Yuan, and X. Liu, "Cutaneous metastatic adenocarcinoma complicated by spontaneous tumor lysis syndrome: A case report," *Oncology Letters*, vol. 8, no. 2, pp. 905–907, 2014.

[6] N. T. Sklarin and M. Markham, "Spontaneous recurrent tumor lysis syndrome in breast cancer," *American Journal of Clinical Oncology*, vol. 18, no. 1, pp. 71–73, 1995.

[7] A. E. Mirrakhimov, A. M. Ali, M. Khan, and A. Barbaryan, "Tumor lysis syndrome in solid tumors: an up to date review of the literature," *Rare Tumors*, vol. 6, article 5389, no. 2, 2014.

[8] E. Vaisban, A. Braester, O. Mosenzon, M. Kolin, and Y. Horn, "Spontaneous tumor lysis syndrome in solid tumors: really a rare condition?" *American Journal of the Medical Sciences*, vol. 325, no. 1, pp. 38–40, 2003.

[9] I. S. Woo, J. S. Kim, M. J. Park et al., "Spontaneous acute tumor lysis syndrome with advanced gastric cancer," *Journal of Korean Medical Science*, vol. 16, no. 1, pp. 115–118, 2001.

[10] H. Goyal, H. Sawhney, S. Bekara, and U. Singla, "Spontaneous Acute Tumour Lysis Syndrome in Gastric Adenocarcinoma: A Case Report and Literature Review," *Journal of Gastrointestinal Cancer*, vol. 45, no. 1, pp. 208–211, 2014.

[11] M. J. Murray, L. E. Metayer, C. L. Mallucci et al., "Intra-abdominal metastasis of an intracranial germinoma via ventriculo-peritoneal shunt in a 13-year-old female," *British Journal of Neurosurgery*, vol. 25, no. 6, pp. 747–749, 2011.

[12] V. D'Alessandro, A. Greco, C. Clemente et al., "Severe spontaneous acute tumor lysis syndrome and hypoglycemia in patient with germ cell tumor," *Tumori*, vol. 96, no. 6, pp. 1040–1043, 2010.

[13] G. Pentheroudakis, V. O'Neill, P. Vasey, and S. Kaye, "Spontaneous acute tumour lysis syndrome in patients with metastatic germ cell tumours: Report of two cases," *Supportive Care in Cancer*, vol. 9, no. 7, pp. 554–557, 2001.

[14] N. Kekre, B. Djordjevic, and C. Touchie, "Cases: Spontaneous tumour lysis syndrome," *CMAJ*, vol. 184, no. 8, pp. 913–916, 2012.

[15] R. Mehrzad, H. Saito, Z. Krahn, and A. Feinstein, "Spontaneous tumor lysis syndrome in a patient with metastatic hepatocellular carcinoma," *Medical Principles and Practice*, vol. 23, no. 6, pp. 574–576, 2014.

[16] J. Feld, H. Mehta, and R. L. Burkes, "Acute spontaneous tumor lysis syndrome in adenocarcinoma of the lung: A case report," *American Journal of Clinical Oncology: Cancer Clinical Trials*, vol. 23, no. 5, pp. 491–493, 2000.

[17] C. Shenoy, "Acute spontaneous tumor lysis syndrome in a patient with squamous cell carcinoma of the lung," *QJM*, vol. 102, no. 1, pp. 71–73, 2009.

[18] V. Kanchustambham, S. Saladi, S. Patolia, and D. Stoeckel, "Spontaneous tumor lysis syndrome in small cell lung cancer," *Cureus*, vol. 9, Article ID e1017, 2017; 9.

[19] M. Abboud and A. Shamseddine, "Maxillary Sinus Squamous Cell Carcinoma Presenting with Fatal Tumor Lysis Syndrome: A Case Report and Review of the Literature," *Case Reports in Oncology*, vol. 2, no. 3, pp. 229–233, 2009.

[20] M. Mouallem, N. Zemer-Wassercug, E. Kugler, N. Sahar, R. Shapira-Frommer, and G. Schiby, "Tumor lysis syndrome and malignant melanoma," *Medical Oncology*, vol. 30, no. 3, article 364, 2013.

[21] T. Grenader and L. Shavit, "Tumor lysis syndrome in a patient with merkel cell carcinoma and provoked pathologic sequence of acute kidney injury, reduced clearance of carboplatin and fatal pancytopenia," *Onkologie*, vol. 34, no. 11, pp. 626–629, 2011.

[22] K. Okamoto, T. Kinoshita, M. Shimizu et al., "A case of spontaneous tumor lysis syndrome in a patient with ovarian cancer," *Case Reports in Obstetrics and Gynecology*, vol. 2015, pp. 1–4, 2015.

[23] R. R. Saleh, J. Rodrigues, and T. C. Lee, "A tumour lysis syndrome in a chemotherapy naïve patient with metastatic pancreatic adenocarcinoma," *BMJ Case Reports*, vol. 2015, article no. 162, 2015.

[24] C.-J. Lin, R.-K. Hsieh, K.-H. Lim, H.-H. Chen, Y.-C. Cheng, and C.-J. Wu, "Fatal spontaneous tumor lysis syndrome in a patient with metastatic, androgen-independent prostate cancer," *Southern Medical Journal*, vol. 100, no. 9, pp. 916-917, 2007.

[25] N. Serling-Boyd, Z. Quandt, and N. Allaudeen, "Spontaneous tumor lysis syndrome in a patient with metastatic prostate cancer," *Molecular and Clinical Oncology*, vol. 6, pp. 589–592, 2017.

[26] S. M. Norberg, M. Oros, M. Birkenbach, and M. Bilusic, "Spontaneous tumor lysis syndrome in renal cell carcinoma: a case report," *Clinical Genitourinary Cancer*, vol. 12, no. 5, pp. e225–e227, 2014.

[27] Y. Zakharia, J. Mansour, S. Vasireddi et al., "Tumor Lysis Syndrome in a Retroperitoneal Sarcoma," *Journal of Investigative Medicine High Impact Case Reports*, vol. 2, no. 3, 2014.

[28] B. Coiffier, A. Altman, C.-H. Pui, A. Younes, and M. S. Cairo, "Guidelines for the management of pediatric and adult tumor lysis syndrome: An evidence-based review," *Journal of Clinical Oncology*, vol. 26, no. 16, pp. 2767–2778, 2008.

[29] R.-L. Chen and S.-S. Chuang, "Transient spontaneous remission after tumor lysis syndrome triggered by a severe pulmonary infection in an adolescent boy with acute lymphoblastic leukemia," *Journal of Pediatric Hematology/Oncology*, vol. 31, no. 1, pp. 76–79, 2009.

[30] S. Yun, N. D. Vincelette, T. Phan, and F. Anwer, "Spontaneous tumour lysis syndrome associated with contrast dye iohexol use in mantle cell lymphoma," *BMJ Case Reports*, 2014.

[31] A. Verma, R. Mathur, M. Chauhan, and P. Ranjan, "Tumor lysis syndrome developing intraoperatively," *Journal of Anaesthesiology Clinical Pharmacology*, vol. 27, no. 4, pp. 561–563, 2011.

[32] E. Farley-Hills, A. J. Byrne, L. Brennan, and P. Sartori, "Tumour lysis syndrome during anaesthesia," *Paediatric Anaesthesia*, vol. 11, no. 2, pp. 233–236, 2001.

[33] E. G. Silva, M. T. Deavers, D. C. Bodurka, and A. Malpica, "Association of low-grade endometrioid carcinoma of the uterus and ovary with undifferentiated carcinoma: A new type of dedifferentiated carcinoma?" *International Journal of Gynecological Pathology*, vol. 25, no. 1, pp. 52–58, 2006.

[34] S. Y. Park, M. H. Park, H. S. Ko et al., "Dedifferentiated endometrioid adenocarcinoma of the uterus: Highly aggressive and poor prognostic tumor," *Korean Journal of Pathology*, vol. 48, no. 4, pp. 327–330, 2014.

[35] S. H. Taraif, M. T. Deavers, A. Malpica, and E. G. Silva, "The significance of neuroendocrine expression in undifferentiated carcinoma of the endometrium," *International Journal of Gynecological Pathology*, vol. 28, no. 2, pp. 142–147, 2009.

33

A Malignant Squeeze: A Rare Cause of Cardiac Tamponade

Elisa Quiroz,[1] Adam Hafeez,[1] Ramy Mando,[1] Zhou Yu,[1] and Feroze Momin[2]

[1]*Department of Internal Medicine, Beaumont Health, Royal Oak, MI, USA*
[2]*Department of Hematology and Oncology, Beaumont Health, Royal Oak, MI, USA*

Correspondence should be addressed to Ramy Mando; ramy.mando@beaumont.org

Academic Editor: Jeanine M. Buchanich

Primary cardiac lymphoma (PCL) is a rare condition described as a lymphoma localized to the heart or pericardium. Although cardiac involvement is seen in 10–20% of non-Hodgkin's lymphomas, PCL is extremely rare. It comprises merely 0.5% of all lymphomas and 1.3–2% of cardiac malignancies. Early detection is essential to avoid potentially fatal complications, and prognosis is highly dependent on the management of cardiac complications. The etiology of PCL is still unknown, and molecular characterization has yet to be studied leaving a great deal of research to be done in order to gain a better understanding of this rare disease process. We discuss the case of an 85-year-old female presenting with dyspnea and chest pain. Computed tomography of the chest revealed a pericardial effusion, and subsequent echocardiogram demonstrated a large circumferential effusion. She underwent emergent pericardiocentesis. Morphologic and immunophenotypic features were consistent with high-grade B-cell lymphoma with $t(8;14)$, and the patient was started on rituximab, cyclophosphamide, doxorubicin, vincristine, and prednisone (R-CHOP) with excellent response.

1. Introduction

Primary cardiac lymphoma (PCL) is a rare condition that is described as a lymphoma localized to the heart or pericardium with no extracardiac involvement. Although cardiac involvement is seen in about 10–20% of non-Hodgkin's lymphomas, PCL is extremely rare. It comprises merely 0.5% of all lymphomas and 1.3–2% of cardiac malignancies [1, 2]. Clinical presentation typically correlates with the region of the heart involved. It is often a clinical emergency as these patients commonly present with heart failure, cardiac tamponade, or arrhythmia [3]. Herein, we describe a rare case of PCL causing cardiac tamponade in an elderly patient.

2. Case Description

An 85-year-old female with past medical history of recurrent deep venous thrombosis, pulmonary embolism on anticoagulation with a vena cava filter in place, rheumatoid arthritis, hypertension, hyperlipidemia, hypothyroidism, and type 2 diabetes mellitus presented to the emergency department with complaint of exertional dyspnea and chest pain. She denied fever, chills, or lower extremity edema and had no history of malignancy, weight loss, or night sweats. Initial vitals revealed BP of 86/62 mmHg that decreased to 79/60 mmHg with inspiration. Initial pulse was 95 bpm, and respiratory rate was 20. White blood cell count was mildly elevated at 11.5, troponins were normal, and electrocardiogram was unremarkable. D-dimer was elevated at 1290. Patient was sent for CT scan to evaluate for pulmonary embolism, and a moderate pericardial effusion was found (Figure 1). Subsequently, an echocardiogram was done to further delineate the effusion which revealed a large circumferential effusion with mild respiratory variation concerning for impending cardiac tamponade (Figure 2). She was admitted to the intensive care unit and underwent emergent pericardiocentesis. Flow cytometry of the pericardial fluid revealed a population of monoclonal B-cells with significant large cell component (Figure 3). The overall morphologic and immunophenotypic features were consistent with high-grade B-cell lymphoma with $t(8;14)$ (Figure 4). Bone marrow biopsy demonstrated monotypic B-cells compatible with the diagnosis of large B-cell lymphoma. The patient was started on rituximab, cyclophosphamide, doxorubicin, vincristine, and prednisone

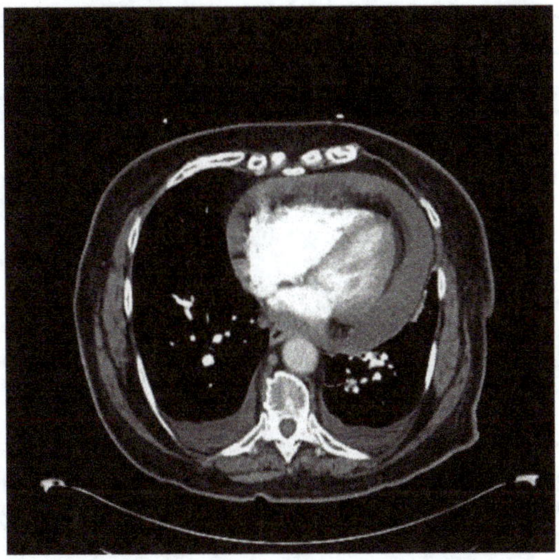

FIGURE 1: Computed tomography of the chest demonstrating pericardial effusion.

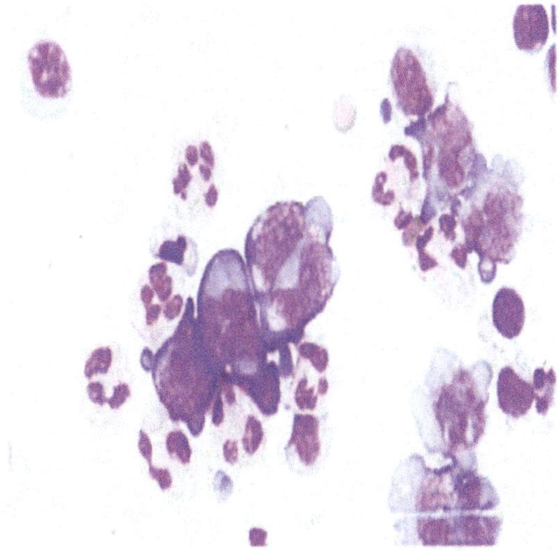

FIGURE 3: Histopathology remarkable for monoclonal B-cells with significant large cell components.

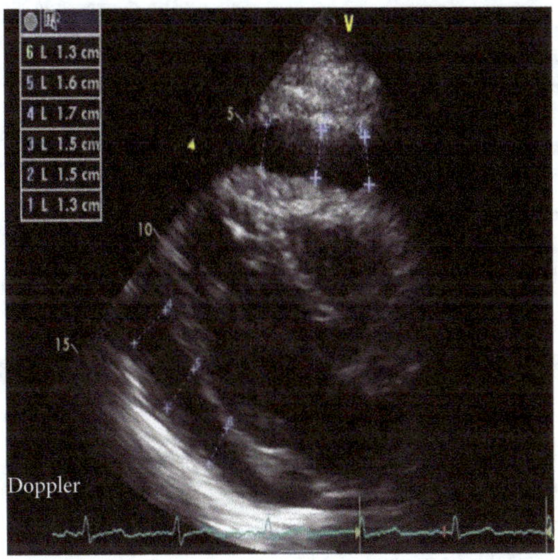

FIGURE 2: Echocardiogram demonstrating a large circumferential effusion (outlined) concerning for impending tamponade.

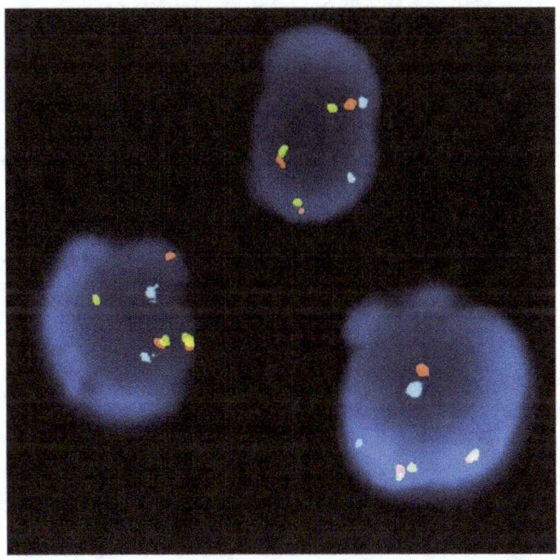

FIGURE 4: Fluorescence in situ hybridization demonstrating $t(8;14)$. This translocation is between IGH on chromasome 8 and MYC on chromosome 14.

(R-CHOP) with an excellent initial response. She was transferred out of the ICU within days and discharged home for outpatient follow-up.

3. Discussion

Primary cardiac tumors are known classically to be rare and benign. Cardiac myxoma is the most frequently reported primary cardiac tumor, but hematologic disease, in rare cases, has been known to orginate in the heart [4]. Lymphomas compromise only 0.5–2% of primary cardiac tumors and occur most often in immunocompromised patients, such as those with human immunodeficiency virus (HIV) [5]. The frequencies of other types of non-Hodgkin's lymphoma are detailed in Figure 5 with diffuse large B-cell lymphoma comprising the majority at 30% [6]. PCL does occur in immunocompetent hosts although infrequently, as it did in

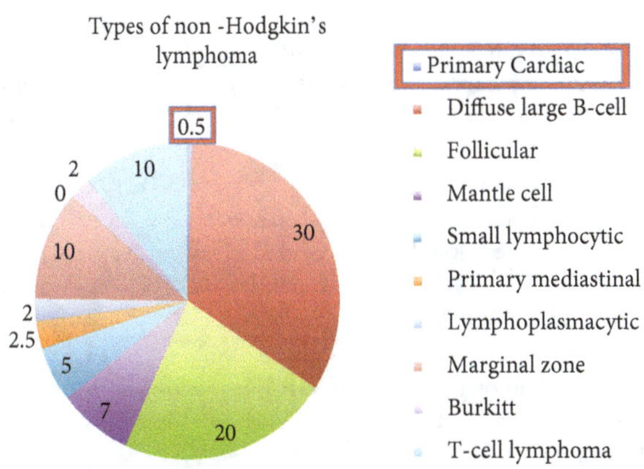

FIGURE 5: Graphical representation of frequencies of subtypes of non-Hodgkin's lymphoma.

Table 1: Reports of primary cardiac lymphoma causing cardiac tamponade.

Article (language, PMID)	Description	Highlights
Parato VM, Muscente F, Scarano M. Primary cardiac lymphoma: a case report. G Ital Cardiol (Rome). 2017 Jan; 18(1): 11–13 (Italian, 28287210)	35-year-old immunocompromised patient presented with signs and symptoms of tamponade. Echocardiography revealed lateral AV mass with large pericardial effusion. Patient had surgical excision of mass followed by chemotherapy that induced complete remission at 6 months.	
Tzachanis D, Dewar R, Luptakova K, Chang JD, et al. Primary cardiac Burkitt lymphoma presenting with abdominal pain (English, 25431699)	44-year-old female presented with abdominal bloating who was found to have a large pericardial effusion with tamponade physiology. Pericardial fluid studies led to diagnosis of cardiac Burkitt lymphoma.	Primary Burkitt lymphoma
Frikha Z, Abid L, Abid D, Mallek S, et al. Cardiac tamponade and paroxysmal third-degree atrioventricular block revealing a primary cardiac non-Hodgkin large B-cell lymphoma of the right ventricle: a case report. J Med Case Rep. 2011 Sep 5; 5: 433 (English, 21892927)	64-year-old immunocompromised male presented with cardiac tamponade as well as paroxysmal third-degree AV block. He was found to have a large RV mass. Following excision, histology confirmed non-Hodgkin large B-cell lymphoma.	Primary non-Hodgkin large B-cell lymphoma 3rd-degree AV block
Houchaymi Z, Helou S, Ballout J. Pericardial tamponade and third-degree atrioventricular block revealing a primary cardiac lymphoma. Rev Med Interne. 2010 Nov; 31 (11): e4-6 (French, 20605278)	78-year-old immunocompetent male presented with pericardial tamponade and third-degree AV block. Biopsy of the cardiac tumor showed non-Hodgkin large B-Cell lymphoma.	Primary non-Hodgkin large B-cell lymphoma 3rd-degree AV block
Chiba Y, Oka K, Saito H, et al. Primary cardiac B-cell lymphoma presented as heart tamponade and atrioventricular block: a case report. Acta Cytol. 2010 Jan–Feb; 54 (1): 79–81 (English, 20306995)	49-year-old male with cardiac tamponade and AV block. Pericardial effusion and transvenous biopsy confirmed diagnosis of diffuse large B-cell lymphoma. He underwent chemotherapy and permanent pacemaker placement.	Diffuse large B-cell lymphoma AV block
Legault S, Couture C, Bourgault C, et al. Primary cardiac Burkitt-like lymphoma of the right atrium	74-year-old male with dyspnea found to have a large pericardial effusion with tamponade physiology. Found on pericardial fluid studies and biopsy to have Burkitt-like PCL.	Burkitt-like PCL
Ling LF, Chai P, Kee AC, et al. Primary cardiac lymphoma presenting with cardiac tamponade. Am Heart Hosp J. 2009 Winter; 7 (2): E125-7 (English, 19279985)	55-year-old immunocompetent man presented with pyrexia initially and was found later to have cardiac tamponade. He was diagnosed with PCL.	
Gosev I, Siric F, Gasparovic H, et al. Surgical treatment of a primary cardiac lymphoma presenting with tamponade physiology (English, 16846425)	67-year-old immunocompetent presented with dyspnea. Found to have tamponade physiology on echocardiography. Surgical biopsy confirmed diffuse large B-cell lymphoma of centroblastic subtype.	Diffuse large B-cell lymphoma of centroblastic subtype Surgical diagnosis, no pericardiocentesis performed
Wilhite DB, Quigley RL. Occult cardiac lymphoma presenting with cardiac tamponade. Tex Heart Inst. J. 2003; 30 (1): 62–4 (English, 12638674)	83-year-old Filipino male with dyspnea found on echocardiogram to have a large, homogenous pericardial effusion with RA collapse. He was treated with subxiphoid pericardiostomy and had the pericardial drain removed the next day as he clinically improved. He returned two weeks later with same symptoms and again found to have reaccumulating pericardial fluid requiring urgent anterior pericardiectomy.	Failure of traditional pericardiostomy
Menotti A, Imperadore F, Pelosi G. et al. Heart rupture at the right atrial level as the first manifestation of malignant lymphoma. Cardiologia. 1996 Jan;41(1):65–7 (Italian, 8697472)	Malignant lymphoma presenting as cardiac tamponade due to right atrial rupture.	Right atrial rupture causing the tamponade
Roller MB, Manoharan A, Lvoff R. Primary cardiac lymphoma. Acta Haematol. 1991; 85 (1): 47–48 (English, 2011932)	Elderly male with cardiac tamponade found on pericardial fluid analysis to have PCL.	

Table 1: Continued.

Article (language, PMID)	Description	Highlights
Nagamine K, Noda H. Two cases cardiac lymphoma presenting with pericardial effusion and tamponade. Jpn Circ. J. 1990 Sep; 54 (9): 1158–64 (English, 2266577)	Two cases of males in their 70s presenting with dyspnea who were found to have pericardial effusion with tamponade physiology on echocardiogram.	
Pozniak AL, Thomas RD, Hobbs CB, et al. Primary malignant lymphoma of the heart. Antemorten cytologic diagnosis. Acta Cytol. 1986 Nov–Dec; 30 (6): 662–4. (English, 3466501)	Patient who presented with ventricular arrhythmias and was found to have pericardial effusion with impairment of LV contraction. Postmortem examination showed malignant lymphoma confined to myocardium.	
Patel J, Melly L, Sheppard MN. Primary cardiac lymphoma: B- and T-cell cases at a specialist UK centre	Case series of six patients presenting with wide spectrum of symptoms. Most cases involved 2 or more chambers of the heart. Presentations included conduction disturbances, effusion, valvular dysfunction, heart failure, stroke, and sudden death.	Clinical presentation of PCL (B- and T-cells)

our patient. In these immunocompetent patients, studies have shown that 80% of PCL are of diffuse B-cell lymphoma [7]. The location of cardiac involvement for PCL is often the right atrium and right ventricle. Clinical presentation can vary depending on the site of involvement of the heart. Most often, an extensive multidisciplinary workup is employed to come up with the correct diagnosis. Imaging modalities such as transthoracic and transesophageal echocardiography, computed tomography (as done in our patient), and magnetic resonance imaging are all utilized in diagnosing this entity. Confirmation of the diagnosis is through cytology of biopsy or pericardial fluid. The combination of chemotherapy and radiation is the treatment of choice. Treatment for B-cell lymphoma is typically an anthracycline-based, such as given in our patient. Our patient was treated with rituximab, cyclophosphamide, doxorubicin, vincristine, and prednisone (R-CHOP). Survival has been demonstrated in some cases up to 5 years with treatment but is less than a month without it [7].

Although PCL is rare, the pathophysiology is classic and detection through a detailed physical exam and directed workup diagnosis can be promptly made, even when presenting as tamponade as did our patient. Patients presenting with signs and symptoms of new-onset acute decompensated heart failure can potentially have this diagnosis. Immediate detection is essential to avoid fatal complications, which include cardiac tamponade, ischemia, and fatal arrhythmia. To our knowledge, only 13 cases have described PCL presenting with tamponade physiology and are highlighted in Table 1. Parato et al. describe a case of a younger patient who presented with cardiac tamponade due to PCL. The patient was treated with management of cardiac tamponade, surgical excision of the mass, and chemotherapy. Complete remission was obtained after six months of chemotherapy [8]. Although there was a large age difference, our patient also responded to chemotherapy following medical stabilization. Interestingly, Frikha et al. describe a case of an elderly immunocompromised patient presenting with cardiac tamponade along with paroxysmal third-degree atrioventricular (AV) block. They hypothesized that electrical compromise occurred via extension of the malignancy into the interatrial septum and the nodal tissue [9]. Similarly, Gowda and Khan and Houchaymi et al. describe a case of an elderly immunocompetent male who was found to have pericardial tamponade along with third-degree AV block. However, pericardial fluid analysis did not reveal the diagnosis until a transvenous biopsy of the cardiac tumor revealed non-Hodgkin large B-cell lymphoma [7, 10]. Gowda and Khan and Chiba et al. report a similar case of a middle-aged male with cardiac tamponade and AV block who was found on right atrial tumor biopsy to have a diffuse large B-cell lymphoma. The patient underwent chemotherapy and required permanent pacemaker placement [7, 11]. On our extensive literature search, we identified one case report in which the cardiac tamponade was not caused by the lymphoma itself, but rather due to the malignant right atrial rupturing causing tamponade [12]. Further cases are described in Table 1.

The etiology of PCL is still unknown, and molecular characterization has yet to be studied leaving a great deal of research to be done to gain a better understanding of this rare disease process. Nevertheless, although extremely rare, PCL can present with severe cardiac dysfunction due to tamponade physiology or impending tamponade physiology and heart failure. Clinical suspicion must remain high, and diagnostic studies of pericardial fluid can help prevent delay in management of an aggressive malignancy.

References

[1] H. Ikeda, S. Nakamura, H. Nishimaki et al., "Primary lymphoma of the heart: case report and literature review," *Pathology International*, vol. 54, no. 3, pp. 187–195, 2004.

[2] G. L. Ceresoli, A. J. M. Ferreri, E. Bucci, C. Ripa, M. Ponzoni, and E. Villa, "Primary cardiac lymphoma in immunocompetent patients: diagnostic and therapeutic management," *Cancer*, vol. 80, no. 8, pp. 1497–1506, 1997.

[3] C. S. Chim, A. C. L. Chan, Y. L. Kwong, and R. Liang, "Primary cardiac lymphoma," *American Journal of Hematology*, vol. 54, no. 1, pp. 79–83, 1997.

[4] J. G. Wang, H. Liu, W. J. Yu, Y. J. Li, and F. J. Xin, "Primary cardiac neoplasms: a clinicopathologic analysis of 81 cases," *Zhonghua Bing Li Xue Za Zhi*, vol. 41, no. 12, pp. 808–12, 2012.

[5] M. Duong, C. Dubois, M. Buisson et al., "Non-Hodgkin's lymphoma of the heart in patients infected with human immunodeficiency virus," *Clinical Cardiology*, vol. 20, no. 5, pp. 497–502, 1997.

[6] American Society of Clinical Oncology (ASCO), "Lymphoma - non-Hodgkin: subtypes," 2016, https://www.cancer.net/cancer-types/lymphoma-non-hodgkin/subtypes.

[7] R. M. Gowda and I. A. Khan, "Clinical perspectives of primary cardiac lymphoma," *Angiology*, vol. 54, no. 5, pp. 599–604, 2003.

[8] V. M. Parato, F. Muscente, and M. Scarano, "Primary cardiac lymphoma: a case report," *Giornale Italiano di Cardiologia*, vol. 18, no. 1, pp. 11–13, 2017.

[9] Z. Frikha, L. Abid, D. Abid et al., "Cardiac tamponade and paroxysmal third-degree atrioventricular block revealing a primary cardiac non-Hodgkin large B-cell lymphoma of the right ventricle: a case report," *Journal of Medical Case Reports*, vol. 5, no. 1, p. 433, 2011.

[10] Z. Houchaymi, S. Helou, and J. Ballout, "Pericardial tamponade and third-degree atrioventricular block revealing a primary cardiac lymphoma," *La Revue de Médecine Interne*, vol. 31, no. 11, pp. e4–e6, 2010.

[11] Y. Chiba, K. Oka, H. Saito, R. Nagayama, M. Murata, and N. Mori, "Primary cardiac B-cell lymphoma presented as heart tamponade and atrioventricular block: a case report," *Acta Cytologica*, vol. 54, no. 1, pp. 79–81, 2010.

[12] A. Menotti, F. Imperadore, G. Pelosi, and M. Disertori, "Heart rupture at the right atrial level as the first manifestation of malignant lymphoma," *Cardiologia*, vol. 41, no. 1, pp. 65–67, 1996.

34

A Patient with Non-Hodgkin Lymphoma and Nonspecific Interstitial Pneumonia during Ibrutinib Therapy

Sven Jungmann,[1] Wolf-Dieter Ludwig,[2] Nicolas Schönfeld,[1] Torsten-Gerriet Blum,[1] Claudia Großwendt,[3] Christian Boch,[1] Beate Rehbock,[4] Sergej Griff,[5] Alexander Schmittel,[6] and Torsten T. Bauer[1]

[1]*Department of Pneumology, Lungenklinik Heckeshorn, HELIOS Klinikum Emil von Behring, Berlin, Germany*
[2]*Drug Commission of the German Medical Association, Herbert-Lewin-Platz 1, Berlin, Germany*
[3]*Department of Radiology, HELIOS Klinikum Emil von Behring, Berlin, Germany*
[4]*Diagnostic Radiology, Thoracic Imaging, Bismarckstr 45-47, Berlin, Germany*
[5]*Institute of Pathology, HELIOS Klinikum Emil von Behring, Berlin, Germany*
[6]*Onkologie Seestrasse, Seestr. 64, 13347 Berlin, Germany*

Correspondence should be addressed to Torsten T. Bauer; torsten.bauer@rub.de

Academic Editor: Kaiser Jamil

We present a 74-year-old male with nonspecific interstitial pneumonia (NSIP) during treatment with ibrutinib for mantle cell lymphoma. Previously, the patient had received six cycles of bendamustine and rituximab and six cycles of R-CHOP, followed by rituximab maintenance therapy. Respiratory tract complications of ibrutinib other than infectious pneumonia have not been mentioned in larger trials, but individual case reports hinted to a possible association with the development of pneumonitis. In our patient, the onset of alveolitis that progressed towards NSIP together with the onset of ibrutinib treatment suggests causality. One week after ibrutinib was discontinued, nasal symptoms resolved first. A follow-up CT showed a reduction in the reticular hyperdensities and ground-glass opacities, suggestive of restitution of the lung disease. To our knowledge, this is the first case showing a strong link between ibrutinib and interstitial lung disease, strengthening a previous report on subacute pneumonitis. Our findings have clinical implications because pulmonary side effects were reversible at this early stage. We, therefore, suggest close monitoring for respiratory side effects in patients receiving ibrutinib.

1. Introduction

Ibrutinib, a selective Bruton's tyrosine kinase inhibitor, was approved initially in November 2013 by the US Food and Drug Administration for the treatment of mantle cell lymphoma and in February 2014 for B-cell chronic lymphocytic leukaemia, and later on also for Waldenström macroglobulinemia, all after first-line treatment [1]. Respiratory tract complications other than infectious pneumonia have not been mentioned in larger trials. However, a single case [2] and a case series [3] of four cases of ibrutinib-induced pneumonitis were published in May 2015 and February 2016, respectively. By November 2016, two cases of pneumonitis were mentioned on http://www.pneumotox.com [4].

2. Patient

We present a 74-year-old male whom we evaluated for a suspected nonspecific interstitial pneumonia (NSIP) under ibrutinib (560 mg QD). He was diagnosed with mantle cell lymphoma (2011) and received six cycles of bendamustine and rituximab (April to August 2011) and later six cycles of R-CHOP (October 2013 to February 2014), followed by rituximab maintenance therapy (February 2014 to January 2015). In February 2015, ibrutinib therapy was initiated because of abdominal progression. He responded well to ibrutinib with a partial remission. The patient felt healthy and denied cough, pain, dyspnoea, fever, night sweats, weight loss, nausea, or fatigue. However, he noted scales in his nasal discharge and frequent nasal bleeding. Medical

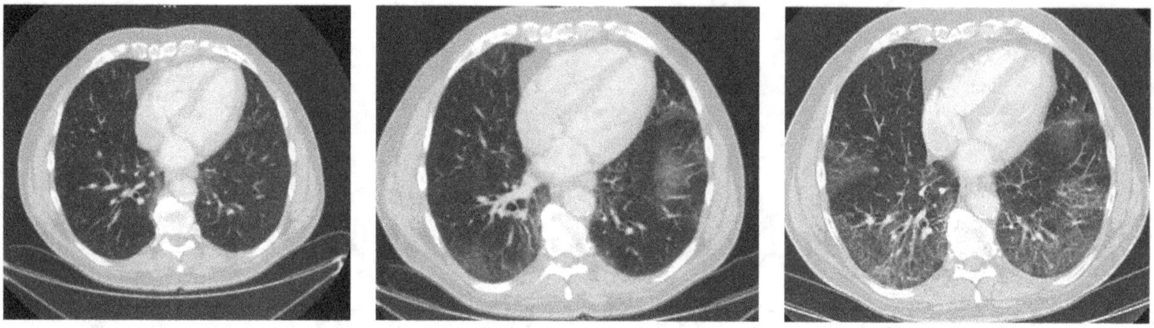

(a) (b) (c)

Figure 1: Computed tomography findings. (a) January 2015: the lower lung shows normal lung structures without signs of interstitial pneumonia or fibrosis. (b) June 2015: the same area now shows a bilateral mild interstitial pneumonia with ground-glass opacities. (c) March 2016: images show a more fibrotic structure with mild reticular abnormalities and ground-glass opacities.

history included hypertension, hyperlipidemia, peripheral artery occlusive disease, benign prostatic hyperplasia, and cigarette smoking (15 pack-years) until 35 years ago. He suffered from pneumonia at age 16 and received coronary artery bypass surgery at 65 years. Additional medication included once-daily doses of acetylsalicylic acid (100 mg), enalapril (10 mg), amlodipine (5 mg), hydrochlorothiazide (25 mg), and simvastatin (40 mg). There was no evidence of existing allergies or toxic exposures.

3. Physical Examination

The male patient was well nourished and was in no apparent distress, alert, and fully oriented. He had normal vital signs and no lymphadenopathy or thyromegaly. Lungs were clear to auscultation. He showed regular heart rate and rhythm without murmurs. He presented with soft abdomen, neither tender nor distended, normal bowel sounds, and no hepatosplenomegaly. No cyanosis, clubbing, rash, lesions, nor oedema were observed. Neurologic examination showed that cranial nerves II–XII were intact, and no focal sensorimotoric deficits were found. Skin examination showed no ulceration or induration, and joints and muscles were unaffected.

4. Diagnostic Findings

An abdominal computed tomography (CT) revealed progressive non-Hodgkin lymphoma so that ibrutinib was initiated (October 2015). All abdominal CT scans included basal lung sections, which were normal until then. Subsequent CT scans depicted progressive ground-glass opacities in the middle and both lower lobes. In April 2015, a discrete fibrotic transition became visible, with radiologic patterns compatible with early fibrotic NSIP (Figure 1). Bronchoscopy revealed mild hypervascularization particularly of the upper lobe and main bronchi. Bronchoalveolar lavage (BAL) showed a lymphocytic alveolitis (47% lymphocytes) with a balanced CD4/CD8 ratio. Sampling of the subcarinal lymph node excluded local progression of the disease. The BAL was sent for a routine bacterial workup including Gram stains, and cultures with no potentially pathogenic microorganisms recovered. Table 1 gives an overview of relevant clinical data and findings.

Table 1: Pulmonary function test and relevant blood values (reference values in parentheses).

Test	Value
One-second forced expiratory volume	2.53 liters (81% of predicted)
Vital capacity	3.17 liters (75% of predicted)
Total lung capacity (single breath)	4.5 liters (62% of predicted)
FEV1/FVC ratio	79.84% (106% of predicted)
Single-breath Krogh transfer factor for carbon monoxide	1.05 mmol/(min kPa l) (84% of predicted)
NT-proBNP	293 ng/l (<229)
Estimated GFR	83 ml/min (>90)
Erythrocytes	4.3 G/l (4.5–5.9)
Haemoglobin	12.9 g/dl (14.0–17.5)
MCHC	32 g/dl (33–36)
Thrombocytes	108 G/l (139–335)
Neutrophils	1.47 G/l, 32% (1.6–7.1, 40–75%)
Monocytes	1.11 G/l, 24% (0.2–0.6, 4–11%)
IgG	5.73 g/l (7–16)
IgG4	0.002 g/l (0.052–1.250)
IgM	0.31 g/l (0.4–2.3)
Capillary pH	7.46 (7.37–7.45)
Capillary pCO_2	34 mmHg (35–46)
INF-gamma	0.49 IU/ml (<0.35)
Relevant normal lab values included	ANA, c-ANCA, p-ANCA, anti-CCP, rheumatoid factor, IgA, IgG1-3, IgE, creatinine, and lactate dehydrogenase

5. Literature Review

Our literature search (PubMed Central) identified articles cited up to November 21, 2016, using the keywords "ibrutinib," "PCI 32765," "imbruvica," or "Bruton's Tyrosine Kinase Inhibitor" in combination with the keywords

(Boolean "AND") "pneumonia," "interstitial lung disease," "fibrotic," or "pneumonitis" in title, abstract, and body, yielding 14 publications. Articles that did not address the issue of respiratory side effects in patients receiving ibrutinib were excluded, leaving seven relevant articles that describe pneumonia [1, 5–11] and one case series that describes pneumonitis as a side effect of ibrutinib [3], which also quotes another case presented in a conference poster publication [2]. However, NSIP has not been described to date. Two cases of pneumonitis but no association of NSIP with ibrutinib were described on http://www.pneumotox.com [4]; however, pneumonitis is mentioned twice. The Drug Commission of the German Medical Association has received 236 reports of adverse effect suspicions for ibrutinib until May 2016, two of which include atypical pneumonia and a total of 21 reported pneumonia [12].

6. Discussion

Only a few ibrutinib-associated lower respiratory tract side effects are known. In seminal phase 2 [13] and phase 3 trials [14], ibrutinib was shown to be effective and well tolerated with no dose-limiting toxicity being observed. Postmarketing adverse effect studies revealed the following pulmonary side effects: a study [6] involving 51 patients with chronic lymphocytic leukaemia receiving ibrutinib described 12% grade 2 and 6% grade 3 pneumonia and pulmonary infiltrates in 2% as treatment-related adverse events and concluded that ibrutinib's safety profile was encouraging. A long-term follow-up [9] of 111 patients reported a favourable benefit-risk profile. While dyspnoea was seen in 32%, two-thirds involved respiratory function, such as chronic obstructive pulmonary disease, respiratory infections, malignant pleural effusion, and pneumonia (8%, grade ≥ 3). Another study [10] including 132 patients concluded that pneumonia was among the most common complications and resumed that ibrutinib is well tolerated. In all studies, complications were well manageable with little or no chronicity.

Our patient's association of the alveolitis that progressed into NSIP pattern after the commencement of ibrutinib treatment suggests causality. One week after the ibrutinib was discontinued, nasal symptoms resolved. In June 2016, a follow-up CT showed a diminution of the reticular hyperdensities and ground-glass opacities with minimal residues in the lingual and lower lobe. To our knowledge, this is the first case showing a link between ibrutinib and fibrotic lung disease, strengthening the previous report on subacute pneumonitis [3]. Similar to our patient, radiographic changes in the four cases presented by Mato et al. [3] were detected after commencement of ibrutinib therapy and resolved after stopping ibrutinib, and respiratory symptoms recurred in the one case that was rechallenged with the drug. Our findings have clinical implications because pulmonary side effects were reversible at this early stage.

Since July 2017, the patient receives lenalidomide after an abdominal progress. Thus far, the patient does tolerate the medication well and is scheduled for restaging. We abstained to reintroduce ibrutinib into the therapeutic regimen due to the lack of information on the repeated reversibility of the pulmonary damage.

Some limitations in the clinical workup apply. We did not look for *Pneumocystis jirovecii* infection and did not exclude viral infection (e.g., CMV) as a cause of pulmonary infiltrates in this patient. However, a normal lactate dehydrogenase and the good clinical improvement with corticosteroids suggest neither one of these infections to be the cause of the clinical deterioration.

We, therefore, suggest monitoring patients receiving ibrutinib for respiratory side effects. Also, more research is required to define the underlying pathways that lead to pulmonary toxicities of signal transduction inhibitors: as Mato et al. point out [3], other targeted therapies such as rapamycin inhibitors [15, 16], phosphatidylinositol 3-kinase inhibitors [17], and spleen tyrosine kinase inhibitors [18] appear to cause similar pulmonary toxicities. Mato et al. suggest that the inhibition of signal transduction enhances the expression of proinflammatory cytokines and the innate immune system [3]. They further propose that Bruton's tyrosine kinase might serve as a mediator of lipopolysaccharide-induced dendritic cell maturation and macrophage polarisation and highlight that several studies have reported an increase in alveolar infiltration of T helper 2 proinflammatory cytokines in Bruton's tyrosine kinase-deficient mice, which results in airway inflammation [19, 20].

Ethical Approval

No ethics committee approval was necessary. The article was written in adherence to the CARE guidelines [21] for clinical case reporting.

Consent

Written informed consent was obtained from the patient described in the case report.

Disclosure

The case was promptly reported to the Drug Commission of the German Medical Association.

Authors' Contributions

Sven Jungmann, Christian Boch, Nicolas Schönfeld, Torsten-Gerriet Blum, Claudia Großwendt, Beate Rehbock, Sergej Griff, Torsten T. Bauer, and Alexander Schmittel performed the case workup. Sven Jungmann, Torsten-Gerriet Blum, Torsten T. Bauer, and Wolf-Dieter Ludwig wrote the article. Christian Boch, Sven Jungmann, Torsten-Gerriet Blum, and Wolf-Dieter Ludwig carried out literature search. Sven Jungmann and Torsten T. Bauer were responsible for administrative and logistical work.

Acknowledgments

The authors thank the radiologists Margit Reichel, MD, and Robert Gehrmann, MD, for their kind permission to publish their radiographic findings.

References

[1] U.S. Food and Drug Administration, Highlights of prescribing information, Reference ID: 3694103, 2016, http://www.accessdata.fda.gov/drugsatfda_docs/label/2015/205552s002lbl.pdf.

[2] M. Mahmoudi, V. Murthy, J. Suh, A.-d. Bradshaw, and M. Sloance, "Ibrutinib-induced rapidly progressive inflammatory pneumonitis," in *Proceedings of the American Thoracic Society International Conference on C51 Toxic Ingestions and Exposure*, Denver, CO, USA, May 2015.

[3] A. R. Mato, P. Islam, C. Daniel et al., "Ibrutinib-induced pneumonitis in patients with chronic lymphocytic leukemia," *Blood*, vol. 127, no. 8, pp. 1064–1067, 2016.

[4] P. Camus, *The Drug-Induced Respiratory Disease Website*, Department of Pulmonary Medicine and Intensive Care, University Hospital, Dijon, France, 2016.

[5] I. E. Ahn, T. Jerussi, M. Farooqui, X. Tian, A. Wiestner, and J. Gea-Banacloche, "Atypical *Pneumocystis jirovecii* pneumonia in previously untreated patients with CLL on single-agent ibrutinib," *Blood*, vol. 128, no. 15, pp. 1940–1943, 2016.

[6] M. Z. H. Farooqui, J. Valdez, S. Martyr et al., "Ibrutinib for previously untreated and relapsed or refractory chronic lymphocytic leukaemia with TP53 aberrations: a phase 2, single-arm trial," *Lancet Oncology*, vol. 16, no. 2, pp. 169–176, 2015.

[7] C. S. Link, R. Teipel, F. Heidenreich et al., "Durable responses to ibrutinib in patients with relapsed CLL after allogeneic stem cell transplantation," *Bone Marrow Transplantion*, vol. 51, no. 6, pp. 793–798, 2016.

[8] K. Tobinai, M. Ogura, K. Ishizawa et al., "Safety and tolerability of ibrutinib monotherapy in Japanese patients with relapsed/refractory B cell malignancies," *International Journal of Hematology*, vol. 103, no. 1, pp. 86–94, 2016.

[9] M. L. Wang, K. A. Blum, P. Martin et al., "Long-term follow-up of MCL patients treated with single-agent ibrutinib: updated safety and efficacy results," *Blood*, vol. 126, no. 6, pp. 739–745, 2015.

[10] J. C. Byrd, R. R. Furman, S. E. Coutre et al., "Three-year follow-up of treatment-naïve and previously treated patients with CLL and SLL receiving single-agent ibrutinib," *Blood*, vol. 125, no. 16, pp. 2497–2506, 2015.

[11] S. O'Brien, J. A. Jones, S. E. Coutre et al., "Ibrutinib for patients with relapsed or refractory chronic lymphocytic leukaemia with 17p deletion (RESONATE-17): a phase 2, open-label, multicentre study," *Lancet Oncology*, vol. 17, no. 10, pp. 1409–1418, 2016.

[12] Drug Commission of the German Medical Association, *Extract from the Adverse Effect Database*, Drug Commission of the German Medical Association, 2016.

[13] M. L. Wang, S. Rule, P. Martin et al., "Targeting BTK with ibrutinib in relapsed or refractory mantle-cell lymphoma," *New England Journal of Medicine*, vol. 369, no. 6, pp. 507–516, 2013.

[14] J. C. Byrd, J. R. Brown, S. O'Brien et al., "Ibrutinib versus ofatumumab in previously treated chronic lymphoid leukemia," *New England Journal of Medicine*, vol. 371, no. 3, pp. 213–223, 2014.

[15] M. Nishino, E. N. Boswell, H. Hatabu, I. M. Ghobrial, and N. H. Ramaiya, "Drug-related pneumonitis during mammalian target of rapamycin inhibitor therapy: radiographic pattern-based approach in Waldenström macroglobulinemia as a Paradigm," *Oncologist*, vol. 20, no. 9, pp. 1077–1083, 2015.

[16] R. Iacovelli, A. Palazzo, S. Mezi, F. Morano, G. Naso, and E. Cortesi, "Incidence and risk of pulmonary toxicity in patients treated with mTOR inhibitors for malignancy. A meta-analysis of published trials," *Acta Oncologica*, vol. 51, no. 7, pp. 873–879, 2012.

[17] R. R. Furman, J. P. Sharman, S. E. Coutre et al., "Idelalisib and rituximab in relapsed chronic lymphocytic leukemia," *New England Journal of Medicine*, vol. 370, no. 11, pp. 997–1007, 2014.

[18] P. M. Barr, G. B. Saylors, E. Forbes Spurgeon et al., "Phase 2 trial of GS-9973, a selective syk inhibitor, and idelalisib (idela) in chronic lymphocytic leukemia (CLL) and non-Hodgkin lymphoma (NHL)," in *ASCO Annual Meeting Proceedings*, Chicago, IL, USA, May–June 2014.

[19] Y. Kawakami, N. Inagaki, S. Salek-Ardakani et al., "Regulation of dendritic cell maturation and function by Bruton's tyrosine kinase via IL-10 and Stat3," *Proceedings of the National Academy of Sciences of the United States of America*, vol. 103, no. 1, pp. 153–158, 2006.

[20] J. Ní Gabhann, E. Hams, S. Smith et al., "Btk regulates macrophage polarization in response to lipopolysaccharide," *PLoS ONE*, vol. 9, no. 1, article e85834, 2014.

[21] J. J. Gagnier, D. Riley, D. G. Altman, D. Moher, H. Sox, and G. S. Kienle, "The CARE guidelines: consensus-based clinical case reporting guideline development," *Deutsches Ärzteblatt International*, vol. 110, no. 37, pp. 603–608, 2013.

35

Radiation-Induced Sarcoma Originating in Recurrent Juvenile Nasopharyngeal Angiofibroma

Smriti Panda,[1] Madhu Rajeshwari,[2] Chirom Amit Singh,[1] Suresh C. Sharma,[1] and Pirabu Sakthivel[1]

[1]Department of Otolaryngology & Head & Neck Surgery, All India Institute of Medical Sciences, New Delhi, India
[2]Department of Pathology, All India Institute of Medical Sciences, New Delhi, India

Correspondence should be addressed to Chirom Amit Singh; amitchirom@gmail.com

Academic Editor: Jeanine M. Buchanich

Juvenile nasopharyngeal angiofibroma is a benign disease affecting young males with a propensity to invade intracranially and into the orbit along preformed pathways. Complete surgical excision is the mainstay of management. Patients with multiple recurrences along with tumour extension into skull base and orbit can be considered for external beam radiation as either adjuvant or definitive treatment. Possibility of radiation-induced malignancy has been speculated by many authors, proof of which exists in only two studies so far. This report focuses on radiation-induced leiomyosarcoma in a patient with recurrent juvenile nasopharyngeal angiofibroma.

1. Introduction

Juvenile nasopharyngeal angiofibroma is a benign tumour originating in the nasopharynx, presenting in adolescent males with nasal mass, epistaxis, nasal obstruction, cheek swelling, and proptosis. Though benign, it has a capacity for local invasion along preformed pathways. Thus, JNA can encroach into critical structures like optic nerve, internal carotid artery and present intracranially. Surgery is the main modality of treatment, preceded by embolisation of arterial feeders in case of extensive tumours involving infratemporal fossa or intracranial involvement. For tumours infiltrating into infratemporal fossa, sphenoid sinus, base of pterygoid, cavernous sinus, foramen lacerum, anterior and middle cranial fossa [1], subtotal tumour excision predisposes to recurrence. Patients with massive intracranial involvement, incomplete resection, and recurrent tumours can be considered for either definitive radiotherapy or radiotherapy in the adjuvant setting [2]. However, use of radiation in the case of a benign tumour in such young patients should be weighed against the possible complications like osteoradionecrosis, panhypopituitarism, temporal lobe necrosis, cataract, radiation keratopathy, and rarely radiation-induced malignancy [3]. This is a report of a case of recurrent JNA postmultiple surgeries developing radiation-induced leiomyosarcoma 3 years after receiving radiation therapy.

2. Case Report

Our patient is a 37-year-old male who was previously diagnosed as a case of juvenile nasopharyngeal angiofibroma. He was diagnosed with the condition at 30 years of age during which he underwent his first surgery by the lateral rhinotomy approach. Tumour was seen to involve the nasopharynx and sphenoid sinus, eroding the basisphenoid. Optic nerve and carotid artery were not involved. He underwent endoscopic excision 2 years later for tumour involving nasopharynx and sphenoid sinus. The patient remained symptom-free for 2 years, following which lateral rhinotomy excision was performed for a recurrent tumour involving nasopharynx, sphenoid sinus, eroding basisphenoid, and vidian canal. Postoperative histopathology confirmed the presence of angiofibroma and ruled out the presence of any sarcomatous element. In view of the frequently recurring nature of the tumour, the patient was given 45 Gy, 25 fractions of conformal radiotherapy. During the routine

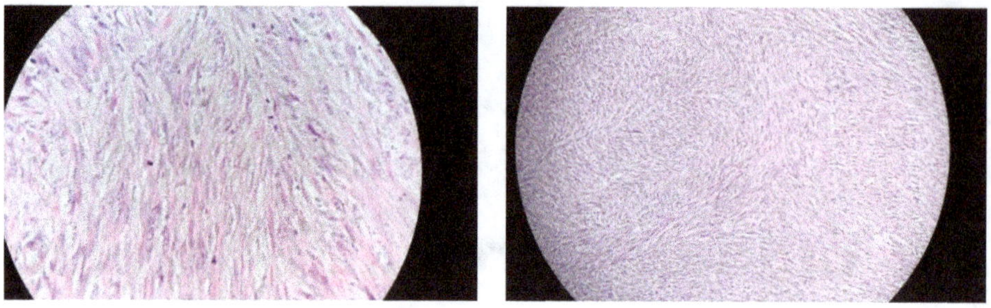

(a) (b)

Figure 1: Histopathology sections showing spindle-shaped tumour cells arranged in long intersecting fascicles, with moderate nuclear pleomorphism and increased mitosis.

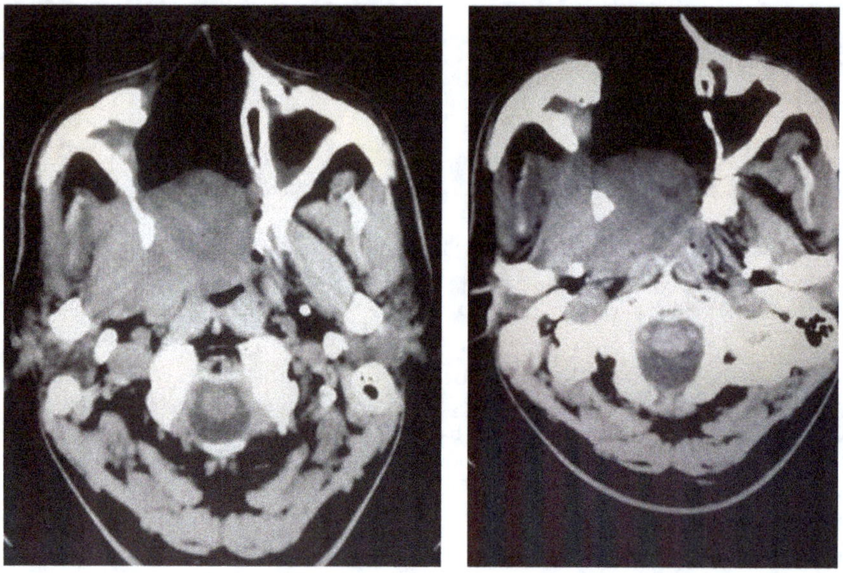

(a) (b)

Figure 2: Enhancing soft tissue mass arising from nasopharynx, destroying pterygoid plates and extending to infratemporal fossa.

follow-up nasal endoscopy after 3 years, a fleshy vascular mass was seen in the nasopharynx. The patient underwent subtotal excision at another centre by lateral rhinotomy.

The specimen block was reviewed. Sections examined showed spindle-shaped tumour cells arranged in long intersecting fascicles, with moderate nuclear pleomorphism and increased mitosis (Figure 1). Tumour cells were immunopositive for smooth muscle actin, while negative for CD34, cytokeratin, CD 56, S100, and HMB 45. MIB-1 labelling index was 25%. Overall features were suggestive of leiomyosarcoma.

Contrast-enhanced computed tomogram showed heterogeneously enhancing soft tissue mass lesion in the right posterolateral wall of nasopharynx measuring $6 \times 3.7 \times 4$ cm with erosion of the adjacent bone with involvement of the pterygoid muscles (Figure 2).

In view of the extensive involvement of skull base, surgery was not considered to be suitable for providing a negative margin. Patient has thus been planned for neoadjuvant chemotherapy (gemcitabine based) followed by chemoradiation.

3. Discussion

Surgery is undoubtedly the definitive treatment option for juvenile nasopharyngeal angiofibroma. Dilemma arises when there are multiple recurrences, extensive intracranial, intraorbital, or infratemporal fossa involvement. There are multiple case series and case reports citing the use of radiation therapy for this benign condition. Cure rates of 80% have been reported for both these modalities of treatment [2]. The recent largest series is that of 32 patients of stage III JNA from India, reviewed over a period of 25 years [4]. Median dose of radiotherapy was 30 Gy, with 14 patients treated with a radical intent. The same authors reported a case of squamous cell carcinoma of the nasal ala developing 15 years after receiving radiotherapy. Notable complications following radiation therapy for JNA reported in the literature include panhypopituitarism, posterior capsular opacification, temporal lobe necrosis, growth retardation, and radiation keratopathy [5]. Numerous other studies have evaluated the role of radiation therapy for JNA [2, 6–9], of which secondary malignancies were reported by Cummings et al. [2] (thyroid carcinoma and basal cell carcinoma of skin, 14 and 13 years after irradiation, resp.) and Reddy et al. [8] (basal cell carcinoma). Conley et al. also reported a case of orbital squamous cell carcinoma [10]. Only two studies have reported sarcomatous change in JNA postirradiation [11, 12], though possibility of the same have been put forth by many studies [4, 13]. As in our patient, radiotherapy has been used in the adjuvant setting as well. Álvarez et al. [1] used stereotactic radiosurgery on residual JNA, showing tumour decrement in 3 out of 7 patients after a follow-up of 3 years.

Radiation-induced malignancy (RIM) is thus the rarest and the most feared complication following irradiation for a benign condition like JNA. Our patient fulfilled the criteria for RIM as stated by Cahan et al. [14] and Murray et al. [15]:

(1) The tumour arose in a previously irradiated field.

(2) The new tumour is histologically different from the original condition.

(3) There was no evidence of the new tumour at the time of radiation therapy.

(4) A latency period existed between irradiation and the development of the new tumour.

RIM in head and neck has an incidence of 0.9% and develops after a mean latency of 22 years with a mean radiation dose of 6035 cGy, most commonly located in paranasal sinuses [16]. The same study showed that sarcomas outnumbered other RIM histological subtypes. Other studies, however, showed pharynx to be the most common location for RIM and squamous cell carcinoma and thyroid cancers being the most common RIMs [17, 18]. There are studies that claim radiation-induced sarcomas to be more sinister in their course and having shorter latency than other RIM [19, 20]. Studies evaluating risk of RIM in intermediate dose radiation given to benign diseases indicate a very small risk but have advised caution in pediatric population in view of long latency of these tumours [21].

The mechanism behind the occurrence of RIM is not well established. One hypothesis as proposed by Brenner and Shuryak et al. [22, 23] include generation of radiation-induced premalignant cells that initially survive low-dose radiation exposure and subsequently repopulate "sterilized area" following radiotherapy. Due to the small number of affected individuals and long latency period associated with RIM, there is currently no level 1 evidence analyzing risk factors predicting the development of RIM. However, McKeown et al. [21] have reviewed the existing literature and have found a trend towards increased risk of RIM with increasing dose, estimated to be 10%/Sv for high-dose rate exposure. The effect was more pronounced in children. That is, the risk of RIM was 15%/Sv in the case of children < 10 years compared with 1%/Sv in the case of adults > 60 years of age.

Surgery is generally the preferred modality for RIM; however, as in our case due to the involvement of critical structures like skull base, nonsurgical modality including radiation have also been employed for management by other authors [24]. But in general, surgically treated patients have better survival outcomes [17, 24].

Though current radiation techniques have been significantly refined in terms of limiting exposure to uninvolved tissues and putative organs at risk, it is essential to bear in mind this small but potentially life-threatening risk while irradiating benign diseases in the case of children.

4. Conclusion

Sarcomatous change in JNA following irradiation is the rarest and the most dangerous complication ever reported. This case report aims to lay emphasis on this aspect of managing JNA which recur frequently. Multiple recurrences and skull base involvement precludes surgery as an option in our patient. Though both the modalities of treatment have equal recurrence rates, morbidity and mortality, use of conformal radiotherapy should be carefully weighed against the possible occurrence of such complications. The long-term effects of IMRT and stereotactic radiosurgery also need to be evaluated in detail before these modalities can be used in this setting without being fraught with such complications.

References

[1] F. L. Álvarez, V. Suárez, C. Suárez, and J. L. Llorente, "Multimodality approach for advanced-stage juvenile nasopharyngeal angiofibromas," *Head & Neck*, vol. 35, no. 2, pp. 209–213, 2013.

[2] B. J. Cummings, R. Blend, T. Keane et al., "Primary radiation therapy for juvenile nasopharyngeal angiofibroma," *The Laryngoscope*, vol. 94, no. 12, pp. 1599–1605, 1984.

[3] J. M. Hodges, A. S. McDevitt, A. I. el-Sayed Ali, and M. E. Sebelik, "Juvenile nasopharyngeal angiofibroma: current treatment modalities and future considerations," *Indian Journal of Otolaryngology and Head & Neck Surgery*, vol. 62, no. 3, pp. 236–247, 2010.

[4] S. Mallick, R. Benson, S. Bhasker, and B. K. Mohanti, "Conformal radiotherapy for locally advanced juvenile nasopharyngeal angiofibroma," *Journal of Cancer Research and Therapeutics*, vol. 11, no. 1, pp. 73–77, 2015.

[5] J. T. Lee, P. Chen, A. Safa, G. Juillard, and T. C. Calcaterra, "The role of radiation in the treatment of advanced juvenile angiofibroma," *Laryngoscope*, vol. 112, no. 7, pp. 1213–1220, 2002.

[6] S. Chakraborty, S. Ghoshal, V. M. Patil, A. S. Oinam, and S. C. Sharma, "Conformal radiotherapy in the treatment of advanced juvenile nasopharyngeal angiofibroma with intracranial extension: an institutional experience," *International Journal of Radiation Oncology, Biology, Physics*, vol. 80, no. 5, pp. 1398–1404, 2011.

[7] W. J. McAfee, C. G. Morris, R. J. Amdur, J. W. Werning, and W. M. Mendenhall, "Definitive radiotherapy for juvenile nasopharyngeal angiofibroma," *American Journal of Clinical Oncology*, vol. 29, no. 2, pp. 168–170, 2006.

[8] K. A. Reddy, W. M. Mendenhall, R. J. Amdur, S. P. Stringer, and N. J. Cassisi, "Long-term results of radiation therapy for juvenile nasopharyngeal angiofibroma," *American Journal of Otolaryngology*, vol. 22, no. 3, pp. 172–175, 2001.

[9] R. J. Amdur, A. R. Yeung, B. M. Fitzgerald, A. A. Mancuso, J. W. Werning, and W. M. Mendenhall, "Radiotherapy for juvenile nasopharyngeal angiofibroma," *Practical Radiation Oncology*, vol. 1, no. 4, pp. 271–278, 2011.

[10] J. Conley, W. V. Healey, S. M. Blaugrund, and K. H. Erzin, "Nasopharyngeal angiofibroma in the juvenile," *Surgery, Gynecology & Obstetrics*, vol. 126, no. 4, pp. 825–837, 1968.

[11] W. R. Hudson, "Discussion," *Laryngoscope*, vol. 86, no. 18, 1976.

[12] K. T. K. Chen and F. W. Bauer, "Sarcomatous transformation of nasopharyngeal angiofibroma," *Cancer*, vol. 49, no. 2, pp. 369–371, 1982.

[13] N. B. Shunyu, A. Thakar, and V. Gupta, "Complete resolution of stage IIIB juvenile nasopharyngeal angiofibroma with radiation therapy," *Indian Journal of Otolaryngology and Head & Neck Surgery*, vol. 60, no. 3, pp. 238–241, 2008.

[14] W. G. Cahan, H. Q. Woodard, N. L. Higinbotham, F. W. Stewart, and B. L. Coley, "Sarcoma in irradiated bone: report of eleven cases," *Cancer*, vol. 1, no. 1, pp. 3–29, 1948.

[15] E. M. Murray, D. Werner, E. A. Greeff, and D. A. Taylor, "Postradiation sarcomas: 20 cases and a literature review," *International Journal of Radiation Oncology, Biology, Physics*, vol. 45, no. 4, pp. 951–961, 1999.

[16] K. A. Sale, D. I. Wallace, D. A. Girod, and T. T. Tsue, "Radiation-induced malignancy of the head and neck," *Otolaryngology-Head and Neck Surgery*, vol. 131, no. 5, pp. 643–645, 2016.

[17] H. Miyahara, T. Sato, and K. Yos, "Radiation-induced cancers of the head and neck region," *Acta Oto-Laryngologica*, vol. 118, no. 533, pp. 60–64, 2009.

[18] B. F. Van der Laan, G. Baris, R. T. Gregor, F. J. Hilgers, and A. J. Balm, "Radiation induced tumours of the head and neck," *The Journal of Laryngology and Otology*, vol. 109, no. 4, pp. 346–349, 1995.

[19] A. D. King, A. T. Ahuja, P. Teo, G. M. K. Tse, and J. Kew, "Radiation induced sarcomas of the head and neck following radiotherapy for nasopharyngeal carcinoma," *Clinical Radiology*, vol. 55, no. 9, pp. 684–689, 2000.

[20] J. Chung, V. Lee, R. Tsang et al., "Treatment outcomes of postradiation second head and neck malignancies managed by a multidisciplinary approach," *Head & Neck*, vol. 37, no. 6, pp. 815–822, 2015.

[21] S. R. McKeown, P. Hatfield, R. J. D. Prestwich, R. E. Shaffer, and R. E. Taylor, "Radiotherapy for benign disease; assessing the risk of radiation induced cancer following exposure to intermediate dose radiation," *The British Journal of Radiology*, vol. 88, no. 1056, article 20150405, 2015.

[22] D. J. Brenner, "Exploring two two-edged swords," *Radiation Research*, vol. 178, no. 1, pp. 7–16, 2012.

[23] I. Shuryak, R. K. Sachs, and D. J. Brenner, "A new view of radiation-induced cancer," *Radiation Protection Dosimetry*, vol. 143, no. 2–4, pp. 358–364, 2011.

[24] A. W. G. Goolden and R. L. Morgan, "Radiation cancer of the pharynx," *Acta Radiologica: Therapy, Physics, Biology*, vol. 3, no. 5, pp. 353–360, 2009.

36

Malignant Spinal Cord Compression Syndrome as an Initial Presentation of Testicular Cancer

Carlos Eduardo Salazar-Mejía, Edio Llerena-Hernández, David Hernández-Barajas, Oscar Vidal-Gutiérrez, Adriana González-Gutiérrez, Rolando Jacob Martínez-Granados, and Blanca Otilia Wimer-Castillo

Centro Universitario Contra el Cáncer, University Hospital "Dr. José Eleuterio González" and Faculty of Medicine, Universidad Autónoma de Nuevo León, Monterrey, Nuevo León, Mexico

Correspondence should be addressed to Carlos Eduardo Salazar-Mejía; drsalazarmejia@gmail.com

Academic Editor: Raffaele Palmirotta

Malignant spinal cord compression syndrome (MSCCS) occurs in 2.5 to 5% of all oncological patients. In 20% of the cases, it is the initial manifestation. This syndrome is a rare event among germ cell tumors (GCT), occurring in only 1.7% of the patients. We present the case of a 24-year-old man who arrived at the emergency department with dysesthesia and paraparesis as well as urinary incontinence. Imaging studies showed an infiltrative lesion in the left testicle, pulmonary and hepatic metastatic disease, and a large retroperitoneal ganglionar conglomerate that infiltrated the spinal cord through the intervertebral foramina of the vertebra level T11 with displacement of the L1 vertebral body. A postoperative biopsy showed a pure embryonal carcinoma. In the initial approach of a young man who presents spinal cord compression, the presence of MSCCS associated with GCT should be considered as a possible cause. A high level of suspicion is required to achieve a timely diagnosis, to grant the patient the best possible outcome.

1. Introduction

Malignant spinal cord compression syndrome (MSCCS) occurs in 2.5 to 5% of all oncological patients. In 20% of the cases, it is the initial manifestation [1]. Detection and intervention within the first 24 hours are essential for therapeutic success [2]. Although several case reports have documented the presence of MSCCS in patients with germ cell tumors (GCT) as an initial presentation or as part of their evolution after primary therapy, there is little evidence on the best therapeutic option in this context. We present a rare case of MSCCS as the initial presentation of a pure testicular embryonal carcinoma.

2. Case Presentation

A 24-year-old man arrived at the emergency department with a four-month history of pain and swelling of the left testicle. A week ago, he developed progressive edema in the lower limbs, which was followed 48 hours before admission by dysesthesia and paraparesis as well as urinary incontinence. He had no previous medical history and did not consume alcohol or use any illicit drug or medication.

Physical examination on admission showed a blood pressure of 100/60 mmHg, a temperature of 36°C, a pulse rate of 90/min, and a respiratory rate of 22/min; his height was 1.75 m, weight 98 kg, and BMI 32 kg/m^2. He referred bilateral paresthesia of the lower limbs and pain on mobilization of the lumbar spine. The left scrotal sac was enlarged and indurated, and there was a mass in the left scrotum that was indistinguishable from the right testis and provoked displacement of the penis and right testis. No inguinal lymphadenopathy was identified. When examining both lower extremities, we found edema without fovea. Neurological examination revealed hypoesthesia, areflexia, and decreased muscle strength.

Laboratory tests revealed normal liver function. Hemoglobin was 9.13 g/dL, MCV was 87.9 fL, WBC was 11.9 K/μL, neutrophil count was 9.81 K/μL, lymphocyte count was 1.59 K/μL, and the platelet level was 252 K/μL. Serum glucose was 148 mg/dL, BUN was 38 mg/dL, creatinine was 1.3 mg/dL, and calcium was 8.9 mg/dL. Serum alpha-fetoprotein (AFP) was 11.28 ng/mL, lactate dehydrogenase was 1687 U/L (normal range 91–180 IU/L), and human chorionic gonadotropin level was 10.05 IU/mL.

A scrotal ultrasound showed a hypoechoic oval-shaped infiltrative lesion in the left testicle of 6.1 × 3.2 × 2.7 cm, associated with a large left hydrocele, with an estimated volume of 450 mL. Microcalcifications were seen in both testis.

A contrasted CT scan of the thorax, abdomen, and pelvis showed bilateral supraclavicular adenopathies and multiple round pulmonary nodules with well-defined edges of bilateral and diffuse distribution. In the liver, there were two hyperdense lesions: one larger lesion of 4.8 × 2 cm located in hepatic segment IV and a second lesion of 1.9 cm in segment VIII, with partially defined borders and enhancement to contrast administration. There was also a large retroperitoneal ganglionar conglomerate of 10 × 6 cm, which infiltrated the spinal cord.

An MRI of the dorsal and lumbar spine showed a large and heterogeneous retroperitoneal conglomerate which invaded the left psoas muscle and infiltrated the spinal cord through the intervertebral foramina of T11 with displacement of the L1 vertebral body (Figure 1). Metastatic infiltration of the vertebral bodies L3–L5 was also seen (Figure 2).

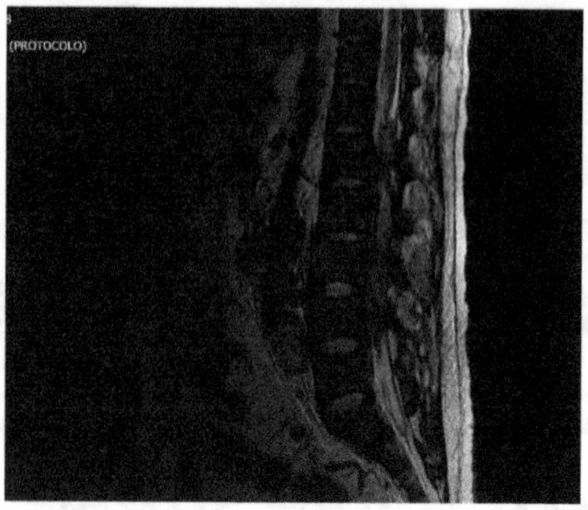

Figure 1

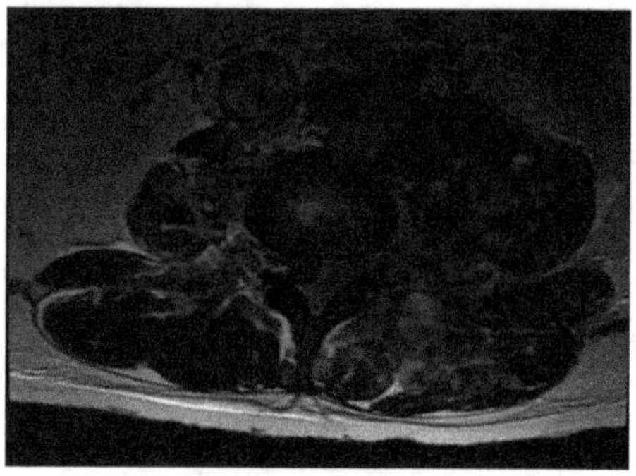

Figure 2

A diagnosis of clinical stage IIIC testicular cancer was established with a poor prognosis due to nonpulmonary visceral metastases. After initial treatment with high-dose intravenous corticosteroids, the case was evaluated by a multidisciplinary oncological team. Three fractions of external beam radiotherapy were given. He then underwent a left radical orchiectomy by an inguinal approach with a left hemiscrotectomy, without complications. A postoperative biopsy showed a pure embryonal carcinoma with invasion of the spermatic cord and necrosis of more than 50% of its surface. After finishing 10 fractions of radiotherapy for a total of 30 Gy, and improving his renal function with intravenous crystalloids, the patient received his first cycle of chemotherapy (CT). We planned a CT regimen based on bleomycin, etoposide, and cisplatin (BEP), repeated every 21 days for a total of four cycles.

After the eighth day of CT, the patient presented sudden dyspnea at rest that progressed to hypoxemic respiratory failure. Due to this condition, we decided to perform orotracheal intubation and the patient was then transferred to the intensive care unit. An angio-CT revealed the presence of bilateral pulmonary thromboembolism. Despite the treatment received, the patient died three days later.

3. Discussion

MSCCS is a devastating manifestation of metastatic cancer that results from compression of the dural sac or its contents by an extradural tumoral mass that manifests clinically by local or radicular pain in 83% to 95% of the cases; this is usually the initial symptom [1]. The presence of motor deficit that incapacitates deambulation is manifested in 50 to 68% of the cases, while sensory or autonomic deficit can be observed in about 60% of these patients [3]. The main oncological pathologies associated with MSCCS are lung (22.9%), breast (19.9%), and prostate cancer (18.4%) [4]. MSCCS is a rare event among GCT, occurring in only 1.7% of the patients [5]. Table 1 summarizes the reported cases of MSCCS as an initial presentation of GCT in the English literature.

GCT are the most common malignancies in men aged 15 to 39 years. Their main origin is the gonads; extragonadal GCT comprise only 5 to 10% of the cases [6]. Within the histological classification of GCT, pure embryonal carcinoma comprises approximately 2% of the cases [7]. Characteristically, these tumors generally predispose only to modest elevation of the AFP [8].

Independent adverse factors in GCT include the degree of elevation of tumor markers, mediastinal primary site, and the presence of nonpulmonary visceral metastases. Regardless of the initial clinical stage and risk stratification, the therapeutic goal is to achieve cure of the disease, since patients with advanced GCT who survive and remain disease-free for more than 2 years after their diagnosis have a great chance of surviving in subsequent years [9]. The standard of treatment for patients with advanced disease and intermediate to high risk, is a CT regimen based on BEP every 21 days for 4 cycles [6, 10].

Table 1: Summary of the reported cases of MSCCS as an initial presentation of GCT in the English literature.

Author/year	Country	Age of presentation	Mechanism of spinal cord injury	Spinal level of metastasis causing cord compression	Histology	Treatment of MSCCS, in chronological order	Outcome, follow-up
Nelson and Ruffolo 1966 [16]	USA	63 years	Extradural compression	T9	Classic seminoma	Laminectomy	Death, 12 days
Arnold et al. 2000 [17]	USA	41 years	Extradural compression	T7	Mixed GCT	Laminectomy, unspecified CT	Good, 1 year
Yee et al. 2007 [18]	Canada	44 years	Extradural compression	T4	Classic seminoma	Steroids, EBRT 20 Gy/5 Fx, BEP	Good, 1 year
Salazar-Mejía et al. 2018	Mexico	24 years	Extradural compression	T11	Pure embryonal carcinoma	Steroids, EBRT 30 Gy/10 Fx, BEP	Death, 3 weeks

CT, chemotherapy; BEP, bleomycin/etoposide/cisplatin; EBRT, external beam radiotherapy.

The management of a patient with MSCCS must be multidisciplinary and integral, taking into account symptomatic control and the primary tumor, as well as possible associated comorbidities. MRI is the imaging study of choice to better characterize the degree of involvement of the spinal cord canal. Initial treatment includes the use of high doses of intravenous corticosteroids and decompression by surgery and/or radiotherapy (RT) [11, 12]. The ASTRO guidelines for palliative RT for bone metastases, in its update of 2017, recommend doses of 8 Gy in a single fraction (Fx), 20 Gy/5 Fx, 24 Gy/6 Fx, or 30 Gy/10 Fx for patients with bone disease not previously treated [13]. CT is the main therapeutic option in GCT, due to the high chemosensitivity exhibited by these tumors [14]. The key prognostic factor for optimal functional outcome is the degree of functional capacity at the time of treatment initiation [3].

The benefit of adding radiotherapy prior to chemotherapy (RT/CT) in this group of patients has been debated for decades. The largest series in this regard is a retrospective analysis of the database of patients with GCT of the Memorial Sloan-Kettering Cancer Center from 1984 to 2009 [5]. Of 1734 patients included, 29 were found to have MSCCS (10 patients with seminoma, 19 nonseminoma). The main spinal cord compression sites were located in the lumbar and thoracic spine and 20% showed involvement in multiple sites. The most used CT regimen was BEP in both groups, and 62% of the patients had not previously received CT. This study showed no difference in symptomatic response between both treatment arms. A significant difference was found in overall survival after diagnosis and first-line treatment of MSCCS between the group treated with RT/CT ($n = 4$) and the group with CT alone ($n = 11$), with a mean overall survival not reached in the CT group versus 22 months in the RT/CT group ($p = 0.04$). An analysis of patients who received 2 or less lines of treatment showed a mean survival of 138 months for the CT group alone compared to 38 months in the RT/CT group ($p = 0.23$).

Based on the results of this analysis, CT could be considered as an appropriate treatment option in patients with newly diagnosed GCT who present MSCCS, as well as those with no more than two previous treatment regimens if the disease is chemosensitive. In patients who have received 2 or more cycles of CT, RT/CT may be an option [5]. Despite the limitations of this study (retrospective design and number of patients included), it is unlikely that a prospective protocol will be carried out in this regard, given the rarity of the presentation.

The event that predisposed to the clinical deterioration and subsequent death of our patient was the development of pulmonary thromboembolism. Cancer patients on active therapy have a higher risk for venous thromboembolism (VTE) and those receiving CT account for as much as 13% of the total burden of VTE. The presence of this complication is strongly associated with an increased early all-cause mortality during the course of CT and reduced long-term survival [15].

Within the initial approach of a young man who presents with spinal cord compression syndrome, the presence of MSCCS associated with GCT should be considered as a possible cause. A high level of suspicion and a complete physical examination, including a genital exam, is required to achieve a timely diagnosis, in order to grant the patient the best possible outcome.

References

[1] F. Estevinho, N. Sousa, Â. Rodrigues et al., "Compressão Medular por Tumor de Células Germinativas do Testículo," *Acta Médica Portuguesa*, vol. 25, no. 6, pp. 461–465, 2012.

[2] D. J. Husband, "Malignant spinal cord compression: prospective study of delays in referral and treatment," *BMJ*, vol. 317, no. 7150, pp. 18–21, 1998.

[3] J. S. Cole and R. A. Patchell, "Metastatic epidural spinal cord compression," *The Lancet Neurology*, vol. 7, no. 5, pp. 459–466, 2008.

[4] D. Loblaw, N. Laperriere, and W. Mackillop, "A population-based study of malignant spinal cord compression in Ontario," *Clinical Oncology*, vol. 15, no. 4, pp. 211–217, 2003.

[5] C. Grommes, G. J. Bosl, and L. M. Deangelis, "Treatment of epidural spinal cord involvement from germ cell tumors with chemotherapy," *Cancer*, vol. 117, no. 9, pp. 1911–1916, 2011.

[6] C. Albany, N. Hanna, and L. H. Einhorn, "Testicular cancer," in *The American Cancer Society's Oncology in Practice*, The American Cancer Society, Ed., pp. 329–343, John Wiley & Sons, Inc., 2018.

[7] F. K. Mostofi, I. A. Sesterhenn, and C. J. Davis Jr., "Developments in histopathology of testicular germ cell tumors," *Seminars in Urology*, vol. 6, no. 3, pp. 171–188, 1988.

[8] A. Talerman, W. G. Haije, and L. Baggerman, "Serum alphafetoprotein (AFP) in patients with germ cell tumors of the gonads and extragonadal sites: correlation between endodermal sinus (yolk sac) tumor and raised serum AFP," *Cancer*, vol. 46, no. 2, pp. 380–385, 1980.

[9] J. J. Ko, B. Bernard, B. Tran et al., "Conditional survival of patients with metastatic testicular germ cell tumors treated with first-line curative therapy," *Journal of Clinical Oncology*, vol. 34, no. 7, pp. 714–720, 2016.

[10] J. Oldenburg, S. D. Fossa, J. Nuver et al., "Testicular seminoma and non-seminoma: ESMO clinical practice guidelines for diagnosis, treatment and follow-up," *Annals of Oncology*, vol. 24, Supplement 6, pp. vi125–vi132, 2013.

[11] D. Prasad and D. Schiff, "Malignant spinal-cord compression," *The Lancet Oncology*, vol. 6, no. 1, pp. 15–24, 2005.

[12] M. Penas-Prado and M. E. Loghin, "Spinal cord compression in cancer patients: review of diagnosis and treatment," *Current Oncology Reports*, vol. 10, no. 1, pp. 78–85, 2008.

[13] S. Lutz, T. Balboni, J. Jones et al., "Palliative radiation therapy for bone metastases: update of an ASTRO evidence-based guideline," *Practical Radiation Oncology*, vol. 7, no. 1, pp. 4–12, 2017.

[14] K. Cooper, D. Bajorin, W. Shapiro, G. Krol, G. Sze, and G. Bosl, "Decompression of epidural metastases from germ cell tumors with chemotherapy," *Journal of Neuro-Oncology*, vol. 8, no. 3, pp. 275–280, 1990.

[15] A. A. Khorana, "Venous thromboembolism and prognosis in cancer," *Thrombosis Research*, vol. 125, no. 6, pp. 490–493, 2010.

[16] J. W. Nelson and E. H. Ruffolo, "Testicular seminoma as a cause of paraplegia: a case report," *The Journal of Urology*, vol. 95, no. 1, pp. 70–73, 1966.

[17] P. M. Arnold, C. J. Morgan, R. A. Morantz, D. A. Eckard, and J. J. Kepes, "Metastatic testicular cancer presenting as spinal cord compression: report of two cases," *Surgical Neurology*, vol. 54, no. 1, pp. 27–33, 2000.

[18] D. Yee, Z. Gabos, S. North, and R. B. Moore, "Malignant spinal cord compression secondary to testicular seminoma at the time of initial presentation and at relapse while on surveillance," *Canadian Urological Association Journal*, vol. 1, no. 1, 2007.

37

A Case of Metastatic Adamantinoma that Responded Well to Sunitinib

Andrew D. Liman,[1] Agnes K. Liman,[2] Jenna Shields,[3] Becky Englert,[4] and Rashmikant Shah[5]

[1]*Hematology and Oncology, VA Pittsburgh Healthcare System, University of Pittsburgh School of Medicine, Pittsburgh, PA 15240, USA*
[2]*Pathology, VA Pittsburgh Healthcare System, University of Pittsburgh School of Medicine, Pittsburgh, PA 15240, USA*
[3]*Pharmacy, VA Pittsburgh Healthcare System, Pittsburgh, PA 15240, USA*
[4]*Hematology and Oncology, VA Pittsburgh Healthcare System, Pittsburgh, PA 15240, USA*
[5]*Radiology, VA Pittsburgh Healthcare System, University of Pittsburgh School of Medicine, Pittsburgh, PA 15240, USA*

Correspondence should be addressed to Andrew D. Liman; andrew.liman@va.gov

Academic Editor: Peter F. Lenehan

Adamantinoma is a rare low-grade malignant bone tumor of epithelial origin. Metastatic adamantinoma has been reported to be resistant to chemotherapy. We report a case of metastatic adamantinoma to the lung, 10 years after the initial diagnosis of tibial mass. The patient received radiation therapy to the lung with partial response. A surveillance PET scan revealed progression of the lung mass and biopsy confirmed to be progressive residual metastatic adamantinoma. He received carboplatin and etoposide for 7 months and achieved a partial response. Four months later, PET scan showed disease progression. We started him on sunitinib, a multikinase inhibitor. He achieved a good partial response for 3 years. He died due to pneumonia at the age of 72.

1. Introduction

Adamantinoma is a low-grade, malignant bone tumor that is predominantly located in the midportion of the tibia [1, 2]. Adamantinoma constitutes 0.1% to 0.5% of all malignant bone tumors. The predilection is mainly involving the midshaft of the tibia which accounts for about 85% of all cases [1]. The initial symptoms of adamantinoma are often indolent and include swelling with or without pain. A history of trauma and fracture may be predated to the diagnosis. This tumor tends to be resistant to chemotherapy. We report a case of metastatic adamantinoma to the lung that responded very well to multitargeted receptor tyrosine kinase inhibitor sunitinib.

2. Case Presentation

A 57-year-old Caucasian male presented to Veterans Affairs Pittsburgh Healthcare System (VAPHS) with a left tibial mass in 1999. He had undergone a resection. Due to the limitation of the immunohistochemical staining at that time it was initially diagnosed as fibrosarcoma. The tumor consists predominantly of spindle neoplastic cells arranged in fascicles with occasional mitoses and stained negative with CAM5.2 and EMA. Two years later, he was found to have an enlarged left inguinal lymph node. Excisional biopsy was read as metastatic fibrosarcoma. Histologically it was similar to the original resected tumor and stained negative with AE1/AE3 and desmin and positive with vimentin. Ten years after the initial diagnosis, he presented with coughing and shortness of breath. CT scan revealed a right perihilar mass (Figure 1(a)) and PET scan showed metabolic activity in the right hilar mass (Figure 1(b)). Bronchoscopy and biopsy of the mass were consistent with metastatic adamantinoma. Histologically it was similar to the specimen that was resected from the left tibia and left inguinal lymph node. The slides from tibia and inguinal lymph node were reviewed again with additional immunohistochemical stains. The tumor has predominantly spindle cell pattern (Figure 2(a)) with focal areas of basaloid

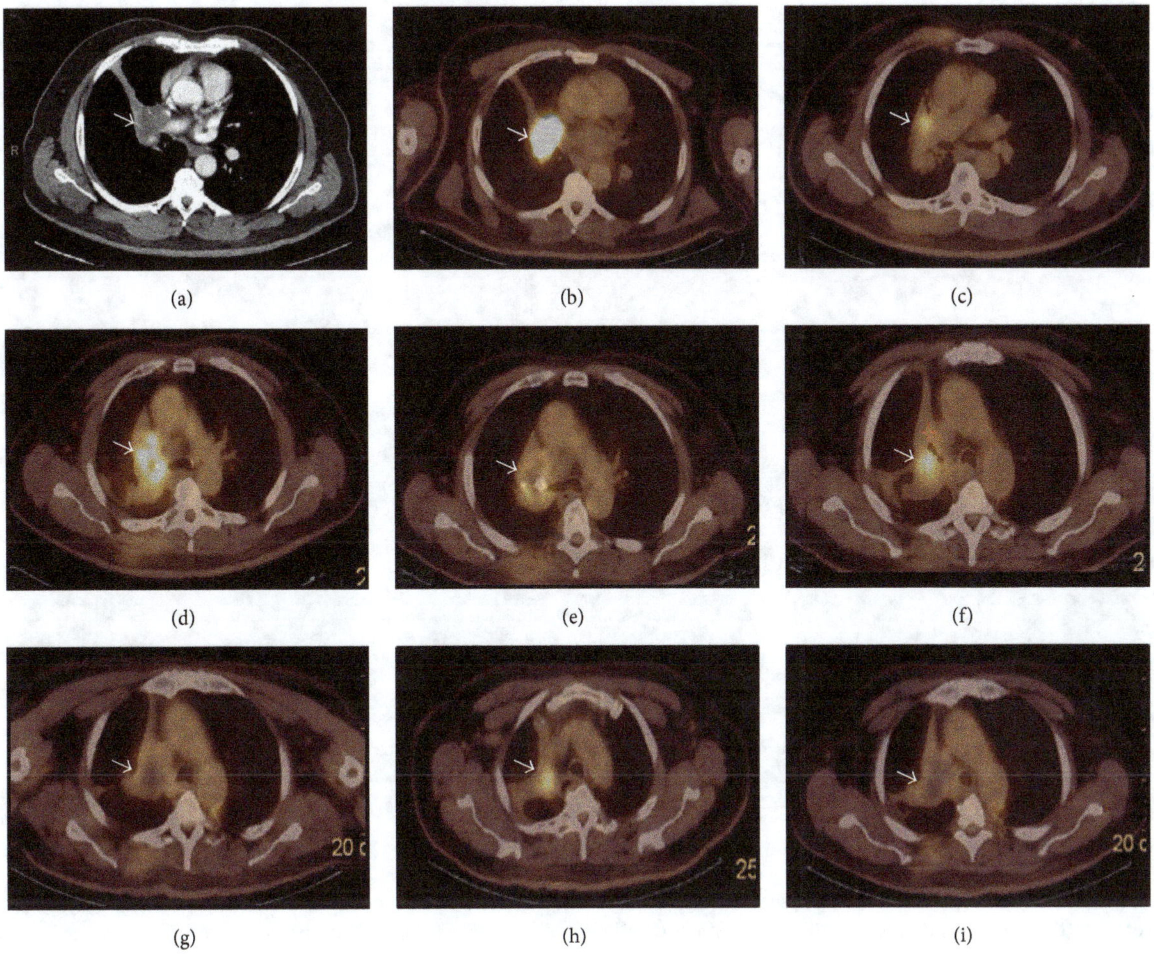

Figure 1: (a) CT scan showed right hilar mass (arrow) in July 2009. (b) PET scan confirmed FDG activity of the mass. (c) Partial response after radiation therapy (October 2009). (d) Extensive disease progression (May 2011). (e) Partial response after chemotherapy (December 2011). (f) Disease progression (March 2012). (g) Reduced metabolic activity after sunitinib (August 2013). (h) Disease progression (September 2014). (i) Complete disappearance of FDG activity with central necrosis after increased dose of sunitinib (February 2015).

pattern showing peripheral palisading (Figure 2(b)) and fibrous stroma. Both the spindle and basaloid components are epithelial that showed immunoreactivity for epithelial markers CAM5.2, CK5/6 (Figure 2(c)), and K903. It was also positive for BCL-2 (Figure 2(d)), p63, p53, and vimentin. Immunostaining for melanoma markers (S-100 and HMB-45), vascular markers (CD34 and CD31), CK7, CK20, CD99, actin, TTF-1, and CD56 were all negative. Pankeratin and c-kit (CD117) showed focal positivity (Figure 2(e)). Ki-67 proliferation marker was approximately 35% in the epithelial component. The slides were reviewed and concurred by a bone pathologist at the University of Pittsburgh Medical Center.

He received radiation therapy to the right hilar mass for a total dose of 7500 cGy, and PET scan revealed a partial response (Figure 1(c)). Follow-up PET scan 19 months later revealed progression of disease in the right hilar mass with atelectasis of the right upper lung (Figure 1(d)) and a new small metastatic focus was detected in the left lung. The case was presented in multidisciplinary tumor board meeting. The consensus was that he needed a repeat biopsy of the right hilar mass to rule out concomitant primary lung malignancy because he was a heavy smoker. The left lung nodule was too small and difficult to approach for a biopsy. Repeat biopsy of the right hilar mass revealed persistent metastatic adamantinoma. Additional immunostaining from the biopsy showed focal positivity for VEGF (Figure 2(f)) and diffuse positivity for EGFR (Figure 2(g)). We started him on chemotherapy in June 2011. Chemotherapy consists of carboplatin with AUC of 6 on day 1 and etoposide 100 mg/m^2 daily on days 1, 2, and 3 every 3 weeks for total of 9 cycles. PET scan in December 2011 showed partial response (Figure 1(e)) but 4 months later a surveillance PET scan showed rapid increase in size and metabolic activity of the right hilar mass (Figure 1(f)). In May 2012 we started him on sunitinib 37.5 mg orally, once daily for 4 weeks, followed by 2 weeks off, in a repeated 6-week cycle. He tolerated the drug very well except mild tiredness. He was diagnosed with hypothyroidism and was placed on levothyroxine. Serial PET scans continue to show improvement with decrease in the size of hilar mass with reduced metabolic activity (Figure 1(g)). PET scan in

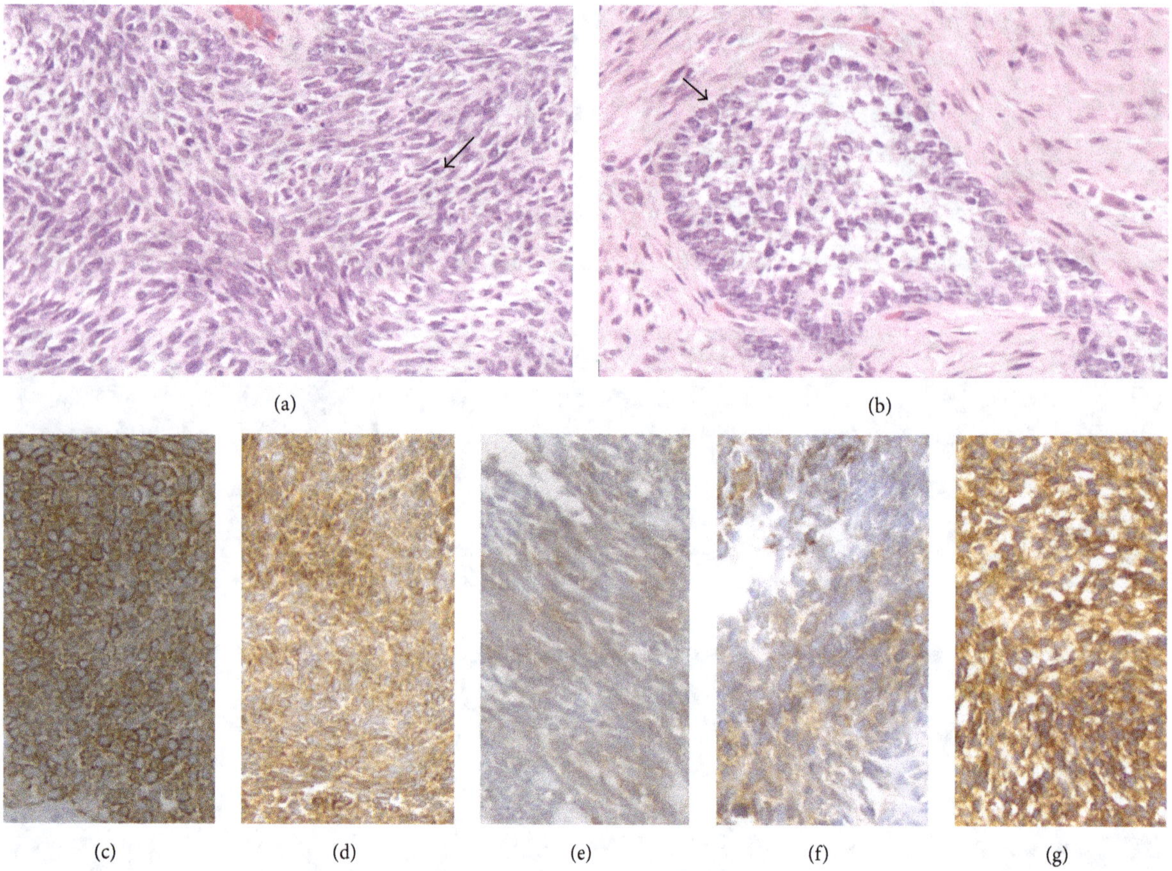

FIGURE 2: (a) Predominant spindle cell pattern; see arrow (H&E). (b) Basaloid pattern with peripheral palisading; see arrow (H&E). (c) CK5/6 strong positive. (d) BCL-2 positive. (e) CD117 focal positive. (f) VEGF focal positive. (g) EGFR diffuse positive.

September 2014 showed progression in metabolic activity (Figure 1(h)). We increased the dose of sunitinib to 50 mg daily. The last PET scan in February 2015 revealed that the hilar mass developed central necrosis without metabolic activity (Figure 1(i)). The patient had continued taking of sunitinib until May 2015 when he developed hemoptysis and was admitted for pneumonia at a local hospital. He died due to complication of pneumonia at the age of 72.

3. Discussion

Adamantinoma is a primary low-grade, malignant bone tumor of epithelial origin. It is a rare neoplasm and comprises only 0.1–0.5% of all primary bone tumors. In 1913, Fischer named the lesion "primary adamantinoma of the tibia" because of its striking histologic resemblance to the "jaw adamantinoma" (ameloblastoma) [3]. This tumor mostly occurs in the second to fifth decades with median age of 25 to 35 years. It is more common in men than women. The tumor has a predilection in the tibia (80 to 85% of cases). In 10 to 15% of cases, the tumor is also found in the ipsilateral fibula and other major limb bones such as humerus, ulna, femur, fibula, radius, ribs, and spine as primary sites [4]. The etiology of this tumor is thought to be from displacement of basal epithelium of skin during embryological development. The theory behind predominantly tibial bone involvement by this tumor is enchondrally formed bone closest to the skin surface of tibia [5]. Adamantinoma is a tumor of epithelial origin based on immunohistochemical and ultrastructural studies. The tumor cells show strong positive staining with pan cytokeratin. In our case the tumor has positive immunoreactivity for epithelial markers CAM5.2, CK5/6, K903, and pankeratin. Ultrastructurally, the tumor cells have epithelial characteristics such as basal lamina, desmosomes, gap junctions, epithelial specific keratin, and extracellular composition similar to epithelial tissue [6].

The initial symptom of adamantinoma is swelling with or without pain involving tibia. The onset is insidious and slow but progressive in nature. Trauma has been reported in about 60% of cases. Pathological fracture may be present. Paraneoplastic manifestations, such as hypercalcemia, have been associated with tibial adamantinoma with lung metastasis. Adamantinoma is most often located in the diaphyseal area of tibia. The bone lesion is usually multilocular with sclerotic margin and overlapping with radiolucencies. These multifocal radiolucencies were surrounded by ring-shaped densities producing the characteristic "soap-bubble" appearance [2]. The differential diagnosis of adamantinoma includes osteofibrosis dysplasia (OFD) and fibrous dysplasia. OFD is located in the cortex without involvement of medullary canal while adamantinoma usually involves anterior cortical bone with extension toward the bone marrow [7].

There are two different types of adamantinoma: classic and differentiated. Classic type usually occurs in patients older than 20 years old, whereas differentiated type such as osteofibrous dysplasia- (OFD-) like adamantinoma occurs in patients younger than 20 years old. Classic type is characterized by admixture of both epithelial and osteofibrous components while OFD-like adamantinoma is predominantly osteofibrous tissue [8]. The term dedifferentiated adamantinoma means complete loss of epithelial differentiation and is usually used for tumor that is transforming to a more sarcomatoid differentiation. Immunohistochemically all adamantinomas have been uniformly positive for cytokeratins 5, 14, and 19 which represents basal epithelial cell keratins. Vimentin has been reported to be positive as well. The immunoreactivity of other bone and soft tissue tumors with known epithelial characteristics such as synovial sarcomas, epithelioid sarcomas, and chordomas has positive cytokeratins 8 and 18 [9].

Bovée et al. studied 25 cases by immunohistochemistry. The expression of fibroblast growth factor type 2 (FGF-2) and its receptor (FGFR) was present in both components of adamantinoma, but predominantly in the epithelial component. The expression of epidermal growth factor (EGF) and its receptor (EGFR) was restricted to the epithelial component. This expression was most intense and in a higher percentage of cells in classic adamantinoma. Proliferative marker Ki-67 was found exclusively in the epithelial component. During progression of adamantinoma, the epithelial cells acquire expression of FGF-2, EGF, and EGFR, accompanied by a higher proliferative activity [10].

Surgery is the main treatment for localized adamantinoma. En bloc tumor resection with wide surgical margin and limb salvage and reconstruction will likely decrease local recurrence. In a review of 70 patients, en bloc tumor resection with wide margins and limb salvage surgery was shown to have 10-year survival rate of 87.2% [11]. Amputation has not been shown to improve survival. Once adamantinoma metastasizes the prognosis is poor. This tumor has been reported to be resistant to radiation therapy and chemotherapy. Cisplatin, carboplatin, and etoposide have been reported with some response, but tumors relapse quickly [12].

Our patient has metastatic adamantinoma to the lung 10 years after the diagnosis of his primary tibial disease. The biopsy from the tibia and the inguinal lymph node metastasis were incorrectly diagnosed as fibrosarcoma due to the spindle cell predominant morphology with occasional mitoses and limited availability of immunohistochemical stains in our institution in 1999. Biopsy on the hilar mass was compared with the biopsy of inguinal lymph node and tibial mass and confirmed to have the same adamantinoma diagnosis. This diagnosis was reviewed and concurred by a bone pathologist at University of Pittsburgh Medical Center. Figures 2(a) and 2(b) showed spindle cell pattern and basaloid pattern with peripheral palisading, respectively. Czerniak et al. reported that, in the basaloid variant, the epithelial cells exhibit solid nests of basaloid cells with distinctive peripheral palisading. The spindled form shows uniform spindling with presence of clefts lined by epithelial cells [2, 7]. The epithelial component of tumor cells in our case showed immunoreactivity for all cytokeratin markers, EGFR, CD117, and VGEF. Ki-67 proliferation marker was approximately 35% in the epithelial component. We elected to start our patient on multikinase inhibitor sunitinib because of his expression of EGFR, CD117, and VGEF. We started at a lower dose of 37.5 mg orally daily for 4 weeks on 2 weeks off schedule in May 2012. The right hilar mass responded very well to therapy. Follow-up PET scan in September 2014 showed progression, so we increased the dose of sunitinib to 50 mg daily with the same schedule. The last PET scan in February 2015 revealed central necrosis and disappearance of FDG activity. He died due to complication of pneumonia in May 2015.

There are only three published case reports in the literature of using VEGFR inhibitor. Dudek et al. reported a patient with right tibial adamantinoma with lung metastasis that responded well to sunitinib 50 mg daily for 4 weeks on and 2 weeks off schedule. The lung metastasis continues to be stable for 11 months of sunitinib therapy. The tumor cells from lung biopsy in this case showed focal positive immunostaining for CD117 (c-kit) and vascular endothelial growth factor receptor-2 (VEGFR-2) and weakly positive for platelet-derived growth factor receptor beta (PDGFR-beta) [13]. Cohen et al. reported a case of metastatic adamantinoma to the lung after 4 years of primary tumor tibial resection. The patient received ifosfamide, mesna, and doxorubicin and subsequently he was treated with gemcitabine and paclitaxel. Two months later the lung metastasis progressed. He then received pazopanib, a multityrosine kinase inhibitor at 800 mg orally per day. After 6 months the lung metastasis progressed radiologically [14]. Unal et al. recently reported a case of metastatic adamantinoma. They used pazopanib and alisertib (a small molecule Aurora kinase inhibitor) with a good response for 5 months [15].

Sunitinib inhibits VEGFR, PDGFR-β, and c-kit. These receptors are responsible for both tumor angiogenesis and tumor cell proliferation. Inhibition of these targets leads to reduced tumor vascularization and induced cancer cell death [16]. In our case, expression of VEGF and c-kit (CD117) may explain the response of this tumor to sunitinib. We did not test VEGFR but considering the excellent response to sunitinib for 3 years the tumor could have been positive for VEGFR as well. The tumor was also focally positive for proliferation marker Ki-67 in the epithelial component. Bovée et al. reported that Ki-67 was mostly found in the epithelial component of the tumor rather than in the osteofibrous component. This epithelial component has expression of FGFR, EGFR, and Ki-67 when they metastasize to other organs just like in our case [10]. Our case is the fourth reported case of metastatic adamantinoma that responded very well to multi-receptor tyrosine kinase inhibitor with the longest survival.

4. Conclusion

Metastatic adamantinoma has been reported to be resistant to chemotherapy. Immunohistochemistry testing of VEGFR, PDGFR, c-kit (CD117), and EGFR is paramount in this disease. Expression of those receptors in the epithelial component of the tumor has been proven to predict a good response and may prolong survival. Our patient received multikinase inhibitor sunitinib and the disease had been stable with a very good partial response for 3 years. He died of pneumonia. This is by far the longest survival for metastatic adamantinoma. We would recommend sunitinib, pazopanib, or other new multikinase inhibitors to treat this disease.

Consent

Verbal consent was documented in the medical chart.

Disclosure

The authors presented the poster at the 9th Annual Meeting of Association of Veteran Affairs Hematology Oncology, Atlanta, GA, USA, on October 4–6, 2013.

References

[1] L. B. Kahn, "Adamantinoma," in *Bone and Soft Tissue Pathology*, A. L. Folpe and C. Y. Inwards, Eds., chapter 22, pp. 414–418, 2010.

[2] D. Jain, V. K. Jain, R. K. Vasishta, P. Ranjan, and Y. Kumar, "Adamantinoma: a clinicopathological review and update," *Diagnostic Pathology*, vol. 3, no. 1, article 8, 2008.

[3] B. Fischer, "Primary adamantinoma of the tibia," *Z Pathology*, vol. 12, pp. 422–441, 1913.

[4] B. Ulmar, G. Delling, M. Werner, K. Huch, and H. Reichel, "Classical and atypical location of adamantinomas—presentation of two cases," *Onkologie*, vol. 29, no. 6, pp. 276–278, 2006.

[5] J. M. Mirra, "Adamantinoma and fibrous dysplasia," in *Bone Tumors*, J. M. Mirra, Ed., pp. 1203–1231, Lea & Febiger, Philadelphia, Pa, USA, 1st edition, 1989.

[6] M. H. Khan, R. Darji, U. Rao, and R. McGough, "Leg pain and swelling in a 22-year-old man," *Clinical Orthopaedics and Related Research*, vol. 448, pp. 259–266, 2006.

[7] B. Czerniak, R. R. Rojas-Corona, and H. D. Dorfman, "Morphologic diversity of long bone adamantinoma. The concept of differentiated (regressing) adamantinoma and its relationship to osteofibrous dysplasia," *Cancer*, vol. 64, no. 11, pp. 2319–2334, 1989.

[8] H. M. Hazelbag, A. H. M. Taminiau, G. J. Fleuren, and P. C. W. Hogendoorn, "Adamantinoma of the long bones. A clinicopathological study of thirty-two patients with emphasis on histological subtype, precursor lesion, and biological behavior," *Journal of Bone and Joint Surgery—Series A*, vol. 76, no. 10, pp. 1482–1499, 1994.

[9] H. M. Hazelbag, G. J. Fleuren, L. J. C. M. V. D. Broek, A. H. M. Taminiau, and P. C. W. Hogendoorn, "Adamantinoma of the long bones: keratin subclass immunoreactivity pattern with reference to its histogenesis," *American Journal of Surgical Pathology*, vol. 17, no. 12, pp. 1225–1233, 1993.

[10] J. V. M. G. Bovée, L. J. C. M. van den Broek, W. I. de Boer, and P. C. W. Hogendoorn, "Expression of growth factors and their receptors in adamantinoma of long bones and the implication for its histogenesis," *The Journal of Pathology*, vol. 184, no. 1, pp. 24–30, 1998.

[11] A. A. Qureshi, S. Shott, B. A. Mallin, and S. Gitelis, "Current trends in the management of adamantinoma of long bones. An international study," *The Journal of Bone & Joint Surgery—American Volume*, vol. 82, no. 8, pp. 1122–1131, 2000.

[12] J. Lokich, "Metastatic adamantinoma of bone to lung: a case report of the natural history and the use of chemotherapy and radiation therapy," *American Journal of Clinical Oncology: Cancer Clinical Trials*, vol. 17, no. 2, pp. 157–159, 1994.

[13] A. Z. Dudek, P. K. Murthaiah, M. Franklin, and A. M. Truskinovsky, "Metastatic adamantinoma responds to treatment with receptor tyrosine kinase inhibitor," *Acta Oncologica*, vol. 49, no. 1, pp. 101–104, 2010.

[14] Y. Cohen, J. E. Cohen, A. Zick et al., "A case of metastatic adamantinoma responding to treatment with pazopanib," *Acta Oncologica*, vol. 52, no. 6, pp. 1229–1230, 2013.

[15] I. Unal, O. David, and A. Z. Dudek, "Metastatic adamantinoma responds to treatment with receptor tyrosine kinase and Aurora A kinase inhibitor," *Journal of Solid Tumors*, vol. 5, no. 2, pp. 27–31, 2015.

[16] A.-M. O'Farrell, T. J. Abrams, H. A. Yuen et al., "SU11248 is a novel FLT3 tyrosine kinase inhibitor with potent activity in vitro and in vivo," *Blood*, vol. 101, no. 9, pp. 3597–3605, 2003.

Primary Pericardial Sarcoma with Right Atrial Invasion and Multiple Bilateral Pulmonary Metastases in a Patient with Hereditary Nonpolyposis Colorectal Cancer

Eugene Wong, Lawrence J. Oh, Kazi Nahar, Adrian Lee, and Stephen Clarke

Royal North Shore Hospital, Reserve Road, St Leonards, NSW 2065, Australia

Correspondence should be addressed to Eugene Wong; eugene.hl.wong@gmail.com

Academic Editor: Peter F. Lenehan

Primary tumours originating from the pericardium are extremely rare. Previous studies have reported that these tumours account for only 6.7–12.8% of all mediastinal tumours with an overall prevalence of 0.001% to 0.007%. The majority of these tumours are benign lipomas or pericardial cysts. The most common pericardial malignancy is mesothelioma. Sarcomas are soft-tissue mesenchymal malignancies originating from various parts of the body but are extremely rare in this area. We report a case of a 52-year-old female who was diagnosed with a primary sarcoma with rhabdoid differentiation originating from the pericardium. The patient presented to her GP with a four-week history of progressive dyspnea and chest pain on exertion. Chest X-Ray demonstrated a prominent pericardial effusion and suspicious chest and pericardial lesions. Biopsies of the effusion and primary tumour identified on FDG/PET scans revealed the diagnosis of primary undifferentiated sarcoma. On thoracotomy, it was noted that the tumour had invaded the right atrium; therefore, pericardial window was aborted and a drain inserted instead. The patient was then started on chemotherapy; however, progression soon occurred and the patient died within 4 months, suggesting there is urgent need for efficacious treatments for sarcomatous lesions.

1. Background

Sarcomas are rare malignant tumours that originate from connective or nonepithelial tissues. They affect many organs in the body, with the most common subtype being a Gastrointestinal Stromal Tumour (GIST) of the stomach. Sarcomas predominantly affect young patients, with a slight preponderance to males [1]. Sarcomas originating from the pericardium are even rarer entities, of which the most described histological subtype being an angiosarcoma, closely followed by undifferentiated sarcomas. A study in 2014 reported only 37 undifferentiated sarcomas that have been described in the literature with common presentations being dyspnea, fever, chest pain, and cough [2, 3].

2. Case Presentation

A 52-year-old female presented with a four-week history of progressive dyspnea on exertion and right-sided chest pain. The only other significant associated history was that she was diagnosed with localised Hereditary Nonpolyposis Colorectal Cancer in 2005 which was treated with colonic resection without adjuvant chemoradiotherapy. There was no asbestos or smoking history.

3. Investigations

A chest X-Ray was performed as the patient initially presented to her local GP, which demonstrated bilateral lung opacifications and a prominent pericardial effusion. This study prompted a high resolution computed tomography (CT) of her chest which demonstrated a large anterior mediastinal mass with extension of the right lower zone and abutting the right heart border. Images of the CT are demonstrated in Figures 1 and 2.

Mediastinal fine needle and core biopsies were then performed on percutaneous approach based on the above scans. Histopathology of a $20 \times 25 \times 6$ mm lesion from biopsy

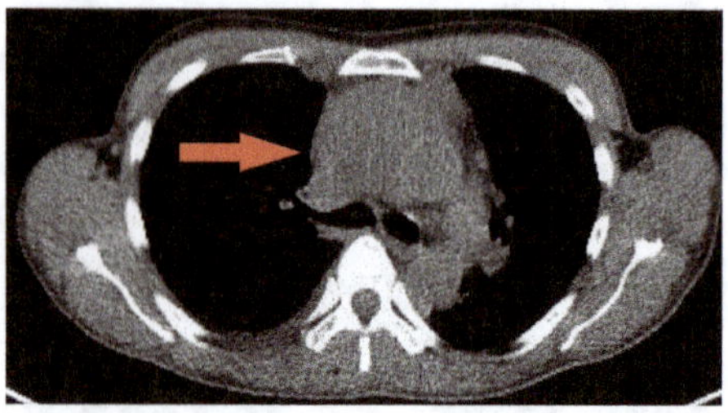

Figure 1: Axial CT demonstrating large anterior mediastinal sarcoma with involvement of the right atrium.

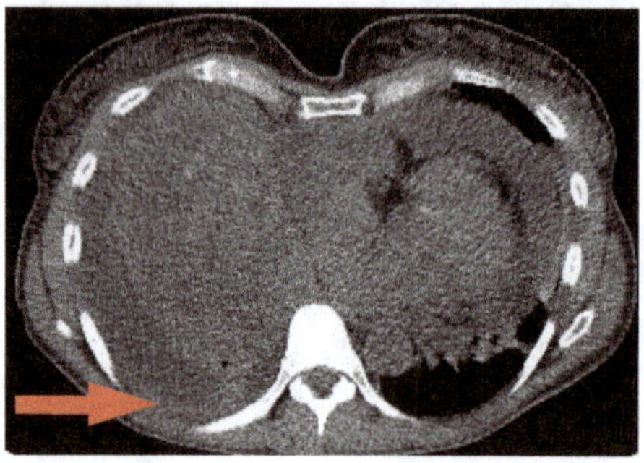

Figure 2: Axial CT demonstrating bilateral pulmonary effusions secondary to sarcoma.

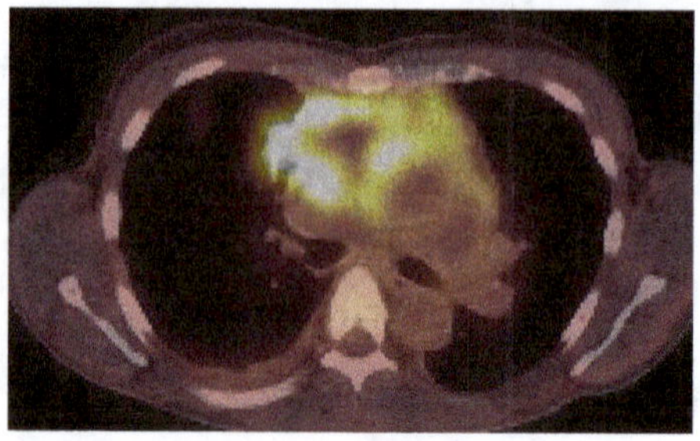

Figure 3: FDG PET demonstrating avid uptake at the pericardium and heart.

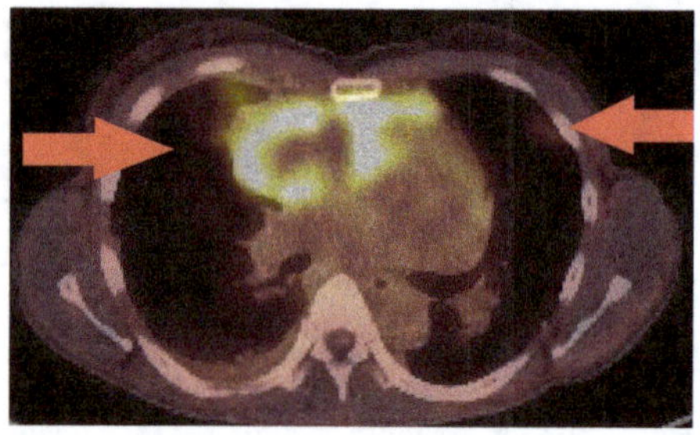

Figure 4: PET demonstrating FDG avid uptake in bilateral lungs, presumed metastases.

revealed a malignant sarcomatoid tumour, with presence of PAX8, myogenin, myoD1, and desmin expression which suggests some skeletal or cardiac muscle differentiation. Flourescent in situ hybridisation studies failed to demonstrate gene rearrangements in SYT, EWSR1, DDIT (CHOP)/FUS, and FOX01/PAX3. INI1 was positive. Given these results, while the tumour represented some rhabdoid differentiation, it could not be further classified.

An FDG/PET scan demonstrated further focally increased uptake superiorly in the pericardial sac and multiple FDG avid pulmonary nodes scattered across all lobes of both lung fields (Figures 3 and 4).

Preoperative transthoracic echocardiography demonstrated a mild right atrial free wall collapse suggestive of early tamponade and a moderately sized pericardial effusion. A well circumscribed round mass was noted abutting the right atrial wall. There was otherwise normal biventricular size, wall thickness and function, and no significant valvular pathology.

4. Treatment

Given the above findings, this patient was at a high risk of tamponade from her pericardial effusion. Therefore, we decided to perform a thoracotomy to facilitate subxiphoid exploration of the pericardium. It was anticipated that a pericardial window procedure would be performed.

On thoracotomy, a solid tumour was identified involving the pericardium with invasion into the right atrium. Transoesophageal echocardiography performed at this time confirmed intra-atrial involvement of the tumour. The procedure was modified from a pericardial window to insertion of a pericardial drain because of these findings. The pericardial catheter was inserted percutaneously through a subxiphoid approach into the pericardial space lateral to the right ventricle.

During the above procedure, the patient developed atrial fibrillation (AF) with fast ventricular response, which was reverted to sinus rhythm after 20 mg of intravenous esmolol. The patient was extubated with no complications; however, on arrival to the Intensive Care Unit, she again developed rapid AF which reverted following administration of 300 mg Amiodarone. The patient thereafter had an uncomplicated recovery.

She then received postoperative first-line single agent Doxorubicin (75 mg/m2) with Pegfilgrastim commencing one week postoperatively, with a plan for continued 3-week treatment for a total of 6 cycles. The patient tolerated the first treatment well with no significant complications.

5. Outcome and Follow-Up

The patient responded well following her second cycle of Doxorubicin chemotherapy and self-reported much improved breathing and quality of life compared to her postoperative level of function.

Unfortunately, three months later, the patient's disease progressed with significant worsening of the right pleural effusion and tumour pressure on the proximal left subclavian vein with development of a thrombus in the superior vena cava. There was also significant progression of the primary

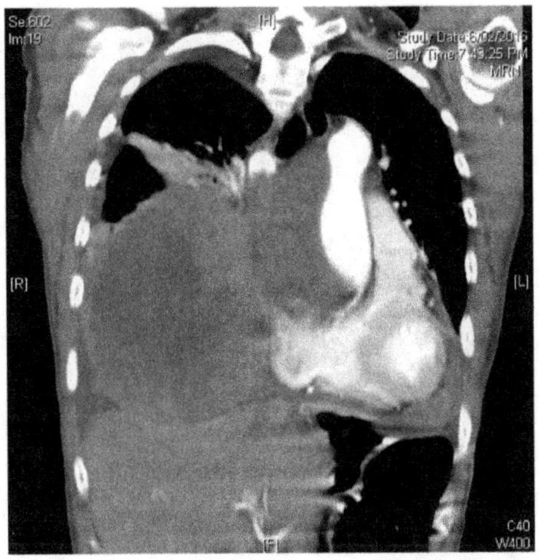

FIGURE 5: CT coronal 3 months following diagnosis demonstrating progression of disease at the Right atrium and Right lung.

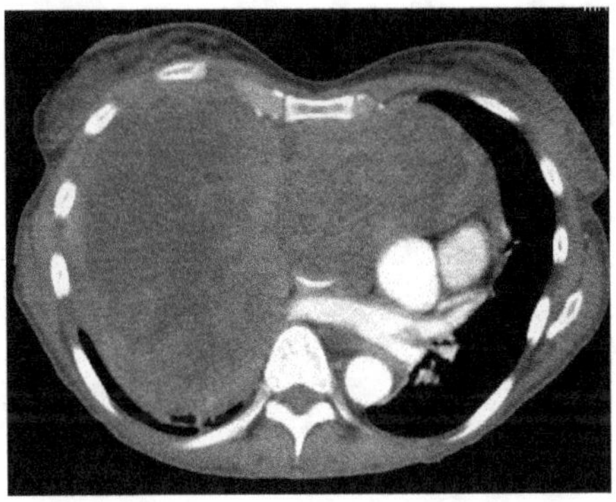

FIGURE 6: Axial CT at 3 months demonstrating progressive disease.

tumour. These findings were demonstrated on high resolution CT as shown in Figures 5 and 6. A decision was made at this stage to cease systemic therapy and for palliation of symptoms and the patient died two weeks later.

6. Discussion

Primary tumours originating from the pericardium or heart are extremely rare, with incidence at autopsy described at around 0.05% [4]. Those primary tumours that are malignant have reported autopsy incidence of around 0.001% [5]. The most common subgroup of malignant pericardial tumours are sarcomas, which are typically histologically mesotheliomas or angiosarcomas. Undifferentiated sarcomas are as such extremely rare, with previous reports suggesting that these may represent only 6-7% of sarcomas in this region. A systematic review published by Butany et al. demonstrated that approximately only 37 cases of undifferentiated sarcoma have been described from articles dating back to 1957 [3].

In our case, the patient presented with a suspected pericardial tumour following investigations of dyspnea secondary to malignant pericardial effusion. The patient underwent both a diagnostic and therapeutic insertion of pericardial drain and postoperatively experienced a recognised complication of cardiac arrhythmia but did not experience other potential complications such as ventricular puncture or pneumothoraxes [6].

This case is interesting for a number of reasons. Firstly, the pathological entity is rare, particularly due to its right-sided pericardial origin and extension into the right atrium, which required modification of surgical intervention from a pericardial window to drain insertion only. Furthermore, this is also the first case to our knowledge of an association between sarcoma of this region and a history of Hereditary Nonpolyposis Colorectal Cancer, although its relevance is uncertain.

The prognosis for metastatic sarcomas of the pericardium and heart is poor, often because of incomplete surgical resection and that radiotherapy and chemotherapy only offer temporary improvement. Gibbs et al. reported that median survival for these patients is around 5 months [6].

Extending the discussion to all localised soft-tissue sarcomas that present in adulthood, there is conflicting evidence surrounding thc efficacy of chemotherapy in the adjuvant setting and remains a controversial topic. As such, wide-local surgical excision with adjuvant radiotherapy remains the cornerstone of treatment in these patients [7]. Unfortunately, our patient had myocardial tumour invasion and distant metastases and therefore neither of these treatment options were amenable.

As this patient was initially experiencing significant shortness of breath for four weeks that limited her function substantially, we felt that she experienced a good response to the early initiation of Doxorubicin chemotherapy. Although there was some symptomatic benefit from initial chemotherapy, progression soon occurred and the patient died within 4 months, suggesting there is urgent need for new treatments for sarcomatous lesions.

References

[1] T. Tran, J. A. Davila, and H. B. El-Serag, "The epidemiology of malignant gastrointestinal stromal tumors: an analysis of 1,458 cases from 1992 to 2000," *The American Journal of Gastroenterology*, vol. 100, no. 1, pp. 162–168, 2005.

[2] I. Burazor, S. Aviel-Ronen, M. Imazio et al., "Primary malignancies of the heart and pericardium," *Clinical Cardiology*, vol. 37, no. 9, pp. 582–588, 2014.

[3] J. Butany, V. Nair, A. Naseemuddin, G. M. Nair, C. Catton, and T. Yau, "Cardiac tumours: diagnosis and management," *The Lancet Oncology*, vol. 6, no. 4, pp. 219–228, 2005.

[4] L. M. Shapiro, "Cardiac tumours: diagnosis and management," *Heart*, vol. 85, no. 2, pp. 218–222, 2001.

[5] A. Pakala, R. Gupta, and R. Lazzara, "Primary pericardial sarcoma: a case report and a brief review," *Cardiology Research and Practice*, vol. 2011, Article ID 853078, 4 pages, 2011.

[6] C. R. Gibbs, R. D. S. Watson, S. P. Singh, and G. Y. H. Lip, "Management of pericardial effusion by drainage: a survey of 10 years' experience in a city centre general hospital serving a multiracial population," *Postgraduate Medical Journal*, vol. 76, no. 902, pp. 809–813, 2000.

[7] A. Le Cesne, M. Ouali, M. G. Leahy et al., "Doxorubicin-based adjuvant chemotherapy in soft tissue sarcoma: pooled analysis of two STBSG-EORTC phase III clinical trials," *Annals of Oncology*, vol. 25, no. 12, pp. 2425–2432, 2014.

39

Sunitinib-Induced Acute Interstitial Nephritis in a Thrombocytopenic Renal Cell Cancer Patient

Ibrahim Azar,[1] Saghi Esfandiarifard,[1] Pedram Sinai,[1] Ali Wazir,[1] Llewellyn Foulke,[2] and Syed Mehdi[3]

[1]*Department of Internal Medicine, Albany Medical Center, 47 New Scotland Ave., Albany, NY 12208, USA*
[2]*Department of Pathology, Albany Medical Center, 47 New Scotland Ave., Albany, NY 12208, USA*
[3]*Division of Hematology and Oncology, Department of Internal Medicine, Stratton Veterans Affairs Medical Center, 113 Holland Ave., Albany, NY 12208, USA*

Correspondence should be addressed to Ibrahim Azar; azari@mail.amc.edu

Academic Editor: Peter F. Lenehan

Sunitinib, a multitargeted tyrosine kinase inhibitor (TKI), is currently the standard of care for patients with metastatic renal cell carcinoma. Renal adverse events associated with sunitinib include proteinuria, renal insufficiency secondary to focal segmental glomerulosclerosis (FSGS), and thrombotic microangiopathy. We describe the second reported instance of biopsy-proven sunitinib-induced acute interstitial nephritis (AIN), in a challenging case complicated by thrombocytopenia. The case illustrates the importance of early diagnosis and intervention in ensuring long-term recovery from renal complications. Four other cases of AIN reported along with inhibition of the vascular endothelial growth factor (VEGF) by either TKI (sunitinib and sorafenib) or antibodies (bevacizumab) suggest a possible class effect. Given our experience, we recommend monitoring renal function with VEGF inhibition, and in the case of renal failure in the setting of an unclear diagnosis, we recommend prompt biopsy.

1. Introduction

Recently, the use of tyrosine kinase inhibitors (TKIs) as antineoplastic agents has increased exponentially. The current National Comprehensive Cancer Network (NCCN) [1] and the European Association of Urology (EAU) [2] guidelines recommend the use of the vascular endothelial growth factor (VEGF) TKI sunitinib [2], among other options (pazopanib, interferon, and bevacizumab), as first-line treatment for metastatic renal cell carcinoma (mRCC). Given their oral availability and their generally well-tolerated side-effects profile, these antiangiogenesis agents have become the standard of care. Despite their widespread use, our understanding of this relatively new class of drugs and their side-effect profile is rudimentary.

Acute interstitial nephritis (AIN) is a characteristic inflammatory infiltrate in the renal tubule-interstitium that is a leading cause of acute renal failure. Drug-induced injuries are thought to be responsible for 60–70% of cases [3], with systemic, autoimmune, and infectious diseases accounting for the rest. In this report, we describe a case of biopsy-proven AIN in an mRCC patient receiving sunitinib.

2. Case Report

A 69-year-old male with a history of stage IV left kidney clear cell carcinoma with metastases to spine and brain presented with a four-day history of gross hematuria, oliguria, fever of 38.5°C, fatigue, and a decreased appetite. He had been started on sunitinib (50 mg daily at bedtime) two weeks ago. Hematuria persisted despite stopping acetylsalicylic acid/dipyridamole prescribed for a previous stroke (for over 5 years), discontinuing sunitinib and a course of amoxicillin for presumed UTI. Upon presentation to ED, vitals were significant for a blood pressure of 160/72 mmHg. A digital rectal exam was negative for occult blood. Laboratory investigations revealed mild anemia (hemoglobin of 11.9 g/dl), thrombocytopenia (platelets of 68,000/mm^3),

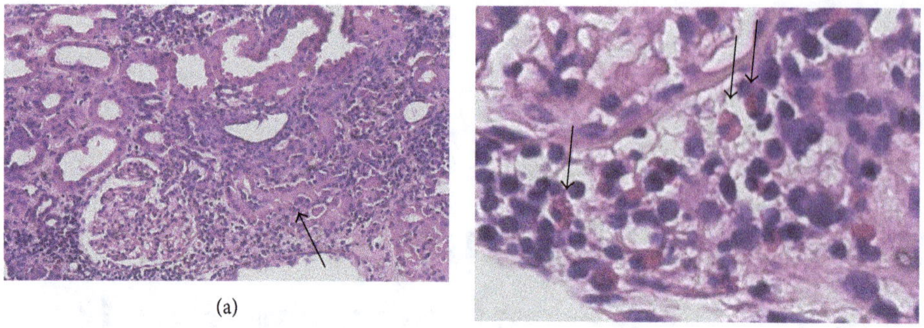

(a) (b)

Figure 1: Renal biopsy demonstrating acute interstitial nephritis (H&E staining): there is edema and an extensive dense interstitial chronic inflammatory infiltrate in the cortex and medulla. (a) In the lower power photomicrograph (left, 100x), the renal cortex shows extensive interstitial chronic inflammation with occasional lymphocytic tubulitis (arrow). In areas of inflammation, there is evidence of acute tubular injury with proximal tubules demonstrating lumenal distension with epithelial flattening. There was no evidence of glomerulitis, vasculitis, or thrombotic microangiopathy. (b) The higher magnification photomicrograph (right, 600x) shows that the interstitial inflammatory cells comprised frequent eosinophils (arrows) as well as lymphocytes and fewer plasma cells.

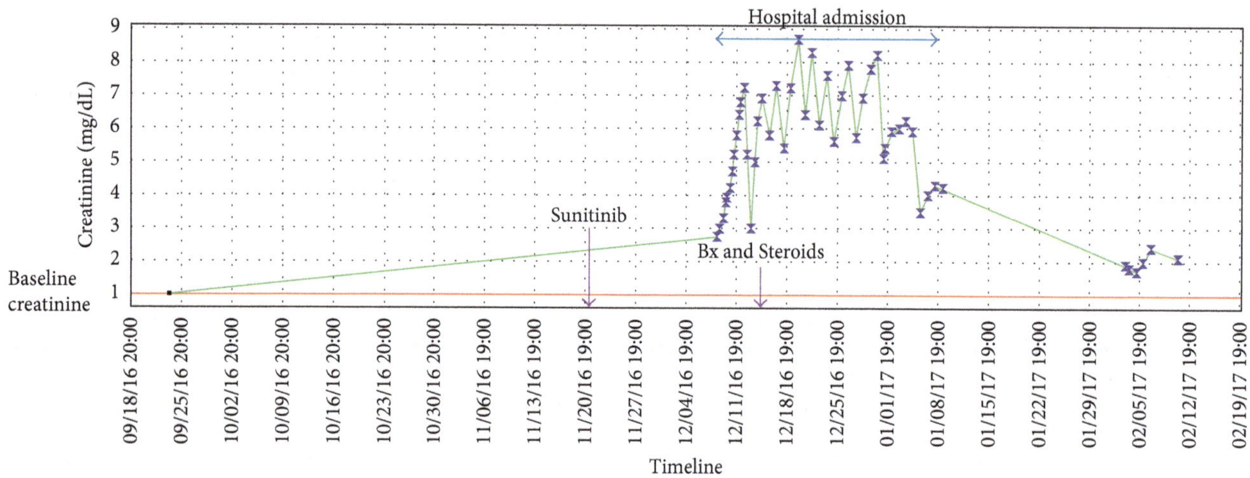

Figure 2: Timeline showing the temporal relationship between the start of sunitinib and the rise of creatinine. Note the normal creatinine at baseline and the decrease of creatinine with steroids and hemodialysis.

hyponatremia (sodium of 120 mEq/L), and acute renal failure (BUN of 41 and creatinine of 2.7 mg/dL with a baseline creatinine of 1.0). Coagulation labs were within normal limits (activated partial thromboplastin time (aPTT) 29, prothrombin (PT) 12.1, and international normalized ratio (INR) 1.1). A urine dipstick was positive for blood and protein. Urine sodium was less than 10 mEq/L, indicating dehydration. Total urine protein collected in 24 hours was 484 mg. Haptoglobin was not decreased, and a peripheral smear examination was negative for schistocytes, ruling out hemolytic uremic syndrome. While nonspecific inflammatory markers (C-reactive protein (CRP) of 55 mg/L and erythrocyte sedimentation rate (ESR) of 80 mm/hr) were elevated, multiple serologies associated with nephritic syndromes (peripheral and cytoplasmic antineutrophilic cytoplasmic antibodies (p- and c-ANCA): antimyeloperoxidase (MPO), antiproteinase 3 (PR3), complement levels, antinuclear antibody (ANA), anti-double-stranded DNA (dsDNA), rheumatoid factor (RF), hepatitis B and C panels, and cryoglobulins) were all negative.

Despite a significant risk of bleeding, a renal biopsy after platelet transfusion was performed to aid in diagnosis. The renal biopsy (Figure 1) showed extensive interstitial inflammation with frequent eosinophils and interstitial edema, consistent with drug-induced acute interstitial nephritis (AIN). The inflammation was more marked in the cortex than in the medulla. There was associated acute tubular injury in regions of inflammation. There were occasional foci of lymphocytic and eosinophilic tubulitis. There was minimal chronicity evident. No evidence of glomerulitis or vasculitis was present. No evidence of immune complex deposits was identified on direct immunofluorescence studies or on ultrastructural analysis. No evidence of thrombotic microangiopathy was present. He was started on oral course of steroids and required intermittent hemodialysis. Throughout his hospital stay, he continued to experience gross hematuria requiring multiple pRBC transfusions. Unfortunately, while the patient's renal function somewhat recovered (Figure 2), he succumbed to hospital-acquired pneumonia 2 months after his diagnosis of AIN.

3. Discussion

This report describes an exceptional diagnostic challenge. The initial presentation of hematuria, thrombocytopenia, and renal failure raised the flag for a thrombotic microangiopathy (TMA), namely, hemolytic-uremic syndrome (HUS), a well-described side effect [4] of VEGF inhibition. However, the absence of schistocytes on the peripheral smear along with the normal haptoglobin pointed away from this diagnosis. Similarly, the constellation of hematuria and mild proteinuria pointed to a possible nephritic disease presentation. However, multiple serologies of systemic diseases associated with nephritic pattern pathology were negative. In the setting of a worsening renal failure requiring dialysis and an uncertain diagnosis, the decision to obtain a kidney biopsy was contemplated. However, the unabating thrombocytopenia exacerbated the risk of retroperitoneal hematoma, the most common side effect of kidney biopsy, to 40% according to one study [5]. After extended discussions between oncology, nephrology, and interventional radiology, the kidney biopsy was performed and revealed the diagnosis of AIN.

Interestingly, when faced with a patient with thrombocytopenia and renal failure following the administration of sunitinib, Khurana [6] decided against performing a biopsy. A notable diagnostic difference between the two cases is that of the classically described AIN triad (rash, fever, and eosinophilia); our case presented with the very nonspecific fever, while the patient seen by Khurana had a peripheral eosinophilia of 40%. The presumed diagnosis of AIN in the Khurana case was further strengthened when renal failure eosinophilia recurred when the patient was rechallenged with sorafenib, another VEGF inhibitor. Unfortunately, despite recovering some kidney function with the course of corticosteroids, our patient succumbed to pneumonia briefly afterwards. Given our experience, we recommend monitoring renal function with VEGF inhibition and advocating a prompter biopsy and treatment in cases of renal failure.

Given the patient use of acetylsalicylic acid/dipyridamole for over five years, interstitial nephritis secondary to acetylsalicylic acid and dipyridamole was on the differential. However, the corresponding biopsy would show evidence of chronic interstitial nephritis, that is, increased interstitial fibrosis and tubular atrophy that is more than what is expected for the patient's age. However, the biopsy demonstrated minimal interstitial fibrosis and tubular atrophy (estimated to be 5–10%) less than the 25–35% expected with a 69-year-old gentleman. As such, acetylsalicylic acid/dipyridamole as the offending drug was ruled out.

This report describes the second known case of biopsy-proven sunitinib-induced acute interstitial nephritis [7]. Current techniques in rational drug design do not allow for the extreme specificity in the era of personalized medicine promised. While sunitinib was ostensibly designed as a VEGF inhibitor, it is in fact a multikinase inhibitor that includes the following receptor tyrosine kinases (RTKs) [8, 9] among its targets: platelet-derived growth factor receptor (PDGFR), stem cell factor receptor c-kit, FMS-like tyrosine kinase 3 (FLT3), and colony-stimulating factor 1 (CSF-1). Similar case reports involving the VEGF-targeting drugs sorafenib (TKI) [6, 10] and bevacizumab (monoclonal antibody) [11, 12] imply a class effect specific to VEGF. No similar case reports were found with other targets. The incidence of AIN with nonrenal cancer [11, 12] indicates that the presence of underlying renal oncogenesis is not associated with AIN.

Previously reported renal adverse events of sunitinib include hypertension, proteinuria, renal insufficiency, and thrombotic microangiopathy; all are present in this case except thrombotic microangiopathy. Thus, thrombocytopenia in this case may be secondary to bone marrow suppression or immunologic in nature [13].

While sunitinib-induced AIN is exceedingly rare, it should be considered in patients with acute renal failure. Given the multiple case reports implicating VEGF-targeting drugs in cases of AIN, further study is required to elicit the link between the VEGF pathway and AIN.

References

[1] National Comprehensive Cancer Network, "Kidney cancer (version 2)," 2017, https://www.nccn.org/professionals/physician_gls/PDF/kidney.pdf.

[2] B. Ljungberg, K. Bensalah, S. Canfield et al., "EAU guidelines on renal cell carcinoma: 2014 update," *European Urology*, vol. 67, no. 5, pp. 913–924, 2015.

[3] M. A. Perazella and G. S. Markowitz, "Drug-induced acute interstitial nephritis," *Nature Reviews Nephrology*, vol. 6, no. 8, pp. 461–470, 2010.

[4] G. Bollée, N. Patey, G. Cazajous et al., "Thrombotic microangiopathy secondary to VEGF pathway inhibition by sunitinib," *Nephrology Dialysis Transplantation*, vol. 24, no. 2, pp. 682–685, 2009.

[5] M. C. Simard-Meilleur, S. Troyanov, L. Roy, E. Dalaire, and S. Brachemi, "Risk factors and timing of native kidney biopsy complications," *Nephron Extra*, vol. 4, no. 1, pp. 42–49, 2014.

[6] A. Khurana, "Allergic interstitial nephritis possibly related to sunitinib use," *American Journal of Geriatric Pharmacotherapy*, vol. 5, no. 4, pp. 341–344, 2007.

[7] S. K. Winn, S. Ellis, P. Savage, S. Sampson, and J. E. Marsh, "Biopsy-proven acute interstitial nephritis associated with the tyrosine kinase inhibitor sunitinib: a class effect?," *Nephrology Dialysis Transplantation*, vol. 24, no. 2, pp. 673–675, 2009.

[8] L. Q. M. Chow and S. G. Eckhardt, "Sunitinib: from rational design to clinical efficacy," *Journal of Clinical Oncology*, vol. 25, no. 7, pp. 884–896, 2007.

[9] G. S. Papaetis and K. N. Syrigos, "Sunitinib: a multitargeted receptor tyrosine kinase inhibitor in the era of molecular cancer therapies," *BioDrugs*, vol. 23, no. 6, pp. 377–389, 2009.

[10] H. Izzedine, I. Brocheriou, O. Rixe, and G. Deray, "Interstitial nephritis in a patient taking sorafenib," *Nephrology Dialysis Transplantation*, vol. 22, no. 8, p. 2411, 2007.

[11] R. K. Barakat, N. Singh, R. Lal, R. R. Verani, K. W. Finkel, and J. R. Foringer, "Interstitial nephritis secondary to bevacizumab treatment in metastatic leiomyosarcoma," *Annals of Pharmacotherapy*, vol. 41, no. 4, pp. 707–710, 2007.

[12] A. J. Lomax, P. A. Hill, and D. M. Ashley, "Case report of interstitial nephritis induced by bevacizumab therapy for glioblastoma multiforme," *Journal of Oncology Pharmacy Practice*, vol. 19, no. 4, pp. 365–368, 2013.

[13] R. Shekarriz, N. Koulaeinejad, A. Nosrati, and E. Salehifa, "Sunitinib induced immune thrombocytopenia," *Iranian Journal of Pharmaceutical Research*, vol. 14, no. 4, pp. 1295–1297, 2015.

40

Breast Implant–Associated Anaplastic Large Cell Lymphoma

Daniel E. Ezekwudo,[1] Tolulope Ifabiyi,[2] Bolanle Gbadamosi,[1] Kristle Haberichter,[3] Zhou Yu,[1] Mitual Amin,[2,3] Kenneth Shaheen,[2] Michael Stender,[1] and Ishmael Jaiyesimi[1,2]

[1]*Department of Hematology and Oncology, Oakland University William Beaumont School of Medicine, William Beaumont Hospital, 3601 W. 13 Mile Rd., Royal Oak, MI 48073, USA*
[2]*Oakland University William Beaumont School of Medicine, 3601 W. 13 Mile Rd., Royal Oak, MI 48073, USA*
[3]*Department of Pathology and Laboratory Medicine, Oakland University William Beaumont School of Medicine, William Beaumont Hospital, 3601 W. 13 Mile Rd., Royal Oak, MI 48073, USA*

Correspondence should be addressed to Daniel E. Ezekwudo; daniel.ezekwudo@beaumont.edu

Academic Editor: Constantine Gennatas

Breast implant–associated anaplastic large T-cell lymphoma has recently been recognized as an entity, with few reports describing the two common subtypes: in situ (indolent) and infiltrative. Recently, the infiltrative subtypes have been shown to be more aggressive requiring adjuvant chemotherapy. We report a rare case of breast implant–associated anaplastic large cell lymphoma (BIA-ALCL) in a 65-year-old Caucasian female following silicone breast implantation and multiple capsulectomies. We discuss the rare presentation of this disease, histopathologic features of the indolent and infiltrative subtypes of ALCL, and their clinical significance. We also review the literature for up-to-date information on the diagnosis and clinical management. Treatment modalities including targeted therapy are also discussed. Although BIA-ALCL is rare, it should always be considered as part of the differential diagnosis especially in women with breast implants. Given the increasing rate of breast reconstruction and cosmetic surgeries, we anticipate a continuous rise in incidence rates of this rare disease; thus, caution must be taken to avoid misdiagnosis.

1. Introduction

Breast lymphoma represents approximately 0.7% of all lymphomas, of which 8% are peripheral T-cell lymphomas (PTCLs) [1]. The majority of reported PTCLs are ALK-negative anaplastic large T-cell lymphomas (ALCLs). Breast implant–associated anaplastic large T-cell lymphoma (BIA-ALCL) has been reported but only recently has gained recognition as a distinct entity. Two different subtypes with a possible histogenetic relationship have been described including in situ BIA-ALCL and infiltrative BIA-ALCL; these subtypes have significantly different prognostic implications with the infiltrative subtype showing worse prognosis [2]. Generally, in situ BIA-ALCL follows an indolent clinical course after breast implant removal, whereas infiltrative BIA-ALCL is more aggressive, requiring additional therapy after implant removal [2]. Thus, accurate histopathologic diagnosis is crucial for risk assessment and therapeutic management. Recent advances in therapeutic approaches have resulted in significant improvement in the overall survival of patients with BIA-ALCL. More recently, targeted therapy utilizing the anti-CD30 antibody brentuximab-vedotin (BV) has shown promising results [3, 4].

2. Case Presentation

A 65-year-old Caucasian female had a past medical history significant for bilateral fibrocystic breast disease resulting in bilateral subcutaneous mastectomy, followed by bilateral cosmetic breast reconstruction with textured silicone gel implants at age 30 (Figure 1). Subsequently, she had multiple complications from the implants including capsule contractures, infections, chronic seroma, and ruptured breast implants, leading to capsulectomy and implant replacements

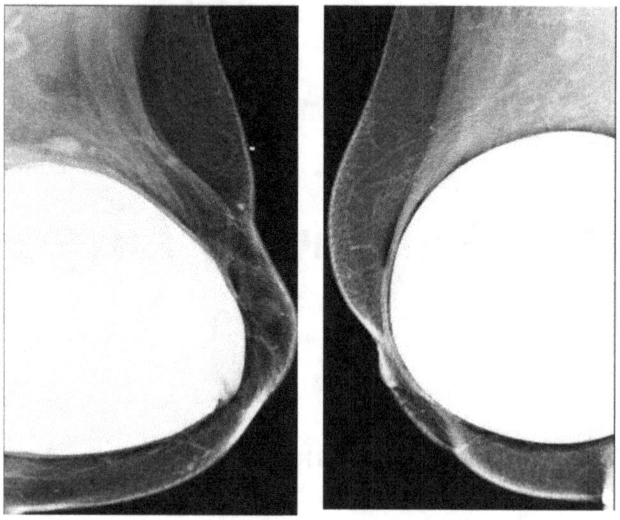

(a) (b)

Figure 1: Mammogram showing silicone implant in the (a) left and (b) right breasts.

15 and 22 years post original implantation. During these periods, the patient was noted to have several areas of calcifications in both breasts (L > R) that had been monitored with routine mammography. The patient noted that at 30 years post original implantation, her left breast became edematous; however, this self-resolved a few months later. Two years later, edema was noted again in the left breast and confirmed by MRI (Figure 2)], resulting in a third replacement of the silicone gel implant. Recently, at 35 years post original surgery, the patient presented with swelling in the left breast which progressively worsened over 2–3 months. A targeted ultrasound examination of the left breast at the approximate twelve o'clock position, left axilla, and of the right breast at the ten o'clock position over areas of concern demonstrated no discrete cystic or solid abnormalities (Figure 3). Unremarkable parenchyma was observed throughout the entire region. However, given the extent of edema in the left breast and associated pain, bilateral total capsulectomy was performed for a fourth time.

Breast tissue obtained during surgery was sent for pathologic evaluation. The left capsulectomy specimen revealed a thickened fibrous capsule with chronic inflammation, consisting of small lymphocytes, eosinophils, plasma cells, and macrophages. The luminal surface of the breast capsule showed fibrin deposition with a thin row of highly atypical cells. The atypical cells were large and pleomorphic, with hyperchromatic nuclei and occasional prominent nucleoli noted along with abundant clear to slightly eosinophilic cytoplasm (Figure 4). Immunohistochemical analysis demonstrated strong CD30, CD43, and MUM1 expression, while EMA was weakly positive (Figure 5). The cells did not express ALK (Figure 5), CD20, CD79a, or estrogen receptor. The overall morphology and immunohistochemical profile were diagnostic for breast implant–associated anaplastic large cell lymphoma.

A bone marrow evaluation, including flow cytometry studies, showed unremarkable trilineage hematopoiesis without evidence of involvement by lymphoma or metastatic malignancy. Cytogenetic examination of the bone marrow revealed twenty metaphase cells with a normal female diploid karyotype with no consistent numerical or structural chromosome aberrations. Computed tomography (CT) scans of the neck, chest, abdomen, and pelvis with IV and oral contrast were essentially negative for any malignancy or lymphadenopathy except for the noted fluid collection in the left breast measuring $12.9 \times 2.8 \times 10.1$ cm (Figure 6). Whole body positron emission tomography–computed tomography (PET/CT) scan with fluorodeoxyglucose (FDG) radiotracer revealed increased FDG uptake along the anterior chest wall, slightly greater on the right than the left, with a maximum SUV of 4.7 and 4.1, respectively. No other area of increased FDG uptake was noted. Given the in situ subtype of ALCL noted in our patient, she underwent capsulectomy with no other local or systemic therapy. She remains clinically well after 12 months follow-up under close surveillance with our clinic.

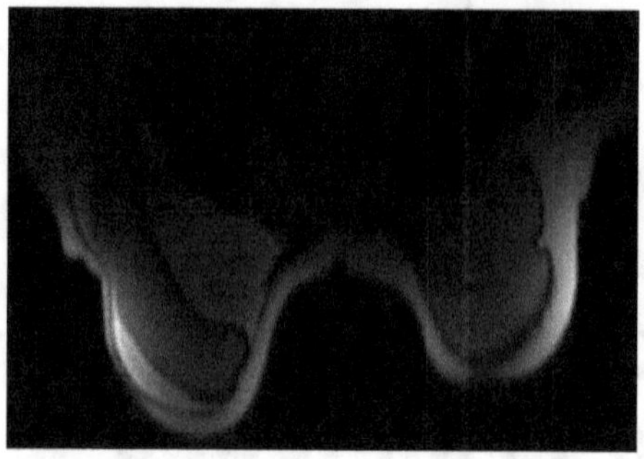

Figure 2: MRI showing fluid accumulation around the left breast subpectoral silicone implant.

3. Discussion

Non-Hodgkin lymphoma of the breast is exceedingly rare; the majority diagnosed are of B-cell origin including diffuse large B-cell lymphoma, extranodal marginal zone lymphoma, follicular lymphoma, primary effusion lymphoma, and lymphoplasmacytic lymphoma [5–7].

Peripheral T-cell lymphoma (PTCL) of the breast is less frequently reported and represents only 10% of all breast lymphomas. In breast implant patients, >90% of these are ALK-negative ALCL, compared to 37% in non–breast implant patients [1, 8]. To date, there are more than 300 reported cases of BIA-ALCL worldwide; however, only about 130 report pathologic markers, the majority of which were in the United States (67.4%) [9, 10]. The US Food and Drug Administration (FDA) estimated the incidence of BIA-ALCL to be 0.6–1.2 per 100,000, based on reported cases of BIA-ALCL among an estimated 5–10 million women with breast implants [11].

Anaplastic large T-cell lymphoma belongs to the spectrum of lymphoproliferative $CD30^+$ disease and can manifest as either cutaneous or systemic disease. There are two known subtypes of ALCL of the breast: (a) in situ, in which disease proliferation is confined to the capsule and is often associated with seroma as in our patient, and (b) infiltrative,

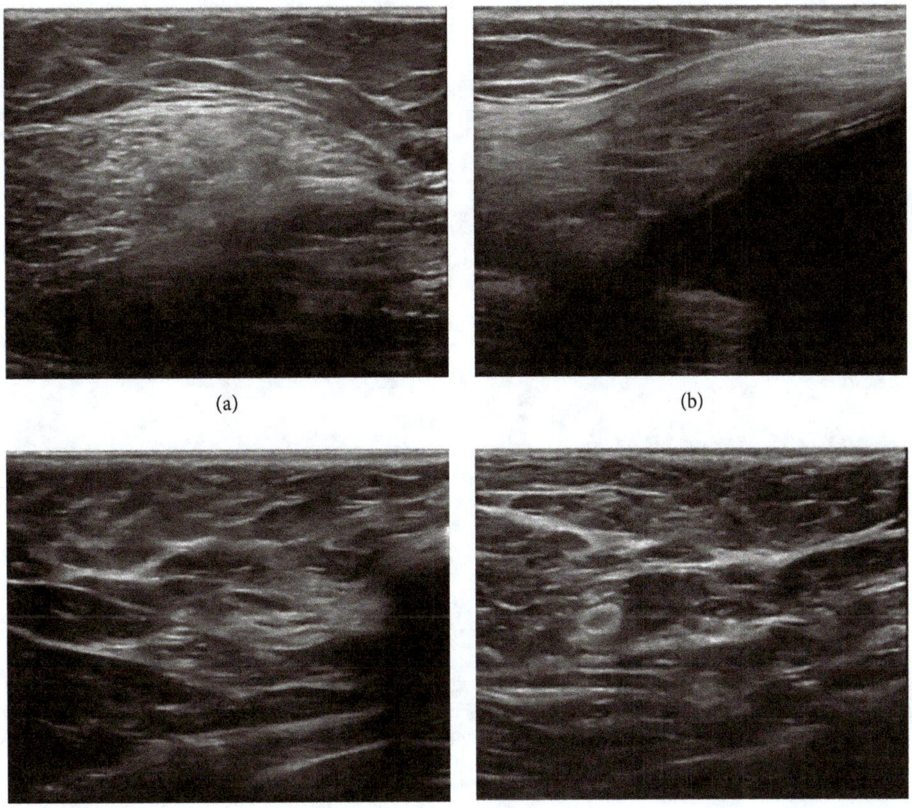

(a) (b) (c) (d)

FIGURE 3: Ultrasound of the left breast ((a) transverse view, (b) sagittal view at 12 : 00 position) and the right breast ((c) transverse view, (d) sagittal view at 10 : 00 position).

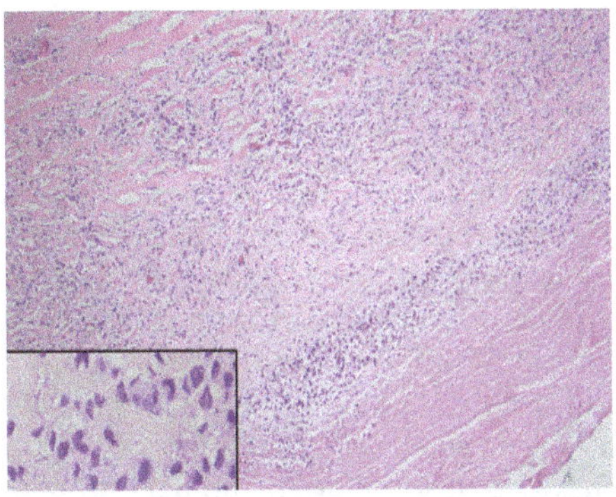

FIGURE 4: Representative sections of the left breast capsule. Larger image: the capsule contains small lymphocytes, macrophages, plasma cells, and occasional eosinophils. In addition, there are clusters of large neoplastic cells throughout the capsule, adjacent to the luminal fibrinoid necrosis (hematoxylin and eosin, 100x). Inset image: the large neoplastic cells are pleomorphic with hyperchromatic nuclei and abundant clear to slightly eosinophilic cytoplasm. Occasional "hallmark" cells with eccentric horseshoe- and kidney-shaped nuclei (hematoxylin and eosin, 1000x).

mostly associated with tumor mass with cells infiltrating the capsule and adjacent tissues [2]. Of the reported cases of BIA-ALCL, approximately 50% have seroma involvement, which is thought to be associated with a better prognosis, although some have argued a histogenetic relationship with the inflammatory subtype of BIA-ALCL [2]. The most common presenting symptom is unilateral swelling related to periprosthetic fluid collection more than a year after implantation [12, 13]. Other symptoms include pain, rash, pruritus, and capsular contracture [13, 14]. Patients present rarely with a mass that protrudes from the fibrous capsule, leading to an implant with an irregular texture [13]. BIA-ALCL has been reported in both silicone and saline (either textured or smooth) implants; for instance, out of the 359 cases of BIA-ALCL reported to the US-FDA in 2017, 28 of the cancers were in women who received breast implants with smooth surfaces, whereas 203 were in women who had breast implant version with a textured surface [15]. Inflammatory TH17 T-cells are found in greater numbers in textured compared to smooth breast implants [9]; however, no causal link between the type of implant and ALCL has been established. Chronic inflammation within the capsule is believed to be the cause of ALCL [16].

Histologically, ALCL may present as epitheloid-like, mimicking poorly differentiated breast carcinoma [12, 13]; thus, accurate immunohistochemical and histopathological evaluation is necessary. Usually, BIA-ALCL has uniform expression of CD30 with atypical cytology and is cytokeratin-negative [8]. Cells are large and pleomorphic with dispersed chromatin and multiple or single prominent nucleoli and have eosinophilic to amphophilic cytoplasm [9, 13]. Hallmark cells can occasionally be observed, with

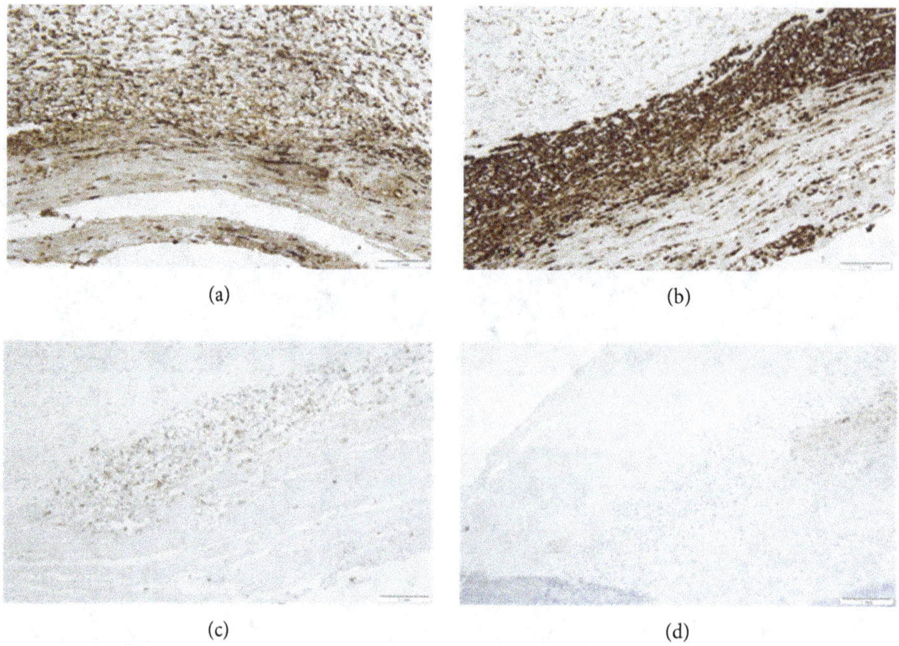

FIGURE 5: Select immunostaining of the region of capsular tissue with atypical cells. (a) Large neoplastic cells stain positive with CD43, confirming T-cell lineage (200x). (b) In addition, the neoplastic cells have uniform membranous and Golgi staining with CD30 (200x). (c) There is weak staining with epithelial membrane antigen (EMA) (200x). (d) The cells lack expression of ALK (200x).

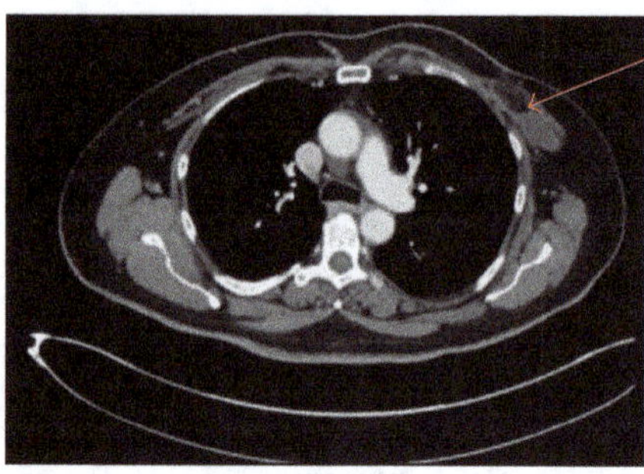

FIGURE 6: CT scan of chest: large fluid collection in the left chest wall measuring $12.9 \times 2.8 \times 10.1$ cm.

horseshoe- or kidney-shaped nuclei and a paranuclear eosinophilic region [5, 13]. Cytogenetically, about two-thirds of BIA-ALCL present with clonal rearrangement of the T-cell receptor gene [17].

Imaging of affected breasts often shows an effusion surrounding the implant with or without a mass [13]. Overall, the lymphoma cells in BIA-ALCL histologically and morphologically resemble that of ALK-negative systemic ALCL. Despite these similarities, the clinical outcome of BIA-ALCL can differ greatly from that of systemic ALCL. A recent report by Laurent et al. [2] indicates that systemic ALCL has an aggressive clinical course closer to the infiltrative subtype of BIA-ALCL than to the in situ subtype. For instance, 2-year overall survival of systemic ALCL and BIA-ALCL are 48% and 52.5%, respectively, whereas the in situ subtype has >95% survival at 2 years [12, 18].

Proposed therapeutic approaches for patients with BIA-ALCL have ranged from surgery with or without standard chemotherapy and with or without radiation to more recent targeted therapy. Gidengil et al. elaborated the use of all these treatment options in a review of 54 cases of BIA-ALCL in which 57% were treated with standard chemotherapy treatment for non-Hodgkin lymphoma including cyclophosphamide, hydroxydaunorubicin, vincristine, and prednisone (CHOP) with or without other chemotherapy agents, 48% received radiation therapy mostly to the chest wall, and 11% received stem cell transplants [14]. Agents such as etoposide have also been reported in treatment therapies for BIA-ALCL [19].

Due to the indolent course of in situ disease, capsulectomy alone without aggressive chemotherapy has been suggested as a more appropriate approach in those patients with disease confined to the capsule [9, 16]. In these patients, removal of implants and capsulectomy treatment alone have favorable outcomes, with the mean duration of remission approximately 16 months [12]. Disease recurrence has also been reported and may present as either localized or metastatic [14]. A more aggressive approach is recommended for patients with the infiltrative subtype of BIA-ALCL. Patients with positive regional lymph node involvement at diagnosis have a higher rate of recurrence, and nodal and/or systemic involvement is often the cause of death [12]. In cases of lymph node involvement with cytogenetic abnormalities, capsulectomy followed by CHOP plus etoposide upon relapse has been suggested [20]. Patients who present with a distinctive mass may have a worse prognosis as this often times indicates the infiltrative subtype of ALCL and require aggressive treatment including chemotherapy and radiation therapy [8, 13]. Other factors such as staging at the time of diagnosis should also be considered. Brody et al. reported nine deaths in patients with BIA-ALCL even after repeated therapies and noted that four out of the nine deaths presented with a mass [9].

Recently, targeted therapy has shown encouraging results. More than 90% of ALCL overexpress CD30 antigen, thus making this a favorable target for future drug designs. The approval of brentuximab-vedotin (BV), a CD30-specific monoclonal antibody conjugated to the tubulin toxin monomethyl auristatin E (MMAE) [21], provides a promising therapy for patients who do not respond to conventional chemotherapy or salvage high-dose chemotherapy and stem cell transplantation [19, 22]. The proposed mechanism of action of BV involves MMAE binding to the CD30 receptor and internalization into the cell, where it induces growth arrest and apoptosis [21]. BV was approved for treatment of Hodgkin lymphoma (HL) and ALCL unresponsive to previous treatment. Peripheral sensory neuropathy is the most common side effect, which has been shown to be dose dependent, and partially reversible following dose reduction or treatment cessation. Other side effects include nausea, fatigue, pyrexia, diarrhea, rash, constipation, and neutropenia [21]. Recent phase II trials reported overall response rates of 75% in patients with HL and 86% in patients with systemic ALCL that have relapsed or were unresponsive to previous treatments. The complete response rates were 34% and 57% for patients with HL and ALCL, respectively [22]. BV has also been shown to be effective as a first line treatment. Oregel et al. reported successful treatment of a critically ill patient with ALK-negative ALCL involving the axillary lymph nodes [23].

The lack of complete response in some patients could be due to development of resistance to BV. Loss of CD30 expression following treatment with BV has been noted in 2 cases of ALK-negative ALCL [3, 4]. Downregulation of CD30 has also been observed in resistant ALCL cell lines [22], supporting this mechanism in the development of resistance to BV. Currently, clinical trials assessing the use of BV with CHOP or CHP (CHOP without vincristine) have shown promising efficacy with tolerable toxicities in CD30$^+$ PTCL [24]. Thus, BV could potentially be an option for treatment of aggressive BIA-ALCL refractory to chemotherapy or even as first line treatment.

Apart from anti-CD30 immunotherapy, emerging studies are revealing other possible targets in patients with ALCL especially those with ALK positivity. For instance, a recent study by Laimer et al. showed that high expression of platelet-derived growth factor receptor (PDGFR a/b) was observed in mouse model effected with human large T cell lymphoma. Their study revealed that combination of standard chemo/immunotherapy plus anti-PDGFR therapy such as imatinib resulted in complete remission in patients with relapsed ALCL after autologous transplantation [25]. Although still in the early stage of research, their results offer great potentials for patients with more aggressive variant of ALCL especially those with ALK expressivity. Currently, a clinical trial (a window of opportunity trial) investigating the therapeutic impact of combination treatment with anti-CD30 plus imatinib is ongoing [26].

4. Conclusion

BIA-ALCL is a rare breast lymphoma that has both indolent (in situ) and aggressive (infiltrative) subtypes. Tumor mass at presentation could be used a marker of the more aggressive type requiring standard chemotherapy with or without radiation plus capsulectomy. Although prognosis for patients with an in situ disease subtype is excellent, the infiltrative subtype has a prognosis similar to systemic ALCL. Early histopathologic diagnosis is crucial to initiating the right treatment course. Patients should continue close surveillance following completion of treatment to monitor for disease recurrence.

Authors' Contributions

Daniel E. Ezekwudo, Tolulope Ifabiyi, Bolanle Gbadamosi, and Zhou Yu prepared the literature review and manuscript drafts. Kristle Haberichter and Mitual Amin obtained and analyzed the pathology slides. Kenneth Shaheen is the operating surgeon. Michael Stender and Ishmael Jaiyesimi provided critical review of the manuscript. All authors read and approved the final manuscript.

References

[1] G. Gualco, L. Chioato, W. J. Harrington, L. M. Weiss, and C. E. Bacchi, "Primary and secondary T-cell lymphomas of the breast: clinico-pathologic features of 11 cases," *Applied Immunohistochemistry and Molecular Morphology*, vol. 17, no. 4, pp. 301–306, 2009.

[2] C. Laurent, A. Delas, P. Gaulard et al., "Breast implant-associated anaplastic large cell lymphoma: two distinct clinicopathological variants with different outcomes," *Annals of Oncology*, vol. 27, no. 2, pp. 306–314, 2016.

[3] R. N. Al-Rohil, C. A. Torres-Cabala, A. Patel et al., "Loss of CD30 expression after treatment with brentuximab vedotin in a patient with anaplastic large cell lymphoma: a novel finding," *Journal of Cutaneous Pathology*, vol. 43, no. 12, pp. 1161–1166, 2016.

[4] H. Arai, S. Furuichi, Y. Nakamura, Y. Nakamura, M. Ichikawa, and K. Mitani, "ALK-negative anaplastic large cell lymphoma with loss of CD30 expression during treatment with brentuximab vedotin," *Rinsho Ketsueki*, vol. 57, no. 5, pp. 634–637, 2016.

[5] S. Li and A. K. Lee, "Silicone implant and primary breast ALK1-negative anaplastic large cell lymphoma, fact or fiction?" *International Journal of Clinical and Experimental Pathology*, vol. 3, no. 1, pp. 117–127, 2010.

[6] P. Validire, M. Capovilla, B. Asselain et al., "Primary breast non-Hodgkin's lymphoma: a large single center study of initial characteristics, natural history, and prognostic factors," *American Journal of Hematology*, vol. 84, no. 3, pp. 133–139, 2009.

[7] G. Martinelli, G. Ryan, J. F. Seymour et al., "Primary follicular and marginal-zone lymphoma of the breast: clinical features, prognostic factors and outcome: a study by the International

Extranodal Lymphoma Study Group," *Annals of Oncology*, vol. 20, no. 12, pp. 1993–1999, 2009.

[8] M. Bizjak, C. Selmi, S. Praprotnik et al., "Silicone implants and lymphoma: the role of inflammation," *Journal of Autoimmunity*, vol. 65, pp. 64–73, 2015.

[9] G. S. Brody, D. Deapen, C. R. Taylor et al., "Anaplastic large cell lymphoma occurring in women with breast implants: analysis of 173 cases," *Plastic and Reconstructive Surgery*, vol. 135, no. 3, pp. 695–705, 2015.

[10] S. Ravi-Kumar, O. Sanaei, M. Vasef, I. Rabinowitz, and M. H. Fekrazad, "Anaplastic large cell lymphoma associated with breast implants," *World Journal of Plastic Surgery*, vol. 1, no. 1, pp. 30–35, 2012.

[11] U.S. Food and Drug Administration, "Anaplastic large cell lymphoma (ALCL) in women with breast implants: preliminary FDA findings and analyses," January 2011, http://www.fda.gov/MedicalDevices/ProductsandMedicalProcedures/ImplantsandProsthetics/BreastImplants/ucm239996.htm.

[12] M. Jewell, S. L. Spear, J. Largent, M. G. Oefelein, and W. P. Adams Jr., "Anaplastic large T-cell lymphoma and breast implants: a review of the literature," *Plastic and Reconstructive Surgery*, vol. 128, no. 3, pp. 651–661, 2011.

[13] J. Xu and S. Wei, "Breast implant-associated anaplastic large cell lymphoma: review of a distinct clinicopathologic entity," *Archives of Pathology and Laboratory Medicine*, vol. 138, no. 6, pp. 842–846, 2014.

[14] C. A. Gidengil, Z. Predmore, S. Mattke, K. van Busum, and B. Kim, "Breast implant–associated anaplastic large cell lymphoma," *Plastic and Reconstructive Surgery*, vol. 135, no. 3, pp. 713–720, 2015.

[15] U.S. Food and Drug Administration, "Anaplastic large cell lymphoma (ALCL) in women with breast implants: preliminary FDA findings and analyses," March 2017, http://www.fda.gov/safety/medwatch/safetyinformation/safetyalertsforhumanmedicalproducts/ucm547622.htm.

[16] X. Ye, K. Shokrollahi, W. M. Rozen et al., "Anaplastic large cell lymphoma (ALCL) and breast implants: breaking down the evidence," *Mutation Research Reviews in Mutation Research*, vol. 762, pp. 123–132, 2014.

[17] T. I. M. Malcolm, P. Villarese, C. J. Fairbairn et al., "Anaplastic large cell lymphoma arises in thymocytes and requires transient TCR expression for thymic egress," *Nature Communications*, vol. 7, article 10087, 2016.

[18] D. Sibon, M. Fournier, J. Brière et al., "Long-term outcome of adults with systemic anaplastic large-cell lymphoma treated within the Groupe d'Étude des Lymphomes de l'Adulte trials," *Journal of Clinical Oncology*, vol. 30, no. 32, pp. 3939–3946, 2012.

[19] W. Delacruz, R. Setlik, A. Hassantoufighi et al., "Novel brentuximab vedotin combination therapies show promising activity in highly refractory CD30+ non-Hodgkin lymphoma: a case series and review of the literature," *Case Reports in Oncological Medicine*, vol. 2016, Article ID 2596423, 7 pages, 2016.

[20] E. V. George, J. Pharm, C. Houston et al., "Breast implant-associated ALK-negative anaplastic large cell lymphoma: a case report and discussion of possible pathogenesis," *International Journal of Clinical and Experimental Pathology*, vol. 6, no. 8, pp. 1631–1642, 2013.

[21] X. Chen, L. A. Soma, and J. R. Fromm, "Targeted therapy for Hodgkin lymphoma and systemic anaplastic large cell lymphoma: focus on brentuximab vedotin," *Onco Targets and Therapy*, vol. 7, pp. 45–56, 2014.

[22] R. Chen, J. Hou, E. Newman et al., "CD30 downregulation, MMAE resistance, and MDR1 upregulation are all associated with resistance to brentuximab vedotin," *Molecular Cancer Therapeutics*, vol. 14, no. 6, pp. 1376–1384, 2015.

[23] K. Z. Oregel, E. Everett, X. Zhang, and G. Nagaraj, "Complete response in a critically ill patient with ALK-negative anaplastic large cell lymphoma treated with single agent brentuximab-vedotin," *Expert Review of Anticancer Therapy*, vol. 16, no. 3, pp. 279–283, 2016.

[24] M. A. Fanale, S. M. Horwitz, A. Forero-Torres et al., "Brentuximab vedotin in the front- line treatment of patients with CD30+ peripheral t-cell lymphomas: results of a phase I study," *Journal of Clinical Oncology*, vol. 32, no. 28, pp. 3137–3143, 2014.

[25] D. Laimer, H. Dolznig, K. Kollmann et al., "PDGFR blockade is a rational and effective therapy for NPM-ALK-driven lymphomas," *Nature Medicine*, vol. 18, no. 11, pp. 1699–1704, 2012.

[26] http://www.agmt.at/files/AGMT_ALCL1_OeGHO_2017_web.pdf.

41

Malignant Phyllodes Tumor of the Breast with Metastasis to the Pancreas

R. A. Amir,[1] Rola S. Rabah,[2] and S. S. Sheikh[2]

[1]*Imam Abdulrahman Bin Faisal University, Dhahran, Saudi Arabia*
[2]*Pathology Services Division, Johns Hopkins Aramco Healthcare, Dhahran, Saudi Arabia*

Correspondence should be addressed to R. A. Amir; r.a.amir793@gmail.com

Academic Editor: Katsuhiro Tanaka

Phyllodes tumor (PT) is a rare tumor of the breast accounting for approximately 1% of all breast neoplasms. In 1838, J. Muller coined the term "cystosarcoma phyllodes" based on the leaf-like projections of the tumor extending into the cystic spaces and sarcomatous stromal growth. However, seeing as up to 70% of phyllodes tumors are benign, "cystosarcoma" was removed, and the tumor is now recognized simply as phyllodes tumor. It is mainly seen in females between the ages of 35 and 55. Although most phyllodes tumors are benign, malignant cases do uncommonly occur, 22% of which have distant metastasis typically to the lungs and bones. Rarely, this tumor metastasizes to other locations. Herein, we report a case of malignant phyllodes tumor with metastasis to the pancreas. According to our knowledge, only 3 case reports of pancreatic metastasis from malignant phyllodes tumor have been reported in literature thus far. We aim to increase awareness among physicians of this rare metastasic potential of the uncommonly encountered malignant phyllodes tumor.

1. Introduction

Phyllodes tumor is a rare tumor of the breast comprising about 1% of all breast tumors. In 1838, Johannes Muller created the term cystosarcoma phyllodes based on the leaf-like projections extending into cystic spaces and sarcoma-like stroma of the tumor. However, seeing as up to 70% of phyllodes tumors are benign, "cystosarcoma" was removed, and the tumor is now recognized simply as phyllodes tumor. This tumor is mainly seen in females between 35 and 55 years of age. Although the vast majority of phyllodes tumors behave in a benign fashion, there are cases in which these tumors are malignant and have even metastasized. Usually, PTs metastasize to the lungs and bones, rarely will they metastasize to other locations. Herein, we report a case of malignant phyllodes tumor with metastasis to the pancreas. This, according to our knowledge, has only been previously reported in 3 case reports in literature.

2. Case Presentation

A 34-year-old female who has no previous clinical illness presented in 2000 with a large irregular mass, estimated clinically to be around 5×6 cm by physical examination, involving the right breast while she was lactating. There were no other signs or symptoms. FNA was done to rule out breast cancer, and the specimen showed few foamy macrophages and rare clusters of ductal cells, with focal secretory lactational changes. Based on that, it was determined that the specimen was negative for malignancy. The tumor continued to grow, and in June 2004, FNA of the right breast was repeated and showed large staghorn-shaped sheets of uniform ductal cells with no cytologic atypia along with myoepithelial cells. There were fragments of fibrotic stroma and bare nuclei scattered in a bloody background, and so, a diagnosis of fibroadenoma was made. Two months later, the patient underwent excision of the tumor in another

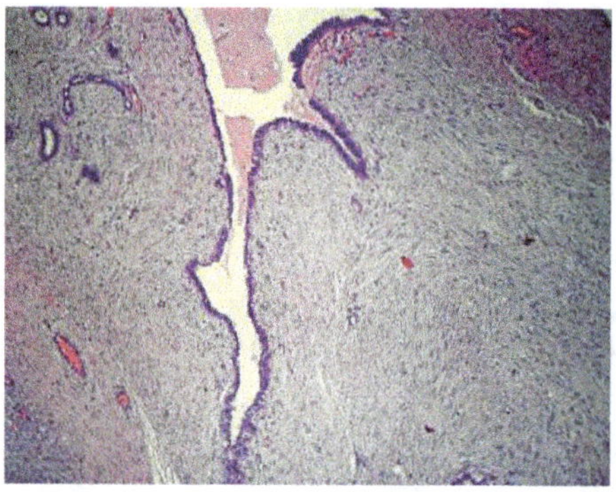

FIGURE 1: Prominent leaf-like pattern of the ducts surrounded by stromal overgrowth.

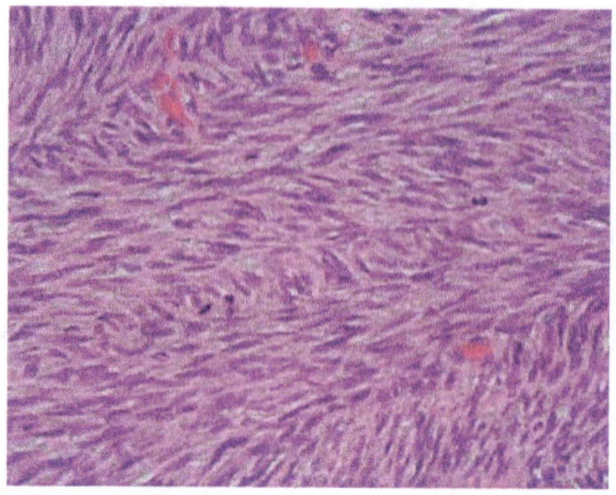

FIGURE 2: Hypercellular stroma with herringbone pattern, marked atypia, increased mitosis, and complete absence of ducts.

healthcare facility. Examination of the slides showed an overgrowth of epithelial and stromal components in pericanalicular and intracanalicular patterns with irregular large cystic spaces showing protruding leaf-like structures (Figure 1). The stromal cells showed plump elongated slightly dysmorphic nuclei with occasional prominent nucleoli. Other areas showed significant cellular growth of the stromal spindle cells which appeared to be arranged in long intersecting fascicles and growing in herringbone pattern (Figure 2). Within the spindle cell growth, extracellular mucin was noted. One focus showed an exclusive spindle cell growth which was moderately atypical with plump elongated hyperchromatic nuclei. Numerous mitosis was found, up to 20 in 10 high power fields in this focus. Entrapped epithelial ductal elements were occasionally seen in other areas exhibiting ductal epithelial hyperplasia. These features were consistent with malignant phyllodes tumor with stromal fibrosarcomatous overgrowth. The patient subsequently underwent mastectomy as the margins were focally involved. During the procedure, a mass measuring around 3-4 cm was found in the most posterior aspect of the breast and there was some indication that it may have invaded the pectoralis major muscle. All the breast tissue, the tumor, and some of the muscle fibers were removed. On gross examination, there were multiple tumor masses in the inner lower and outer upper quadrants, the largest being 3 cm. On microscopy, there was proliferation of atypical spindle and elongated plump cells with pleomorphic nuclei and occasional prominent nucleoli. Extracellular mucin was also identified. The atypical stromal cells formed herringbone fascicular growth pattern reminiscent to fibrosarcoma and numerous mitosis averaging around 14 mitosis in 10 high power fields. No residual phyllodes tumor elements were identified. The tumor nodules had a well-demarcated margin with focal infiltration of surrounding breast and adipose tissue. No lymphovascular invasion, necrosis, or heterologous differentiation was seen. All surgical margins and muscle fibers were not involved by the tumor. The skin and nipple did not show any involvement either. All these histological features were identical to those identified in her previous lumpectomy except that there was more pronounced atypia and no residual epithelial component of phyllodes tumor identified. No lymph nodes were identified. A year later, the patient began to suffer from acute bouts of pancreatitis and was admitted several times for this. In March of 2006, abdominal CT was performed and showed a heterogenous low attenuation soft tissue mass involving the head and body of the pancreas and was extending upwards. The celiac vessels and its branches were going through this mass but did not show any significant narrowing. There was obvious atrophy of the pancreatic tail and dilatation of the pancreatic duct. The mass was in contact with the anterior aspect of the inferior vena cava (IVC) with no clear fat plane in between (Figure 3(a)). Biopsy of the pancreatic mass showed uniform proliferation of elongated spindly cells which had coarse chromatin and mild to moderate nuclear pleomorphism. Some cells had plump hyperchromatic nuclei. Numerous mitotic figures were identified (Figure 4). The background showed variable amounts of collagen and stroma with focal areas of myxoid appearance. Immunohistochemical staining showed strong positivity for vimentin; however, the cells were negative for actin, S100, and cytokeratin (Figure 5). These findings were consistent with metastatic fibrosarcoma of the pancreas secondary to her primary breast lesion. Due to the location, extent, and nature of the condition, the case was deemed unresectable. Chemotherapy was initiated; and in the little chance that the tumor shrunk enough, the possibility of resecting the metastasis would be entertained. In January 2007, the patient presented to the ER with severe epigastric pain, where she collapsed, was hypotensive, and subsequently admitted. On examination, a tender mass in the epigastric area was felt. Urgent CT of the abdomen and pelvis with and without contrast showed a pseudoaneurysm in the splenic artery measuring around 3.5 cm. There was also expansion of the retroperitoneal mass and blood in the intraperitoneal cavity. There was heterogenous enhancement in the liver most probably indicating liver infarct. In addition, there were areas of the IVC which had markedly thinned wall and areas suspicious for active bleeding, especially from the proximal splenic artery (Figure 3(b)). The pancreatic fibrosarcoma had grown and eroded branches of the celiac artery with bleeding pseudoaneurysm along with infarct of the liver, spleen, and adjacent organs. The patient continued to be hypotensive with abdominal distention due to severe intra-abdominal bleeding and developed multiorgan failure and hemorrhagic shock leading to her death.

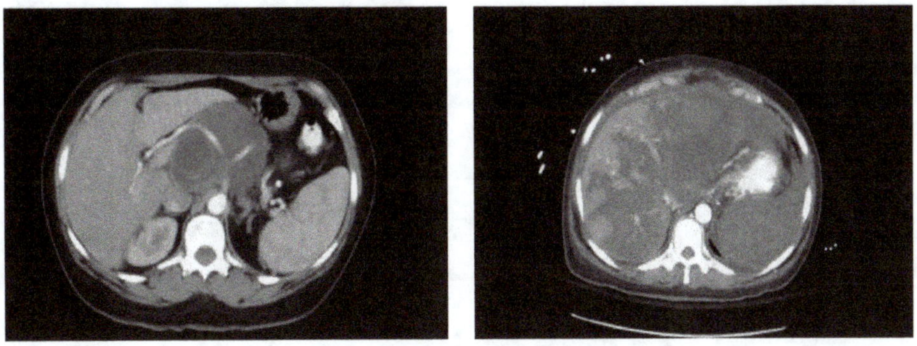

(a) (b)

FIGURE 3: Abdominal CT scan showing (a) pancreatic mass involving the head of the pancreas, surrounding the celiac artery, in contact with the anterior aspect of the inferior vena cava, and (b) greatly enlarged pancreatic mass, extravasation of contrast from proximal splenic artery, and multiple heterogenous enhancements of the liver most likely indicating liver infarcts.

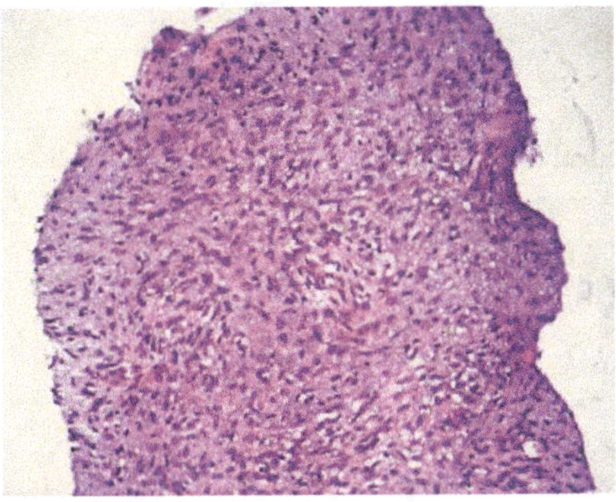

FIGURE 4: Spindle cell proliferation with focal herringbone pattern, cellular atypia, and increased mitosis.

3. Discussion

PTs are benign breast tumors found predominantly in females between the ages 35 and 55 (median 45). The incidence is higher in Caucasians and is highest in Latino women [1]. Few cases of PTs have been reported during pregnancy. In general, these tumors are unilateral and unifocal, but can occasionally present as bilateral and multifocal. In the case series done by Barrio et al., only 3.4% of the 293 cases studied were bilateral PTs while the majority was unilateral [2].

Clinically, the tumor often presents as a well-circumscribed oval painless mobile lump in the breast. It has a biphasic growth pattern: the initial phase of slow growth followed by the second phase of rapidly accelerating growth over a period of weeks to months. It may be associated with changes of overlying skin including atrophy, skin thinning, bloody nipple discharge, or nipple retraction if the areolar region is involved. The mean size of PTs is around 4-5 cm, but cases of PTs up to 40 cm in size have been reported in literature [3]. The larger the tumor the more likely it is to be malignant.

On mammography and ultrasound, PTs lack distinguishing characteristics, and, thus, findings are not specific [4]. Preoperative diagnosis of PTs is extremely difficult as the only imaging findings suggestive of PTs are the rapid growth rate and/or very large size of what looks like a fibroadenoma. On mammography, PTs are seen as well-circumscribed round or oval-shaped lobulated masses which on occasion could contain some calcifications [5, 6]. On sonography, they appear as well-defined solid masses with heterogenous internal echos, with no posterior acoustic attenuation [7]. If a solid mass containing clefts or elongated fluid-filled spaces is seen on sonography, PT should be considered. With the abovementioned imaging techniques, it is difficult to distinguish a fibroadenoma from a PT, and it is impossible to differentiate a benign from a malignant PT. The full extent of the tumor and metastatic sites can be delineated using magnetic resonance imaging prior to surgical excision.

Histologically, PTs are biphasic fibroepithelial tumors consisting of epithelial and stromal elements. The epithelial ducts are organized in cleft-like and cystic structures surrounded by stroma arranged in leaf-like pattern. The stromal component has various histological appearances. Generally speaking, benign PTs' stroma shows regular fusiform fibroblasts, while the stroma of malignant PTs usually shows high cellular atypia, increased stromal cellularity, and increased mitotic count. On occasion, degenerative changes can be seen including bleeding, cystic degeneration, and necrosis [8].

Since 2003, PTs have been classified by the WHO into three main categories: benign, borderline, and malignant, based on various histological findings. These features include margin characteristics (permeative versus circumscribed), mitotic activity, degree of cellular atypia, stromal cellularity, and stromal overgrowth (proliferation of stroma in relation to the glandular component with the presence of stroma and no epithelium in at least one 40 power fields) [9]. Benign PTs are well circumscribed with an increase in stromal cellularity, mild to moderate atypia, mitosis $< 4/10$ hpfs, and no signs of stromal overgrowth. Borderline PTs have an even larger increase in stromal cellularity and atypia, mitosis of 4-9/10 hpfs, but no stromal overgrowth. Malignant PTs on the other hand present with permeative margins, significant increase in both stromal cellularity and atypia, mitotic count of 10/10 hpfs, and signs of stromal overgrowth as opposed to the previous two categories [10]. In a review of 19 series of PTs, 35–85% were categorized as benign, 7–40% borderline, and 7–45% malignant showing variable incidence reporting [11].

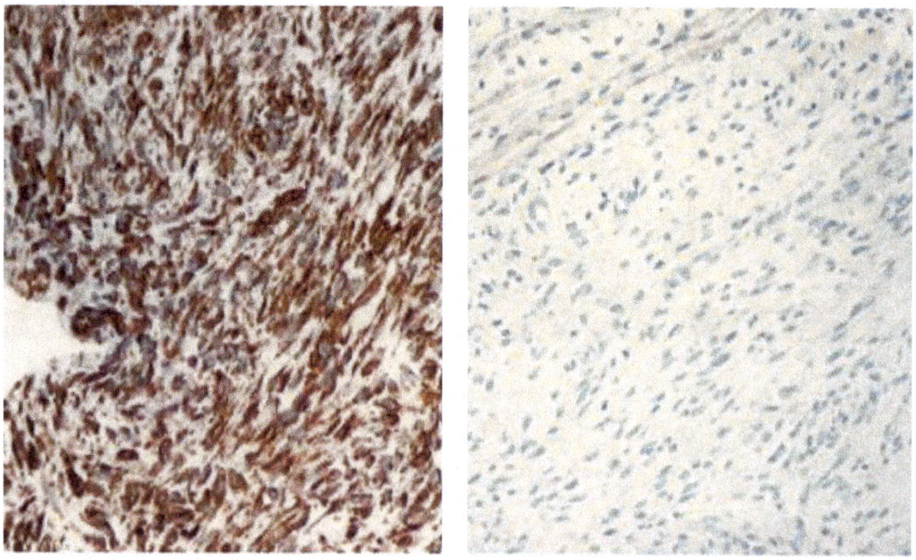

(a) (b)

FIGURE 5: Immunohistochemistry staining showing (a) neoplastic cells strongly positive for vimentin and (b) malignant cells negative for cytokeratin, actin, and s100.

Metastasis of the PTs is seen in 5–20% of all patients with PTs [12]. The timing of metastasis appearance has been studied in multiple publication and ranged from as little as 1 month after primary therapy to as long as a decade posttreatment with an average of around 15 to 26 months. Most patients with metastasis die within 3 years of primary diagnosis [13]. It is important to note that a defining factor in the occurrence of metastasis is the primary tumor size [14].

Malignant PTs tend to metastasize hematogenously with lymph node metastasis seen only rarely. However, in the cases of malignant PT, axillary lymph nodes must be dissected. The main site of metastasis is the lungs (66–84.5%) followed by bones (28–39%) and less commonly the liver and brain. Other reported sites of metastasis include the skin, nasal and oral cavity, salivary gland, larynx, thyroid gland, pleura, heart, kidneys, adrenal glands, stomach, small and large intestine, spleen, and pancreas.

In our case, the patient had metastasis only to the pancreas. Metastasis of PT to the pancreas is uncommon with frequency of secondary pancreatic tumors varying between 3% and 12% of all pancreatic malignancies. Clinical symptoms of pancreatic metastasis are similar to primary pancreatic tumors. Often the patient presents with jaundice, abdominal or back pain, weight loss, poor appetite, nausea, vomiting, pale greasy stool, hypercoagulability (e.g., DVT), abnormalities and unevenness of fatty tissue due to fat necrosis, or diabetes. The most common primary tumors to give rise to metastasis to pancreas are carcinoma of lung, breast, gastrointestinal tract, prostate, and kidney. Less commonly metastasis from soft tissue sarcomas to the pancreas has been reported. As for phyllodes tumor metastasizing to the pancreas, there are only three previous case reports to date in literature indicating its rarity.

Disclosure

This case has previously been presented in the "3rd Euro-Global Experts Meeting on Medical Case Reports" in Spain, in July 2016.

References

[1] M. Reinfuss, J. Mituś, K. Duda, A. Stelmach, J. Ryś, and K. Smolak, "The treatment and prognosis of patients with phyllodes tumor of the breast: an analysis of 170 cases," *Cancer*, vol. 77, no. 5, pp. 910–916, 1996.

[2] A. V. Barrio, B. D. Clark, J. I. Goldberg et al., "Clinicopathologic features and long-term outcomes of 293 phyllodes tumors of the breast," *Annals of Surgical Oncology*, vol. 14, no. 10, pp. 2961–2970, 2007.

[3] R. Khajotia, S. Poovaneswaran, T. Pavadai, S. Sabaratnam, and H. Khairan, "Unusually large breast tumour in a middle-aged woman," *Canadian Family Physician*, vol. 60, no. 2, pp. 142–146, 2014.

[4] O. H. Lifshitz, G. J. Whitman, A. A. Sahin, and W. T. Yang, "Radiologic—pathologic conferences of the University of Texas M. D. Anderson Cancer Center. Phyllodes tumor of the breast," *American Journal of Roentgenology*, vol. 180, no. 2, p. 332, 2003.

[5] S. J. Parker and S. A. Harries, "Phyllodes tumours," *Postgraduate Medical Journal*, vol. 77, no. 909, pp. 428–435, 2001.

[6] D. M. Farria, D. P. Gorczyca, S. H. Barsky, S. Sinha, and L. W. Bassett, "Benign phyllodes tumor of the breast: MR imaging features," *American Journal of Roentgenology*, vol. 167, no. 1, pp. 187–189, 1996.

[7] S. Abdelkrim, A. Trabelsi, M. Bouzrara, M. Boudagga, D. Bakir, and M. Mokni, "Phyllodes tumors of the breast: a review of 26 cases," *World Journal of Oncology*, vol. 1, no. 3, pp. 129–134, 2010.

[8] B. Kraemer, J. Hoffmann, C. Roehm, C. Gall, D. Wallwiener, and U. Krainick-Strobel, "Cystosarcoma phyllodes of the breast: a rare diagnosis: case studies and review of literature," *Archives of Gynecology and Obstetrics*, vol. 276, no. 6, pp. 649–653, 2007.

[9] C. J. C. Moffat, S. E. Pinder, A. R. Dixon, C. W. Elston, R. W. Blamey, and I. O. Ellis, "Phyllodes tumours of the breast: a clinicopathological review of thirty-two cases," *Histopathology*, vol. 27, no. 3, pp. 205–218, 1995.

[10] C. Atalay, V. Kinas, and S. Celebioglu, "Analysis of patients with phyllodes tumor of the breast," *Turkish Journal of Surgery*, vol. 30, no. 3, pp. 129–132, 2014.

[11] R. Z. Karim, S. K. Gerega, Y. H. Yang et al., "Phyllodes tumours of the breast: a clinicopathological analysis of 65 cases from a single institution," *The Breast*, vol. 18, no. 3, pp. 165–170, 2009.

[12] B. C. B. C. Karczmarek-Borowska, A. Bukala, K. Syrek-Kaplita, M. Ksiazek, J. Filipowska, and M. Gradalska-Lampart, "A rare case of breast malignant phyllodes tumor with metastases to the kidney," *Medicine*, vol. 94, no. 33, article e1312, 2015.

[13] H. L. Brooks, S. Priolo, J. Waxman, and W. F. Pizzi, "Cystosarcoma phyllodes: a case report of an 11-year survival and review of surgical experience," *Contemporary Surgery*, vol. 53, p. 169, 1998.

[14] S. P. Mishra, S. K. Tiwary, M. Mishra, and A. K. Khanna, "Phyllodes tumor of breast: a review article," *ISRN Surgery*, vol. 2013, Article ID 361469, 10 pages, 2013.

42

Extramedullary Plasmacytoma Mimicking Pancreatic Cancer: An Unusual Presentation

Daniela Sciancalepore,[1] Sergio Musci,[2] Maria Rosaria Fracella,[3] Grazia D'Alesio,[3] Azzurra Sportelli,[1] Giuseppe Ingravallo,[4] Angelo Vacca,[1] and Roberto Ria[1]

[1] *Department of Biomedical Sciences and Human Oncology, Section of Internal Medicine and Clinical Oncology, University of Bari, Bari, Italy*
[2] *Cardiology Unit, San Paolo Hospital, Contrada Caposcardicchio, Bari, Italy*
[3] *Radiology Unit, San Paolo Hospital, Contrada Caposcardicchio, Bari, Italy*
[4] *Department of Pathology, University of Bari, Bari, Italy*

Correspondence should be addressed to Roberto Ria; roberto.ria@uniba.it

Academic Editor: Jose I. Mayordomo

Multiple myeloma is a plasma cell tumor that homes to and expands in the bone marrow and that, despite the new available drugs, remains incurable. Extramedullary plasmacytoma is a not frequent manifestation during the natural history of multiple myeloma and is frequently associated with plasma cell bone marrow infiltration. The most common locations for an EMP include the gastrointestinal tract, pleura, testis, skin, peritoneum, liver, endocrine glands, and lymph nodes. Primary involvement of the gallbladder fossa is exceedingly rare. In this report, we describe a patient with multiple myeloma who achieved a clinical and serological remission after autologous transplant but progressed rapidly at extramedullary site mimicking a second cancer (i.e., pancreatic or biliary cancer). In this case, the extramedullary localization was refractory to standard therapy, differently from bone marrow localization, but responded to lymphoma-like therapy. In this patient (i) the particular site of developing plasmacytoma is the gallbladder fossa, (ii) the timing of onset of this neoplasm is immediately after autologous transplant, and (iii) its disjunction from primary myeloma is that it appears in clinical and serological remission phase which may be confounding during the diagnostic approach simulating a different tumor (solid tumor).

1. Introduction

Extramedullary plasmacytomas (EMP) represent a rare manifestation in the course of multiple myeloma (MM) [1]. During the last years, however, their incidence has increased predominately in patients who undergo bone marrow transplantation due to the selection of resistant clones after intensified therapy [1] and in patients who receive thalidomide-containing regimens, probably due to dedifferentiation of bone marrow plasma cells or alterations in the expression of adhesion molecules [2].

Moreover, extramedullary progression of MM has consistently been associated with a poorer disease prognosis [3]. This poorer prognosis is not clearly related to the type or intensity of prior treatments and cannot always be explained by occurrence of this progression in very advanced disease stages. There is increasing evidence that extramedullary relapse is associated with secondary changes in the myeloma clone, aggressive disease progression, poor prognostic histological and biological factors (plasmablastic morphology, higher proliferative index, and p53 expression), and treatment resistance [4, 5].

It has also been reported that extramedullary progression or relapse is often associated with the "escape" phenomenon of the monoclonal component [6].

2. Case Presentation

A 62-year-old man had come to our observation in December 2013 because of the onset of a monoclonal component (MC)

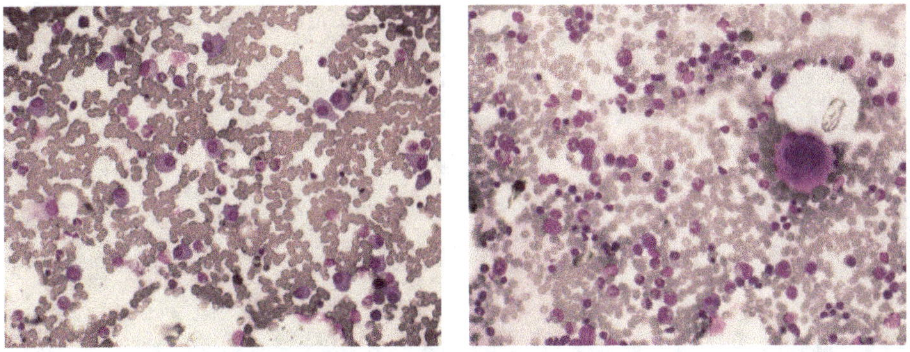

(a) (b)

FIGURE 1: (a) May-Grunwald-Giemsa stain of bone marrow aspirate at diagnosis showing infiltrate of atypical plasma cells and (b) May-Grunwald-Giemsa stain after ASCT at VGPR showing reduction of the infiltration.

of about 51 gr/L typing as IgG-k at immunofixation in absence of anamnestic evidence of hematologic and extrahematologic diseases. Blood tests were normal: Hb 131 g/L, platelets 176000/μL, and leucocytes 5400/μL. Leucocyte differential count, calcium, and LDH serum level were normal. β2-Microglobulin was 4.47 mg/L; albumin was 37 g/L; k/λ free light chain ratio was 29.03. No Bence Jones proteinuria was detected. Bone marrow plasma cell infiltration was 38% (Figure 1(a)). Skeleton X-rays and spine MRI did not visualise osteolyses. The physical examination was negative for objective evidence of disease but the patient complains of vertigo, unsteadiness in walking, muscle pain, paresthesias. The fundus oculi examination showed papilloedema. Patient was diagnosed as "*symptomatic multiple myeloma IgG-k D&S IIA, ISS 2 with hyperviscosity syndrome*" and has undergone first-line therapy consisting of induction therapy with bortezomib, thalidomide, and dexamethasone (VTD) per 4 cycles, stem cell mobilization with cyclophosphamide 4 gr/m^2 and G-CSF, and autologous stem cell transplant (ASCT) with melphalan 200 mg/m^2. At the evaluation of response after ASCT the patient achieved a very good partial response (VGPR); patient refused the second ASCT and consolidation therapy was started with the VTD schema.

In November 2014, after the first consolidation cycle, patient developed fever, mild abdominal pain, and jaundice. The new evaluation of myeloma showed persistence of response with MC of 3 gr/L, Hb 12 g/L, platelets 195000/μL, and leucocytes 8140/μL. Leucocyte differential count, β2-microglobulin, calcium, and LDH serum level were normal. Albumin was 30 g/L and k/λ free light chain ratio was 4.41, with 2% bone marrow plasma cell infiltration (Figure 1(b)) and absence of Bence Jones proteinuria as well as osteolyses at skeleton X-rays and spine MRI. Total bilirubin was of 11.9 mg/dL and direct bilirubin was of 10.03 mg/dL. Gamma-glutamyl transferase was of 892 U/L, alkaline phosphatase was of 405 U/L, alanine aminotransferase was of 51 U/L, aspartate aminotransferase was of 119 U/L, pancreatic amylase was of 130 U/L, lipase was of 2675 U/L, and CA19.9 was of 996.9 U/mL.

MR cholangiopancreatography showed a tumor mass localized at the hepatic hilum without cleavage plane with the head of the pancreas and blood vessels of about 8.35 × 8.7 × 8.9 cm (Figures 2(a) and 2(b)). The site of tumor mass and its occurrence during the remission phase of myeloma, immediately after autologous transplant, made us think of a second cancer, a solid cancer starting from pancreas or extrahepatic biliary tract, so, for that suspicion, the patient was referred to surgeon for biopsy. Histological examination evidenced massive plasmoblastic localization (Figures 2(c) and 2(d)) that, at immunohistochemical staining, was positive for kappa light chain, CD138 (Figure 2(e)), and CD79a, with KI67 > 50% (Figure 2(f)). These histological findings are indicative of the selection of a clone resistant to standard myeloma therapy whose behaviour is similar to an aggressive lymphoma that quickly affected extramedullary tissues.

During the diagnostic period, since the patient had discontinued the specific therapy for myeloma for about one month, it has highlighted also a serological progression of disease with increase of the MC to 24 g/L, decrease of Hb (100 g/L) and albumin (17 g/L), alteration of k/λ free light chain ratio (34.12), and increase of bone marrow plasma cell infiltration to 30%.

Final diagnosis was "multiple myeloma progression with associated extramedullary plasmocytoma" and the patient underwent new therapy with bendamustine, prednisone, and lenalidomide (BPR) in December 2014.

The evaluation after eight cycles of BPR (August/September 2015) showed a new serological response of the disease (CM: 13 g/L, Hb 119 g/L, albumin 34 g/L, normal free light chain ratio, and clonal bone marrow plasma cells 3%) but progression of extramedullary disease because of the increase of the dimension of the primary plasmocytoma (Figures 3(a) and 3(b)) and because of the appearance of new lesions in the liver (Figures 3(c) and 3(d)), at peritoneum and subcutaneous level.

Patient underwent salvage therapy with D-PACE (dexamethasone, cis-platinum, adriamycin, cyclophosphamide, and etoposide) and after two cycles of therapy (February 2016) obtained a good serological disease response and regression of extramedullary plasmacytoma. From March 2016 patient underwent continuous treatment with pomalidomide and dexamethasone.

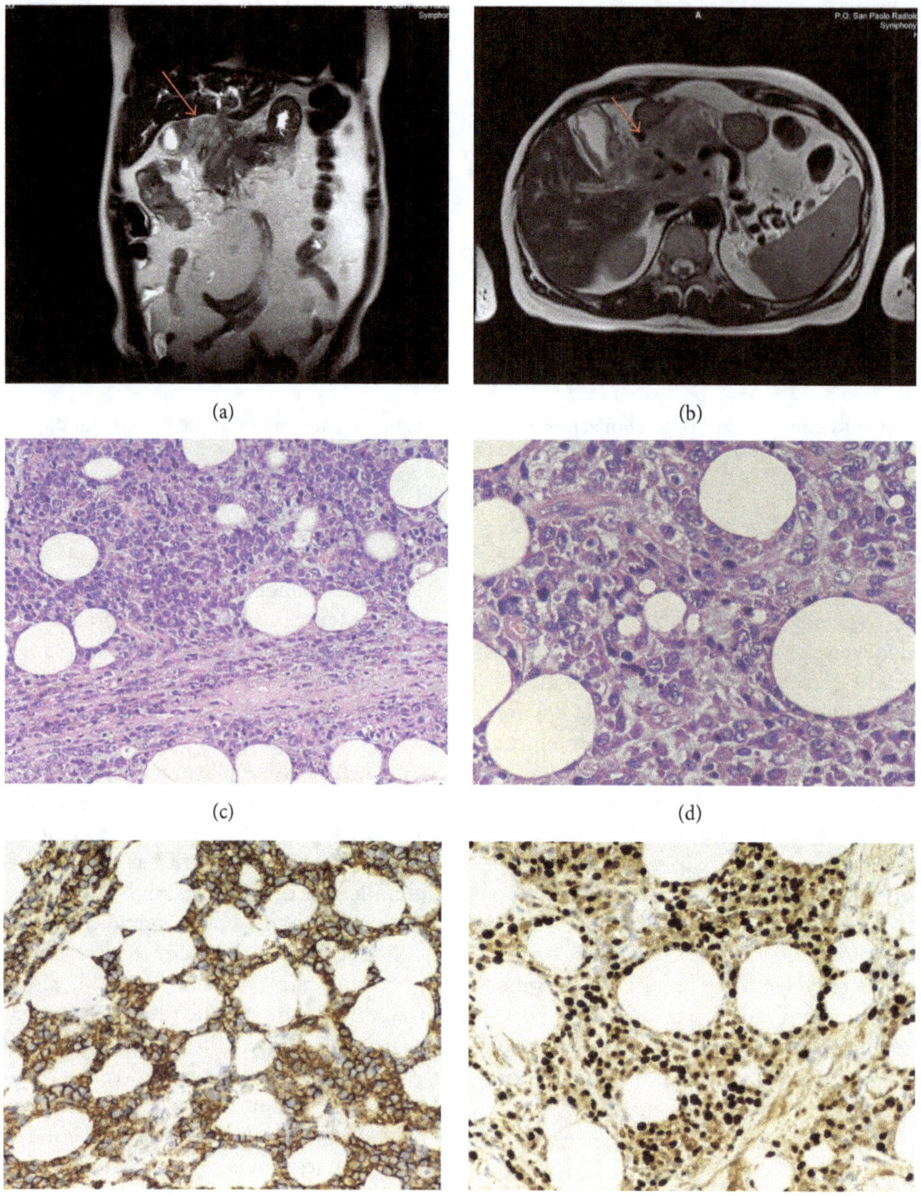

(a) (b) (c) (d) (e) (f)

FIGURE 2: MR cholangiopancreatography before VBD therapy. (a) and (b) show a tumor mass localized at the hepatic hilum without cleavage plane with the head of the pancreas and blood vessels of about 8.35 × 8.7 × 8.9 cm. ((c) and (d)) Hematoxylin and eosin stain. Original magnification ×100 and ×200. The myeloma cell size and nucleus are polymorphic. Many cells have large eccentric nuclei, prominent nucleoli, and abundant basophilic cytoplasm (i.e., nuclear and cytoplasmic maturation asynchrony). (e) The neoplastic cells are positive for CD138. (f) The ki67 labeling index exceeds 50%.

3. Discussion

The clonal evolution theory has been refined to include the concepts of cancer stem cell and intermediate subclones with cancer stemness properties, the importance of genomic instability, the role of epigenetics, and the impact of cancer microenvironment on clonal selection [7, 8]. In fact, the Darwinian behavioural characteristics of cancer stem cells are applicable to MM. Following its initiation, the myeloma propagating cell, which should be considered as the unit of evolutionary selection in Darwinian terms [9], becomes heterogeneous, allowing the transition from a normal plasma cell to the final stage of the transformation process, plasma cell leukaemia (PCL) or extramedullary myeloma [7]. MM cells presented with a significant number of karyotypic aberrations, suggesting that genomic instability plays a major role in MM clonal heterogeneity and evolution [10].

Moreover, growing evidence supports a pivotal role of the microenvironment in guiding clonal evolution and heterogeneity in MM [11, 12]. MM cells and mesenchymal/stromal cells spatially interact via adhesion molecules, communicate

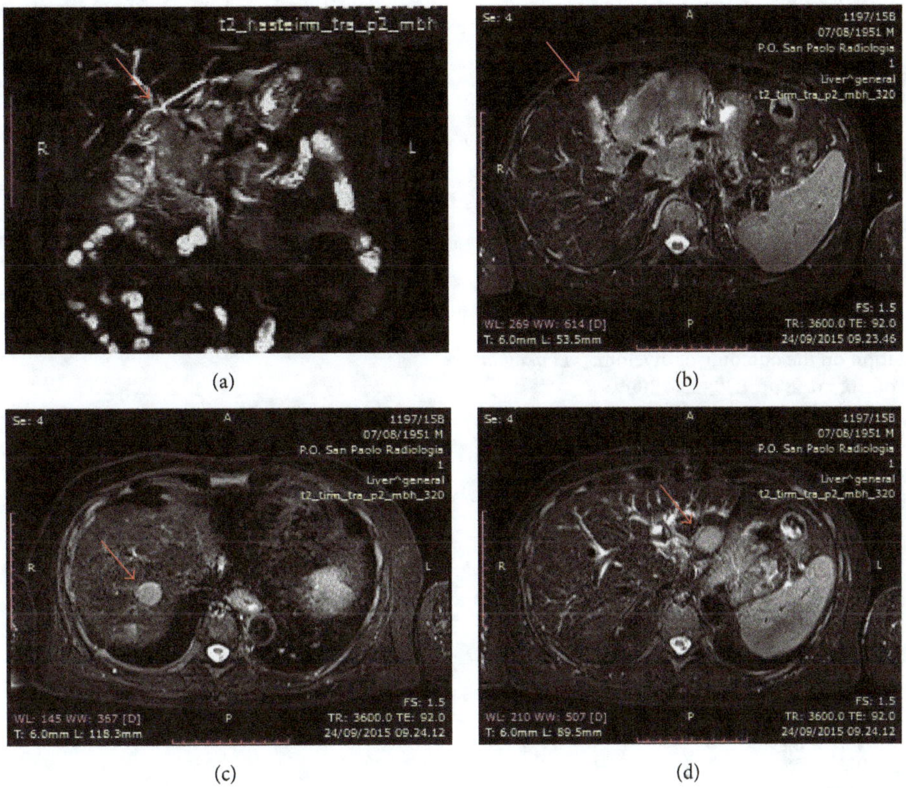

FIGURE 3: MR cholangiopancreatography after VBD therapy. Panels (a) and (b) show progression of extramedullary disease in the primary site (increase of dimension) and panels (c) and (d) show the appearance of new lesions in the liver.

by cytokines and growth factors, and exchange macromolecules such as nucleic acid and proteins via microvesicles and exosomes with subsequent bidirectional signalling, typically resulting in a survival advantage for MM cells [13–15]. Finally, clinical and biological findings indicate that the disappearance and dominance of different clones in MM patient appeared to be determined also by selective pressure from treatment [16].

Our case is indicative of the selection of almost two different clones in this patient with different biological and clinical behaviour. The different response to therapy of medullary and extramedullary disease indicate that, immediately after ASCT, under the pressure of therapy, an aggressive and refractory clone has been selected. This clone, resistant to new drugs, rapidly spread at extramedullary sites and progressed under proteasome inhibitors and immunomodulatory therapy. Only an aggressive treatment induced a response of both clones with remission of bone marrow disease and extramedullary spread.

The knowledge that intraclonal heterogeneity is an important feature of MM biology has changed our way of addressing cancer, now considered as a composite mixture of clones and not as a linear evolving disease. In this variable therapeutic landscape, it is of primary importance for clinicians and researchers to consider the impact that evolutionary biology and intraclonal heterogeneity have on the treatment of myeloma and the emergence of resistance clones. Only by doing so will we be able to effectively use all of the new tools we have at our disposal to cure myeloma and to use treatment in the most effective way possible. All this evidence provides a strong biologic rationale for using combinatory chemotherapy in an attempt to eradicate all clones and avoid selection of aggressive ones.

Authors' Contributions

Roberto Ria prepared the draft and Daniela Sciancalepore, Sergio Musci, Maria Rosaria Fracella, Grazia D'Alesio, Azzurra Sportelli, Giuseppe Ingravallo, Angelo Vacca, and Roberto Ria contributed to the care of patient and all reviewed and contributed to the final manuscript.

Acknowledgments

This work was supported by the Italian Association for Cancer Research (AIRC, Milan), Investigator Grant 2013 (no. 14095) and the 5 per thousand Molecular Clinical Oncology Special Program (Grant no. 9965 to Angelo Vacca), and Grants from MIUR PRIN 2009WCNS5C_004 (to Roberto Ria) and 2010NECHBX (to Angelo Vacca).

References

[1] A. Alegre, A. Granda, C. Martínez-Chamorro et al., "Different patterns of relapse after autologous peripheral blood stem cell transplantation in multiple myeloma: clinical results of 280 cases from the Spanish Registry," *Haematologica*, vol. 87, no. 6, pp. 609–614, 2002.

[2] E. Balleari, R. Ghio, A. Falcone, and P. Musto, "Possible multiple myeloma dedifferentiation following thalidomide therapy: a report of four cases," *Leukemia and Lymphoma*, vol. 45, no. 4, pp. 735–738, 2004.

[3] P. Wu, F. E. Davies, K. Boyd et al., "The impact of extramedullary disease at presentation on the outcome of myeloma," *Leukemia and Lymphoma*, vol. 50, no. 2, pp. 230–235, 2009.

[4] E. Katodritou, V. Gastari, E. Verrou et al., "Extramedullary (EMP) relapse in unusual locations in multiple myeloma: is there an association with precedent thalidomide administration and a correlation of special biological features with treatment and outcome?" *Leukemia Research*, vol. 33, no. 8, pp. 1137–1140, 2009.

[5] N. Sheth, J. Yeung, and H. Chang, "p53 nuclear accumulation is associated with extramedullary progression of multiple myeloma," *Leukemia Research*, vol. 33, no. 10, pp. 1357–1360, 2009.

[6] M. A. Dawson, S. Patil, and A. Spencer, "Extramedullary relapse of multiple myeloma associated with a shift in secretion from intact immunoglobulin to light chains," *Haematologica*, vol. 92, no. 1, pp. 143–144, 2007.

[7] M. Greaves and C. C. Maley, "Clonal evolution in cancer," *Nature*, vol. 481, no. 7381, pp. 306–313, 2012.

[8] R. A. Burrell, N. McGranahan, J. Bartek, and C. Swanton, "The causes and consequences of genetic heterogeneity in cancer evolution," *Nature*, vol. 501, no. 7467, pp. 338–345, 2013.

[9] G. J. Morgan, B. A. Walker, and F. E. Davies, "The genetic architecture of multiple myeloma," *Nature Reviews Cancer*, vol. 12, no. 5, pp. 335–348, 2012.

[10] S. B. Baylin and P. A. Jones, "A decade of exploring the cancer epigenome—biological and translational implications," *Nature Reviews Cancer*, vol. 11, no. 10, pp. 726–734, 2011.

[11] D. F. Quail and J. A. Joyce, "Microenvironmental regulation of tumor progression and metastasis," *Nature Medicine*, vol. 19, no. 11, pp. 1423–1437, 2013.

[12] T. Hideshima, C. Mitsiades, G. Tonon, P. G. Richardson, and K. C. Anderson, "Understanding multiple myeloma pathogenesis in the bone marrow to identify new therapeutic targets," *Nature Reviews Cancer*, vol. 7, no. 8, pp. 585–598, 2007.

[13] G. Camussi, M. C. Deregibus, and C. Tetta, "Tumor-derived microvesicles and the cancer microenvironment," *Current Molecular Medicine*, vol. 13, no. 1, pp. 58–67, 2013.

[14] V. R. Martins, M. S. Dias, and P. Hainaut, "Tumor-cell-derived microvesicles as carriers of molecular information in cancer," *Current Opinion in Oncology*, vol. 25, no. 1, pp. 66–75, 2013.

[15] C. Yang and P. D. Robbins, "The roles of tumor-derived exosomes in cancer pathogenesis," *Clinical and Developmental Immunology*, vol. 2011, Article ID 842849, 11 pages, 2011.

[16] J. J. Keats, M. Chesi, J. B. Egan et al., "Clonal competition with alternating dominance in multiple myeloma," *Blood*, vol. 120, no. 5, pp. 1067–1076, 2012.

43

A Case of Lenvatinib-Induced Focal Segmental Glomerulosclerosis (FSGS) in Metastatic Medullary Thyroid Cancer

Kathryn Fleming,[1] James McGuinness,[1] David Kipgen,[2] Hilary Glen,[1] and Pavlina Spiliopoulou[1,3]

[1]*Beatson West of Scotland Cancer Centre (BWoSCC), Glasgow, UK*
[2]*Queen Elizabeth University Hospital, Glasgow, UK*
[3]*Imperial College London, Hammersmith Hospital, London, UK*

Correspondence should be addressed to Pavlina Spiliopoulou; p.spiliopoulou@imperial.ac.uk

Academic Editor: Raffaele Palmirotta

We describe a case of lenvatinib (E7080) associated focal segmental glomerulosclerosis (FSGS) encountered during the treatment of metastatic medullary thyroid cancer. Proteinuria is a relatively common side effect of VEGF-targeted treatments and can occasionally result in treatment discontinuation. Here, we describe a patient who developed secondary FSGS necessitating discontinuation of treatment at first but who was subsequently rechallenged with anti-VEGF-targeted treatment without recurrence of proteinuria. Lenvatinib was a novel experimental agent at the time the treatment took place; however, its recent licensing for the treatment of thyroid malignancies in the UK makes reporting of these adverse effects all the more important now.

1. Introduction

Angiogenesis is an imperative process for the survival and growth of cancer cells with the most important mediator of angiogenesis being vascular-endothelial growth factor (VEGF) and its associated downstream effectors—VEGF receptors (VEGFRs). These can normally be found on the surface of endothelial cells and endothelial cell precursors, fibroblasts, and macrophages as well as renal epithelial cells such as podocytes [1–3].

VEGF is produced in large amounts by the glomerular podocyte and guides endothelial cells in the developing kidney. Moreover, in adult life, VEGF maintains integrity of the glomerular filtration barrier [4–7]. VEGF/VEGFR axis can be therapeutically targeted either with antibodies aimed at the soluble extracellular ligands or with small molecule inhibitors (tyrosine kinase inhibitors, TKIs) which block the intracellular domains of VEGFRs. Bevacizumab, a humanized monoclonal antibody against VEGF-A is approved for use in combination with chemotherapy in patients with metastatic colorectal cancer and ovarian cancer [8, 9]. Aflibercept (a recombinant fusion protein that blocks the activity of VEGF-A, VEGF-B, and placental growth factor PlGF) has also been approved for use in patients with metastatic colorectal cancer [10]. Small molecule tyrosine kinase inhibitors, pazopanib and sunitinib, are both approved for use as first-line treatment in metastatic renal cell carcinoma and inhibit, amongst others, VEGFR1-3, PDGFRα/β, and the receptor c-KIT [11, 12]. Sorafenib is currently used in advanced hepatocellular carcinoma [13] whereas regorafenib in colorectal and gastrointestinal stromal tumours [14, 15].

2. Case Report

In June 2002, a 36-year-old woman presented to her primary health care doctor with a history of flushing, diarrhoea, night sweats, and a clinically detectable mass in her left medial supraclavicular fossa. Her past medical history consisted only of essential hypertension for which she did not require prescribed therapy. Her family history included a brother with a diagnosis of sarcoma and two other non-first-degree relatives with primary brain malignancies.

Fine needle aspiration confirmed the diagnosis of medullary thyroid cancer, and in July 2002, she underwent total thyroidectomy with left-sided modified radical neck dissection and central compartment clearance. At this point, concerns were raised regarding optimal cytoreduction as the appearances of the central compartment, level 4 and level 5 nodes, were that of extensive disease. In order to maximise local disease control, she received adjuvant radical radiotherapy delivering 60 Gy to the thyroid bed.

Two years after completion of treatment, in February 2004, follow-up repeat imaging reported a recurrent nodule at level 4 of her neck. Subsequent resection confirmed this to be recurrent medullary thyroid cancer with no evidence of distant spread at the time. She continued to be monitored at the oncology clinic and remained disease-free until four years later, in May 2008, when computer tomography (CT) imaging revealed new pulmonary parenchymal metastases. These were closely monitored for the next 2 years with repeat imaging and measurement of calcitonin levels. In May 2010, it was decided that the patient should embark on systemic anticancer treatment.

She was offered participation in a phase 2 clinical trial with the agent lenvatinib (E7080) and she commenced treatment with 24 mg once daily in May 2010. One week into therapy, it was noted that she was marginally hypertensive with a blood pressure of 140/100 mmHg. No proteinuria was identified at this point, but she was commenced on 5 mg of amlodipine to manage hypertension. Monitoring of blood pressure and urinalysis continued as per study protocol.

After two completed cycles of lenvatinib, CT imaging reported a reduction in size of all lesions. Further tumour assessment after 4 months confirmed a partial response to treatment with a 50% reduction of the sum of the long diameters of target lesions. She was experiencing various grade 1 toxicities throughout this time but was keen to maintain treatment given the good response. Due to the multiple low-grade toxicities, the dose of lenvatinib was initially reduced to 20 mg and thereafter to 14 mg.

In December 2011, 19 months after starting lenvatinib, she developed mild ankle oedema. Urinalysis carried out at the time identified proteinuria. A subsequent 24-hour urine collection identified 3.1 g/litre of proteinuria, equating to a urinary protein creatinine ratio (UPCR) of 625. The patient had not started any other medications and the incidence of proteinuria was felt to be lenvatinib related. Treatment with lenvatinib was ceased; however, due to concerns regarding possible intrinsic renal disease, she underwent screening for glomerulonephritis which was negative.

A subsequent renal biopsy showed focal segmental glomerulosclerosis (FSGS) in two of twelve viable glomeruli, with tuft-capsule adhesion, hyalinosis, segmental intracapillary hypercellularity, and segmental splitting of capillary walls, predominantly in regions of segmental sclerosis. There was mild tubular atrophy, interstitial fibrosis, mild/moderate arterial intimal fibroelastic thickening, and mild arteriolosclerosis. Immunofluorescence showed no staining in glomeruli. Electron microscopy showed mild patchy reduplication of the basement membrane and effacement of only 20% of podocyte foot processes. There were no widespread electron dense deposits and no endothelial cell tubule-reticular inclusions. The endothelial cells showed no evidence of activation or damage. The appearances were consistent with a diagnosis of focal segmental glomerulosclerosis (FSGS). The lack of widespread podocyte foot process effacement suggests a secondary form of FSGS, which in the context of anti-VEGF treatment, could be mediated by microangiopathy. Whilst there was no histological evidence of acute thrombotic microangiopathy, it is possible that some of the pathological changes seen (splitting of glomerular capillary walls and mild arteriosclerosis) could be related to chronic low-grade endothelial cell damage. Based on histology, it is not possible to be certain whether the FSGS was caused by direct podocyte injury or whether it was related to endothelial cell injury. Histological slides are illustrated below in Figures 1, 2, and 3.

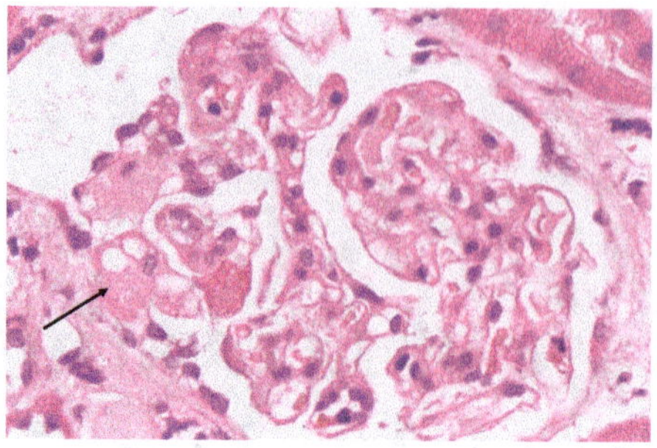

Figure 1: Glomerulus showing segmental sclerosis (arrow). H + E, ×40.

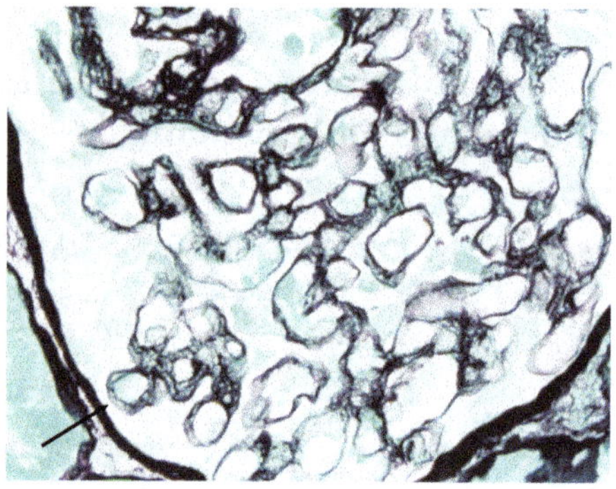

Figure 2: Glomerulus showing segmental splitting of capillary walls (arrow). PA Meth Ag, ×60.

Throughout this time, excretory function remained stable. Treatment with an ACE-inhibitor (ACEi) was introduced but due to poor tolerance and the quick improvement of the proteinuria after cessation of lenvatinib, the ACEi was stopped and patient's blood pressure was monitored closely.

Withdrawal of lenvatinib had a marked effect on the levels of proteinuria, as illustrated in Figure 4.

The patient continued follow-up at the renal clinic on a regular basis until July 2013, when she was discharged with no evidence of proteinuria, normotensive and with normal excretory renal function.

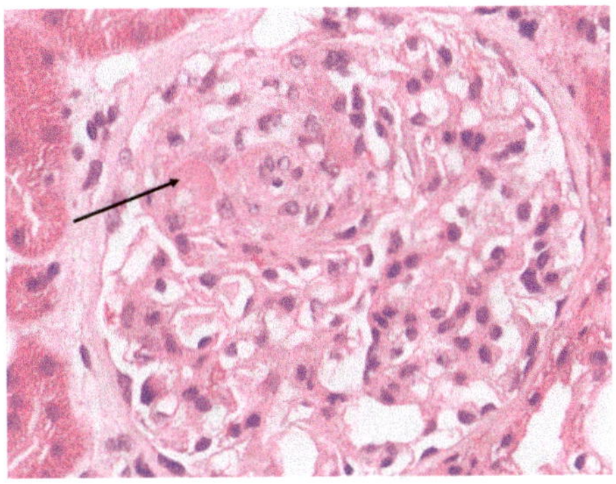

FIGURE 3: Glomerulus showing segmental hyalinosis (arrow). H + E, ×40.

After her discharge from the renal clinic and between 2013 and 2017, the patient was treated with vandetanib, nintedanib, and cabozantinib with no evidence of recurrent renal disease.

2.1. Lenvatinib (E7080). E7080, also known as lenvatinib, is a potent inhibitor of the receptor protein kinases VEGFR-2 and VEGFR-3 but also displays inhibitory binding properties against VGFR-1, FGFR-1, and PDGFRα/β, albeit at significantly higher IC_{50} (half maximal inhibitory concentration, IC_{50}). Its ability to restrain angiogenesis was shown on human umbilical vein endothelial cells (HUVEC) where E7080 inhibited VEGFR-2 phosphorylation and thereby capillary tube formation [16]. Apart from angiogenesis, E7080 decreased lymphangiogenesis in both the primary tumour of human breast adenocarcinoma cells in xenografts as well as in metastatic nodules in the lymph nodes of nude mice bearing these tumours [17]. Glen et al. showed in preclinical experiments that abrogation of FGFR and PDGFR signalling by E7080 inhibited invasion and migration of human melanoma cells lines (DX3) and human osteosarcoma epithelial cells (U2OS) [18]. Its potency against FGFR-1 differentiates E7080 from other currently approved tyrosine kinase inhibitors with antiangiogenesis properties [16, 19].

The preclinical data above were confirmed in several early phase human trials with E7080 in 2011 and 2012 in US, Europe, and Japan. Whilst establishing pharmacokinetic and pharmacodynamic properties of the drug, safety and preliminary efficacy was also well described. Lenvatinib was well tolerated at doses from 10 mg BID to 25 mg OD [20–24] and was associated with a reduction in disease activity biomarkers [23], partial response, and stable disease according to response evaluation criteria in solid tumours [21]. These findings were further established in phase 2 trials and notably responses were demonstrated in thyroid cancer [25–27].

Approval in thyroid cancer was granted in light of significant improvement in progression-free survival (PFS) compared with placebo in patients with radioiodine-refractory differentiated thyroid cancer in a phase 3 study (SELECT study) [28]. Lenvatinib improved median PFS over placebo by almost 15 months (HR 0.21; $p < 0.01$) and induced an objective response rate of 64.8%. The median survival results were diluted due to crossover of the patients from the placebo arm to the treatment arm; nevertheless, a subgroup analysis on patients stratified by age showed that older patients (>71 years old) had a survival advantage when treated with lenvatinib compared to placebo (HR, 0.53; $p = 0.02$), and the younger subgroup achieved a PFS of 20.2 months versus 3.7 m ($p < 0.001$) [29].

2.2. VEGF-Mediated Renal Toxicity. Proteinuria and hypertension are the two most commonly reported side-effects of VEGF inhibitors and frequently the cause for therapy discontinuation. Proteinuria is used as a surrogate marker for glomerular damage and hypertension often accompanies and aggravates this.

The pathophysiology of proteinuria and glomerular damage in anti-VEGF therapy remains complex and far from well understood. Biopsy-proven cases of glomerular disease in anti-VEGF therapy are few; however, most have demonstrated changes in keeping with glomerular thrombotic microangiopathy (TMA) histology, with predominant endotheliosis and membranoproliferative changes [30, 31]. Other histological changes documented include cryoglobulinaemic glomerulonephritis, acute interstitial nephritis, collapsing and crescentic glomerulonephropathies, and FSGS plus TMA [32–35].

It has been theorized that hypertension is caused by decreased vascular production of nitrous oxide induced by inhibiting VEGF. This leads to renal haemodynamic compromise and subsequent proteinuria (much akin to exercise-related proteinuria) [30]. However, a mouse model study showed that glomerular injury preceded hypertension [36] and many cases document glomerular injury in the absence of hypertension [37], indicating that it cannot be the only trigger for proteinuria in anti-VEGF treated patients.

Inhibition of VEGF in podocytes (by injection of anti-VEGF antibodies or VEGF gene deletion) results in loss of endothelial fenestrations in glomerular capillaries, proliferation of glomerular endothelial cells, loss of podocytes, and proteinuria in mice [4, 5]. VEGF appears to be a crucial endothelial survival factor and its inhibition often manifests as TMA, a histology strikingly similar to that of severe preeclampsia—as placenta overproduces a soluble VEGF receptor (fms-like tyrosine kinase 1) that acts as a VEGF antagonist.

Izzedine et al.'s 8-year follow-up study results from 2014 shed great light in anti-VEGF-related renal injury. It showed that in 100 patients who developed renal disease whilst on anti-VEGF treatment, the main histology associated with TKIs was minimal change disease and/or collapsing-like focal segmental glomerulosclerosis (MCN/cFSGS), a FSGC variant which is considered a separate entity to FSGS. In the same analysis, TMA histology was most frequently associated with VEGF-ligand targeted therapy (such as bevacizumab and aflibercept) suggesting two, possibly distinct pathophysiologies [37, 38] between renal damage caused by targeting the VEGF ligand as opposed to targeting the VEGFR tyrosine kinase domain. This could potentially be explained by considering the associations and signal

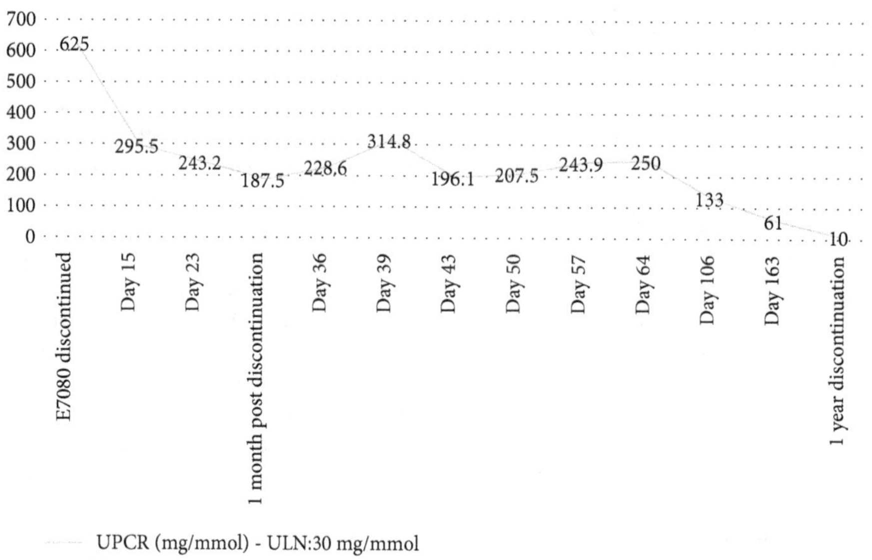

Figure 4: Withdrawal of lenvatinib and subsequent improvement of UPCR.

transduction pathways between podocytes, endothelial cells, and VEGF. Podocytes produce vascular endothelial growth factor (VEGF), whereas VEGF receptor tyrosine kinases (RTKs) are expressed by both podocytes and glomerular endothelial cells.

Our case demonstrates a secondary form of FSGS pathology which cannot confidently be attributed to TMA but could potentially represent the end result of chronic low-grade endothelial cell damage. The moderate histological findings were in keeping with a less-severe clinical course of the FSGS, with fast resolution of proteinuria and hypertension. More significantly, rechallenging the patient with additional three agents blocking the VEGF axis did not result in recurrence of the renal damage.

3. Conclusion

Fortunately, as in our case, cessation of anti-VEGF inhibitors in most cases significantly improves proteinuria and hypertension. In practice, in patients with dipstick detectable proteinuria and BP >130/80, ACE inhibitors are often utilised [30]. In most cases where ACE inhibition fails to control proteinuria, anti-VEGF therapy is ceased. It is interesting to note that a drug holiday followed by reinitiation of anti-VEGF therapy might not result in recurrence of proteinuria [39] which was the experience with our patient. At present, there is unlikely to be any other way of safely continuing anti-VEGF therapy where there is significant proteinuria with or without hypertension (such as immunosuppressive therapy as may be done for other causes of TMA and FSGS). Our understanding of the mechanisms of damage needs to be improved before we can safely continue anti-VEGF treatment in the presence of proteinuria without compromising the prognostic outcome of patients with renal syndromes secondary to anti-VEGF treatment [40, 41].

References

[1] N. Ferrara, H. P. Gerber, and J. LeCouter, "The biology of VEGF and its receptors," *Nature Medicine*, vol. 9, no. 6, pp. 669–676, 2003.

[2] M. H. W. Kappers, J. H. M. van Esch, S. Sleijfer, A. H. J. Danser, and A. H. van den Meiracker, "Cardiovascular and renal toxicity during angiogenesis inhibition: clinical and mechanistic aspects," *Journal of Hypertension*, vol. 27, no. 12, pp. 2297–2309, 2009.

[3] Y. Dor, R. Porat, and E. Keshet, "Vascular endothelial growth factor and vascular adjustments to perturbations in oxygen homeostasis," *American Journal of Physiology. Cell Physiology*, vol. 280, no. 6, pp. C1367–C1374, 2001.

[4] V. Eremina, M. Sood, J. Haigh et al., "Glomerular-specific alterations of VEGF-A expression lead to distinct congenital and acquired renal diseases," *Journal of Clinical Investigation*, vol. 111, no. 5, pp. 707–716, 2003.

[5] H. Sugimoto, Y. Hamano, D. Charytan et al., "Neutralization of circulating vascular endothelial growth factor (VEGF) by anti-VEGF antibodies and soluble VEGF receptor 1 (sFlt-1) induces proteinuria," *The Journal of Biological Chemistry*, vol. 278, no. 15, pp. 12605–12608, 2003.

[6] W. Risau, "Development and differentiation of endothelium," *Kidney International. Supplement*, vol. 67, pp. S3–S6, 1998.

[7] M. J. Karkkainen, T. Makinen, and K. Alitalo, "Lymphatic endothelium: a new frontier of metastasis research," *Nature Cell Biology*, vol. 4, no. 1, pp. E2–E5, 2002.

[8] L. B. Saltz, S. Clarke, E. Díaz-Rubio et al., "Bevacizumab in combination with oxaliplatin-based chemotherapy as first-line therapy in metastatic colorectal cancer: a randomized phase III study," *Journal of Clinical Oncology*, vol. 26, no. 12, pp. 2013–2019, 2008.

[9] A. M. Oza, A. D. Cook, J. Pfisterer et al., "Standard chemotherapy with or without bevacizumab for women with newly diagnosed ovarian cancer (ICON7): overall survival results of a phase 3 randomised trial," *The Lancet Oncology*, vol. 16, no. 8, pp. 928–936, 2015.

[10] E. Van Cutsem, J. Tabernero, R. Lakomy et al., "Addition of aflibercept to fluorouracil, leucovorin, and irinotecan improves survival in a phase III randomized trial in patients with metastatic colorectal cancer previously treated with an oxaliplatin-based regimen," *Journal of Clinical Oncology*, vol. 30, no. 28, pp. 3499–3506, 2012.

[11] C. N. Sternberg, I. D. Davis, J. Mardiak et al., "Pazopanib in locally advanced or metastatic renal cell carcinoma: results of a randomized phase III trial," *Journal of Clinical Oncology*, vol. 28, no. 6, pp. 1061–1068, 2010.

[12] R. J. Motzer, T. E. Hutson, P. Tomczak et al., "Sunitinib versus interferon alfa in metastatic renal-cell carcinoma," *The New England Journal of Medicine*, vol. 356, no. 2, pp. 115–124, 2007.

[13] J. M. Llovet, S. Ricci, V. Mazzaferro et al., "Sorafenib in advanced hepatocellular carcinoma," *The New England Journal of Medicine*, vol. 359, no. 4, pp. 378–390, 2008.

[14] A. Grothey, E. V. Cutsem, A. Sobrero et al., "Regorafenib monotherapy for previously treated metastatic colorectal cancer (CORRECT): an international, multicentre, randomised, placebo-controlled, phase 3 trial," *The Lancet*, vol. 381, no. 9863, pp. 303–312, 2013.

[15] G. D. Demetri, P. Reichardt, Y. K. Kang et al., "Efficacy and safety of regorafenib for advanced gastrointestinal stromal tumours after failure of imatinib and sunitinib (GRID): an international, multicentre, randomised, placebo-controlled, phase 3 trial," *The Lancet*, vol. 381, no. 9863, pp. 295–302, 2013.

[16] J. Matsui, Y. Yamamoto, Y. Funahashi et al., "E7080, a novel inhibitor that targets multiple kinases, has potent antitumor activities against stem cell factor producing human small cell lung cancer H146, based on angiogenesis inhibition," *International Journal of Cancer*, vol. 122, no. 3, pp. 664–671, 2008.

[17] J. Matsui, Y. Funahashi, T. Uenaka, T. Watanabe, A. Tsuruoka, and M. Asada, "Multi-kinase inhibitor E7080 suppresses lymph node and lung metastases of human mammary breast tumor MDA-MB-231 via inhibition of vascular endothelial growth factor-receptor (VEGF-R) 2 and VEGF-R3 kinase," *Clinical Cancer Research*, vol. 14, no. 17, pp. 5459–5465, 2008.

[18] H. Glen, S. Mason, H. Patel, K. Macleod, and V. G. Brunton, "E7080, a multi-targeted tyrosine kinase inhibitor suppresses tumor cell migration and invasion," *BMC Cancer*, vol. 11, no. 1, p. 309, 2011.

[19] M. W. Karaman, S. Herrgard, D. K. Treiber et al., "A quantitative analysis of kinase inhibitor selectivity," *Nature Biotechnology*, vol. 26, no. 1, pp. 127–132, 2008.

[20] S. Nakamichi, H. Nokihara, N. Yamamoto et al., "A phase 1 study of lenvatinib, multiple receptor tyrosine kinase inhibitor, in Japanese patients with advanced solid tumors," *Cancer Chemotherapy and Pharmacology*, vol. 76, no. 6, pp. 1153–1161, 2015.

[21] D. S. Boss, H. Glen, J. H. Beijnen et al., "A phase I study of E7080, a multitargeted tyrosine kinase inhibitor, in patients with advanced solid tumours," *British Journal of Cancer*, vol. 106, no. 10, pp. 1598–1604, 2012.

[22] D. S. Hong, R. Kurzrock, J. J. Wheler et al., "Phase I dose-escalation study of the multikinase inhibitor lenvatinib in patients with advanced solid tumors and in an expanded cohort of patients with melanoma," *Clinical Cancer Research*, vol. 21, no. 21, pp. 4801–4810, 2015.

[23] K. Yamada, N. Yamamoto, Y. Yamada et al., "Phase I dose-escalation study and biomarker analysis of E7080 in patients with advanced solid tumors," *Clinical Cancer Research*, vol. 17, no. 8, pp. 2528–2537, 2011.

[24] M. Nishio, T. Horai, A. Horiike et al., "Phase 1 study of lenvatinib combined with carboplatin and paclitaxel in patients with non-small-cell lung cancer," *British Journal of Cancer*, vol. 109, no. 3, pp. 538–544, 2013.

[25] S. Takahashi, M. Tahara, N. Kiyota et al., "995PD phase II study of lenvatinib (LEN), a multi-targeted tyrosine kinase inhibitor, in patients (PTS) with all histologic subtypes of advanced thyroid cancer (differentiated, medullary and anaplastic)," *Annals of Oncology*, vol. 25, Supplement 4, pp. iv343–iv344, 2014.

[26] M. E. Cabanillas, M. Schlumberger, B. Jarzab et al., "A phase 2 trial of lenvatinib (E7080) in advanced, progressive, radioiodine-refractory, differentiated thyroid cancer: a clinical outcomes and biomarker assessment," *Cancer*, vol. 121, no. 16, pp. 2749–2756, 2015.

[27] M. Schlumberger, B. Jarzab, M. E. Cabanillas et al., "A phase II trial of the multitargeted tyrosine kinase inhibitor lenvatinib (E7080) in advanced medullary thyroid cancer," *Clinical Cancer Research*, vol. 22, no. 1, pp. 44–53, 2016.

[28] M. Schlumberger, M. Tahara, L. J. Wirth et al., "Lenvatinib versus placebo in radioiodine-refractory thyroid cancer," *The New England Journal of Medicine*, vol. 372, no. 7, pp. 621–630, 2015.

[29] M. S. Brose, F. P. Worden, K. L. Newbold, M. Guo, and A. Hurria, "Effect of age on the efficacy and safety of lenvatinib in radioiodine-refractory differentiated thyroid cancer in the phase III SELECT trial," *Journal of Clinical Oncology*, vol. 35, no. 23, pp. 2692–2699, 2017.

[30] H. Izzedine, C. Massard, J. P. Spano, F. Goldwasser, D. Khayat, and J. C. Soria, "VEGF signalling inhibition-induced proteinuria: mechanisms, significance and management," *European Journal of Cancer*, vol. 46, no. 2, pp. 439–448, 2010.

[31] C. Vigneau, N. Lorcy, T. Dolley-Hitze et al., "All anti-vascular endothelial growth factor drugs can induce 'pre-eclampsia-like syndrome': a RARe study," *Nephrology, Dialysis, Transplantation*, vol. 29, no. 2, pp. 325–332, 2014.

[32] S. R. Hayman, N. Leung, J. P. Grande, and V. D. Garovic, "VEGF inhibition, hypertension, and renal toxicity," *Current Oncology Reports*, vol. 14, no. 4, pp. 285–294, 2012.

[33] H. Izzedine, I. Brocheriou, O. Rixe, and G. Deray, "Interstitial nephritis in a patient taking sorafenib," *Nephrology, Dialysis, Transplantation*, vol. 22, no. 8, p. 2411, 2007.

[34] A. Khurana, "Allergic interstitial nephritis possibly related to sunitinib use," *The American Journal of Geriatric Pharmacotherapy*, vol. 5, no. 4, pp. 341–344, 2007.

[35] O. Costero, M. L. Picazo, P. Zamora, S. Romero, J. Martinez-Ara, and R. Selgas, "Inhibition of tyrosine kinases by sunitinib associated with focal segmental glomerulosclerosis lesion in addition to thrombotic microangiopathy," *Nephrology, Dialysis, Transplantation*, vol. 25, no. 3, pp. 1001–1003, 2010.

[36] V. Eremina, J. A. Jefferson, J. Kowalewska et al., "VEGF inhibition and renal thrombotic microangiopathy," *The New England Journal of Medicine*, vol. 358, no. 11, pp. 1129–1136, 2008.

[37] H. Izzedine, B. Escudier, C. Lhomme et al., "Kidney diseases associated with anti-vascular endothelial growth factor (VEGF): an 8-year observational study at a single center," *Medicine (Baltimore)*, vol. 93, no. 24, pp. 333–339, 2014.

[38] H. Izzedine, M. Mangier, V. Ory et al., "Expression patterns of RelA and c-mip are associated with different glomerular diseases following anti-VEGF therapy," *Kidney International*, vol. 85, no. 2, pp. 457–470, 2014.

[39] V. Eremina and S. E. Quaggin, "Biology of anti-angiogenic therapy-induced thrombotic microangiopathy," *Seminars in Nephrology*, vol. 30, no. 6, pp. 582–590, 2010.

[40] B. R. Forzley and W. F. Clark, "TTP/HUS and prognosis: the syndrome and the disease(s)," *Kidney International. Supplement*, vol. 75, no. 112, pp. S59–S61, 2009.

[41] C. M. Stirling, P. Mathieson, J. M. Boulton-Jones et al., "Treatment and outcome of adult patients with primary focal segmental glomerulosclerosis in five UK renal units," *QJM*, vol. 98, no. 6, pp. 443–449, 2005.

44

Chemotherapy used to Halt Lower GI Bleeding in a Rare Case of Metastatic Choriocarcinoma to the GI Tract

Ralph Kamel,[1] Talal Seoud,[2] Teniola Oluwadamilola,[3] Michael Karass,[4] Emily Grossniklaus,[5] Gabriela Oprea-Ilies,[5] Daniel A. Goldstein,[5] and Sanjay Jain[3]

[1]*Saint Joseph University, Beirut, Lebanon*
[2]*American University of Beirut, Beirut, Lebanon*
[3]*Morehouse School of Medicine, Atlanta, GA 30310, USA*
[4]*New York Medical College, Valhalla, NY 10595, USA*
[5]*Emory University, Atlanta, GA 30322, USA*

Correspondence should be addressed to Michael Karass; karass.michael@gmail.com

Academic Editor: Raffaele Palmirotta

Choriocarcinoma, a nonseminomatous germ cell tumor, is a rare type of testicular malignancy that tends to occur in young males. It is, however, exceedingly rare for choriocarcinoma to involve the GI tract. In this article, we present a rare case of a 31-year-old male, diagnosed with choriocarcinoma of the left testes, along with several metastases to distant sites. The patient presented with headaches and severe lower GI bleeding due to metastases to the GI tract, which was eventually controlled with systemic chemotherapy, while requiring several units of packed RBCs during his admission to the hospital. An extensive literature review found very few cases of the occurrence of GI bleeding as a consequence of choriocarcinoma due to metastases to the GI tract.

1. Introduction

Testicular cancers are a rare type of cancer but are unique in the sense that they are largely curable. In 2014, there were approximately 8,820 new cases of testicular cancer in the USA [1], with peak incidence between 20 and 34 years of age [2]. Testicular carcinoma most commonly presents as a painless testicular mass. However, approximately 20% to 40% of patients with primary testicular cancer present with pain, swelling, hardness of the testicle, or a combination of these symptoms [3].

A type of testicular cancer that is of particular concern is choriocarcinoma, given that it often appears with diffuse metastatic disease and progresses very quickly [2]. Testicular choriocarcinoma is a rare, nonseminomatous germ cell tumor that represents less than 1% of testicular neoplasms and presents as a rapidly growing and aggressive tumor of young males. Notably, the disease is metastatic in nearly half of patients at the time of diagnosis [4]. Choriocarcinomas disseminate via blood and lymphatics with early hematogenous dissemination to lungs, liver, brain, and other visceral sites. Because the average diagnostic delay is 4 to 6 months after symptom onset, patients often present initially with acute disorders resulting from hemorrhage or necrosis of the primary tumors or their metastases [5]. Delayed treatment contributes to increased mortality and morbidity [2]. Although choriocarcinoma was one of the first malignancies for which treatments and complete cure were accomplished with aggressive chemotherapy, the outcomes for metastatic choriocarcinoma remain guarded [2].

In this case report, we will discuss a case of choriocarcinoma in a patient who presented with extensive metastatic disease, notably involving the GI tract. We will review his presentation and imaging, and we will discuss the particular challenges faced when treating this patient.

2. Case Presentation

A 31-year-old male with past medical history of asthma presented with headache, melena, and nonbloody nonbilious vomiting, 30 pound (13.6 kg) weight loss, and painful

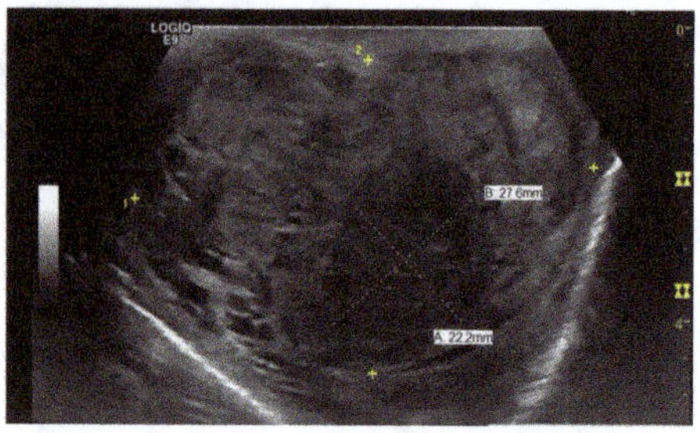

FIGURE 1: Ultrasound of the L testicle, revealing a heterogeneous infiltrating solid mass.

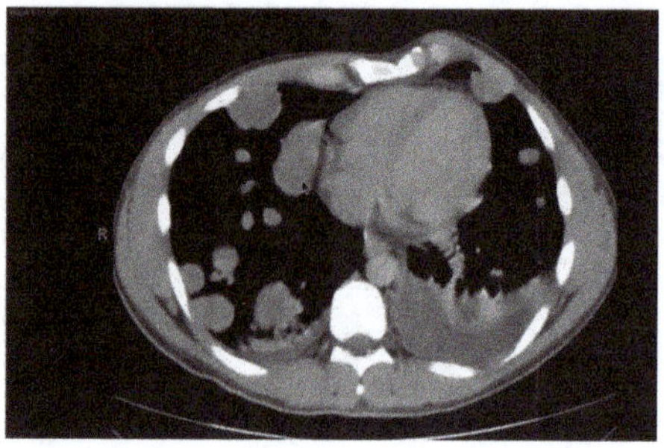

FIGURE 2: CT of the chest, revealing extensive metastatic disease with numerous pulmonary nodular masses and bilateral pleural effusions.

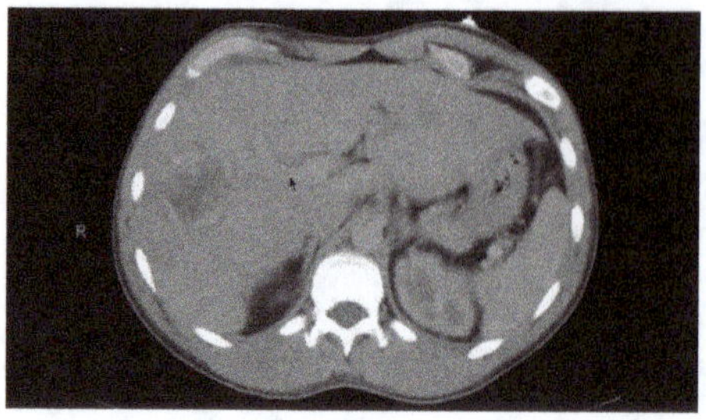

FIGURE 3: CT of the abdomen, revealing a single hypodense lesion with irregular foci and wall thickening in the right hepatic lobe.

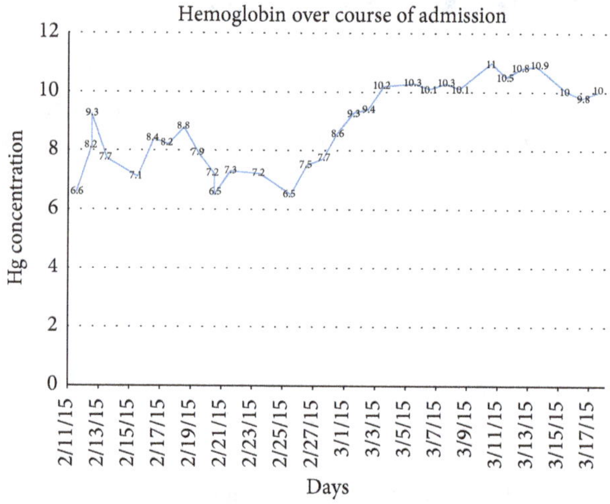

FIGURE 4: Hemoglobin concentration through patient's admission. The first day of chemotherapy coincides with 2/25. The last day of transfusion was 3/3.

left-sided testicular mass. Patient was found to be anemic with a hemoglobin of 7.0 g/dL (Ref.: 13.5–17.5 g/dL) on admission. Computed Tomography (CT) of head done at the time of admission showed no acute intracranial abnormalities and minimal paranasal sinus disease. Ultrasound (US) of the scrotum showed near completely infiltrated left testicle highly concerning for a malignancy (Figure 1). Due to rising concerns of metastatic disease a CT of chest, abdomen, and pelvis was done. Imaging revealed metastatic lesions to the lungs (Figure 2) and liver (Figure 3) and a left testicular mass. Further investigations revealed that beta-HCG was 217,671 IU (Ref.: 0–3 mIU/mL), Alpha Fetoprotein 2.5 ng/mL (Ref.: <9.0 ng/dL), Estradiol 760 (Ref.: 20–47 pg/mL), and lactate dehydrogenase (LDH) 370 U/L (Ref.: 91–180 U/L). Magnetic Resonance Imaging (MRI) was also done 4 days after admission due to patient's recurrent headaches and was consistent with late subacute lacunar infarct, but there were no findings suggestive of metastatic disease. CT angiogram was subsequently done due to persistent headaches, and this did show metastatic disease involving the subcortical white matter. An echocardiogram was also done that showed likely metastasis in the left ventricle.

The patient subsequently had two endoscopies to evaluate for a GI source of bleeding. He was noted to have duodenitis, while a follow-up colonoscopy was within normal limits. Capsular endoscopy performed during the admission showed actively bleeding lesions in the distal small intestine. Radiology guided embolization of the actively bleeding sites was deemed not to be feasible. A biopsy of lung lesion, in the meantime, confirmed metastatic nonseminomatous testicular cancer.

The patient was initiated on chemotherapy on day 14 of his admission with cisplatin, bleomycin, and etoposide with the intent to control the bleeding primarily, as well as overall tumor burden. Patient received a total of 18 blood transfusions over a 19-day period. During this time his hemoglobin concentration continued to fluctuate between 6.5 and 11 (Figure 4). He received his last transfusion 14 days prior to discharge and 6 days after start of chemotherapy. His hemoglobin levels remained on average above 10 g/dL several days before discharge, suggesting adequate control of metastases involving the gastrointestinal tract. In addition a repeat MRI two weeks after admission was noted to have interval hemorrhagic and nonhemorrhagic metastases within the bilateral parietal lobes (Figure 5), left occipital lobe, and right lateral eye. Ophthalmology was consulted and recommended outpatient follow-up without the need for immediate interventions. Palliative XRT to the brain, although initially considered, was deferred, since the patient had a relatively small tumor burden involving his brain and was significantly symptomatic from GI bleeding.

At the time of discharge patient had received 1 cycle of chemotherapy and was to receive a total of 4. He recovered

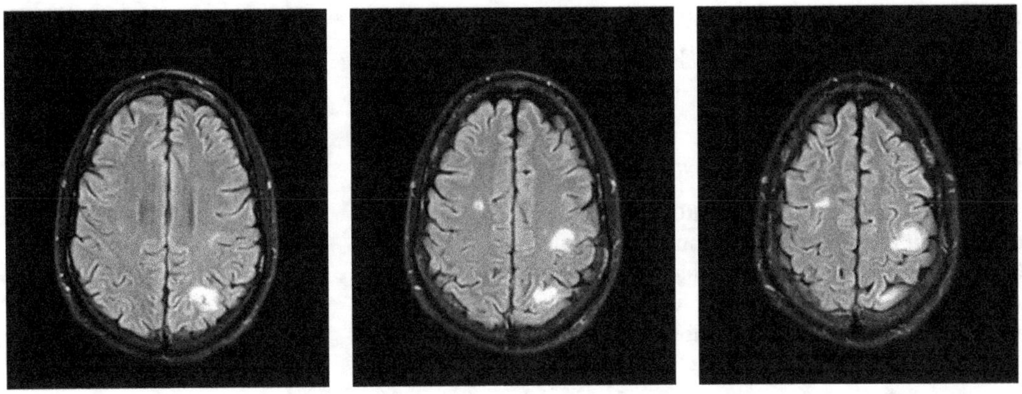

FIGURE 5: MRI of the brain revealing new interval hemorrhagic and nonhemorrhagic metastases within the bilateral parietal lobes and left occipital lobe visible on T2 FLAIR. This was found after starting chemotherapy with 4 cycles of bleomycin, etoposide, and cisplatin.

from his neutropenia and his pain and headaches were significantly improved. MRI done two months after discharge showed favorable treatment response with no definite new or residual enhancing lesions and his hemoglobin remained above 10 g/dL.

3. Discussion

We report the rare clinical presentation of a metastatic testicular choriocarcinoma involving the small bowel, diagnosed after an episode of lower gastrointestinal bleeding and severe headaches. Upon diagnosis, the patient was found to have disseminated disease to the liver, lungs, heart, and brain.

In the setting of testicular choriocarcinoma, metastasis to the gastrointestinal tract is exceedingly rare. Around 0.95% to 5% of the cases present in the small bowel, the duodenum being the most usual site followed by the esophagus, stomach, and colon [6]. Within this group of patients, the most common symptom is hemorrhage presenting as melena or hematemesis. On physical examination, signs of anemia, such as orthostatic hypotension and pale conjunctiva, can be identified in some patients.

In regard to staging and treatment, the patient was diagnosed as having stage IIIC disease, given the presence of visceral metastases involving the liver and brain, and was categorized as a poor-risk patient. The standard chemotherapy regimen for poor-risk patients is 4 cycles of BEP (bleomycin, etoposide, and cisplatin). However, it should be noted that between 20% and 30% of poor-risk patients are not cured with conventional cisplatin-based therapy and less than one-half experience a durable complete response [7].

The patient presented in this case report was admitted with severe gastrointestinal bleeding. Initial surgical management of the intestinal metastatic lesion was deferred because of the identification of multiple sites of metastases, including the lungs and the brain. Systemic chemotherapy was immediately started to control the bleeding while managing the other metastatic foci. Radiation therapy to the brain was also delayed because diffuse metastatic GI disease was considered to be the most life-threatening finding in this patient, as compared to the relatively small secondary brain lesions not accompanied by signs suggestive of increased intracranial pressure and impending herniation (lack of papilledema, no signs of ventricular shifts). The headaches may have been attributable to evolving metastatic disease, as evidenced by a subsequent MRI, while the nausea and vomiting were likely secondary to metastatic involvement of the gastrointestinal tract. The GI bleeding ceased during the first cycle of chemotherapy, an important clinical course adding to the efficacy of chemotherapy in managing systemic disease as well as acute complications of bowel metastases.

The patient was closely monitored for the early detection of treatment complications. The start of chemotherapy can complicate the course of the disease by the development of a very rare, life-threatening syndrome called the choriocarcinoma syndrome, which is characterized by hemorrhage into the metastatic sites accompanied by a significant rise in beta-HCG levels [4]. Given the extent of the disease spread and its aggressive nature, tumor lysis syndrome was a concern as documented cases in the literature were found. However, in this patient, no laboratory or clinical evidence of tumor lysis syndrome was noted. Given the cardiac involvement in this patient, the team was concerned about the development of life-threatening cardiac arrhythmias and embolic cerebral ischemia; however, these complications were luckily avoided during the first round of chemotherapy. The only neurologic symptom that was noted was severe headache that was attributed to the brain metastases and no focal deficits appeared during his hospital stay.

In conclusion, our patient was diagnosed with diffuse metastatic testicular choriocarcinoma that presented with acute gastrointestinal hemorrhage complicated by anemia. However, the therapeutic priority was to address the disseminated disease rather than the localized secondary small bowel lesions or that of his brain disease. The patient was treated with transfusions of packed red blood cells (pRBCs) and the chemotherapy proved efficient in controlling the gastrointestinal hemorrhage while controlling extraintestinal metastatic disease.

This case highlights the importance of considering the rare possibility of a metastatic testicular cancer in a young male patient presenting with acute gastrointestinal bleeding. The management should be based on aggressive chemotherapy with a curative intent.

Acknowledgments

The authors would like to thank their mentors who have guided them throughout the writing process and they would like to thank Grady Memorial Hospital for offering them the opportunity to treat and learn from many different patients with complicated conditions, including the case they present in this article.

References

[1] C. E. DeSantis, C. C. Lin, A. B. Mariotto et al., "Cancer treatment and survivorship statistics, 2014," *CA—A Cancer Journal for Clinicians*, vol. 64, no. 4, pp. 252–271, 2014.

[2] M. J. Reilley and L. C. Pagliaro, "Testicular choriocarcinoma: a rare variant that requires a unique treatment approach," *Current Oncology Reports*, vol. 17, no. 2, article 2, 2015.

[3] Y. Kabir, R. L. Kleynberg, M. D. Rotblatt, J. M. Miller, and N. R. Feldman, "The case of the missed physical examination: testicular carcinoma presenting as a GI bleed," *Journal of Clinical Oncology*, vol. 31, no. 20, pp. e338–e340, 2013.

[4] K. Baagar, F. Y. Khan, and E. AlKuwari, "Choriocarcinoma syndrome: a case report and a literature review," *Case Reports in Oncological Medicine*, vol. 2013, Article ID e697251, 4 pages, 2013.

[5] R. J. Motzer, N. Agarwal, C. Beard et al., "Testicular cancer," *Journal of the National Comprehensive Cancer Network*, vol. 10, no. 4, pp. 502–535, 2012.

[6] Y. Yazgan, K. Öncü, M. Kaplan et al., "Upper gastrointestinal bleeding as an initial manifestation of metastasis secondary to choriocarcinoma," *The Turkish Journal of Gastroenterology*, vol. 24, no. 6, pp. 565–567, 2013.

[7] A. Worster, S. Sharma, F. Mookadam, and J. Opie, "Acute presentation of choriocarcinoma: a case study and review of the literature," *Canadian Journal of Emergency Medicine*, vol. 4, no. 2, pp. 111–114, 2002.

45

Poor Outcomes in Hepatic Amyloidosis: A Report of 2 Cases

Brandon Yim,[1] Elizabeth Kertowidjojo,[2] Yue Zhang,[3] and Pruthvi Patel[4]

[1] *Department of Medicine, Stony Brook University Hospital, Stony Brook, NY, USA*
[2] *Department of Pathology, Stony Brook University Hospital, Stony Brook, NY, USA*
[3] *Division of Hematology and Oncology, Department of Medicine, Stony Brook University Hospital, Stony Brook, NY, USA*
[4] *Division of Gastroenterology, Department of Medicine, Stony Brook University Hospital, Stony Brook, NY, USA*

Correspondence should be addressed to Brandon Yim; brandon.yim@stonybrookmedicine.edu

Academic Editor: Peter F. Lenehan

Hepatic amyloidosis is a rare disease entity that results from insoluble amyloid protein deposition in the liver. The disease often presents with vague, nonspecific clinical features. Currently, there is little literature describing treatment outcomes for biopsy-proven hepatic amyloidosis and current treatment guidelines recommend that patients enroll in a clinical trial due to insufficient evidence to suggest an optimal treatment regimen. Here, we present two cases of hepatic amyloidosis at an academic medical center and describe their presentation, treatment, and outcomes. These cases highlight the poor outcomes and difficult management of hepatic amyloidosis. Further understanding and investigation of this rare disease are warranted.

1. Introduction

Amyloidosis is a rare disease characterized by the deposition of insoluble, fibril-forming amyloid proteins in the extracellular space of organs, which can result in end-organ dysfunction [1, 2]. Systemic light chain (AL) amyloidosis is the most common form of amyloidosis and results from a plasma cell dyscrasia which produces abnormal amounts of immunoglobulin light chains that can deposit in organs such as the heart, kidney, peripheral nerves, and liver [3]. Liver involvement of amyloidosis usually presents with nonspecific clinical symptoms such as weight loss and fatigue; however, prompt diagnosis is critical as liver-biopsy-proven amyloidosis is known to have a poor prognosis, with a median survival of only 8.5 months [4]. Although established systemic chemotherapy is often used for light chain amyloidosis, current guidelines still recommend that patients enroll in a clinical trial as there is currently insufficient data to suggest an optimal treatment regimen [5]. Therefore, further investigation and reporting of the treatment outcomes are needed. Two biopsy-proven liver amyloidosis cases were identified in the past ten years at Stony Brook University Medical Center. Here we report their presentation, treatment, and outcomes.

2. Case 1

A 45-year-old man with a past medical history of hypertension, dyslipidemia, and normocytic anemia presented with a 3-hour history of dull, crampy left lower quadrant abdominal pain. He had an unintentional weight loss of 18 pounds over the course of 5 weeks and also reported generalized fatigue. One month prior to admission, the patient underwent esophagogastroduodenoscopy (EGD), colonoscopy, and video capsule study to evaluate his anemia, all of which were unremarkable. His physical examination was significant for macroglossia and hepatomegaly. Laboratory work revealed a hemoglobin level of 10.8, platelet count of 553, creatinine of 0.8, AST of 119, ALT of 95, total bilirubin of 1.1 (direct bilirubin 0.6), alkaline phosphatase level of 1043, and INR of 1.4. Autoimmune markers and viral hepatitis lab work were negative.

A computed tomography (CT) scan of his abdomen revealed hepatosplenomegaly. A transcutaneous ultrasound-guided liver biopsy was performed to further elucidate the etiology of his hepatomegaly. Biopsy tissue showed deposits that stained with Congo red and produced apple-green

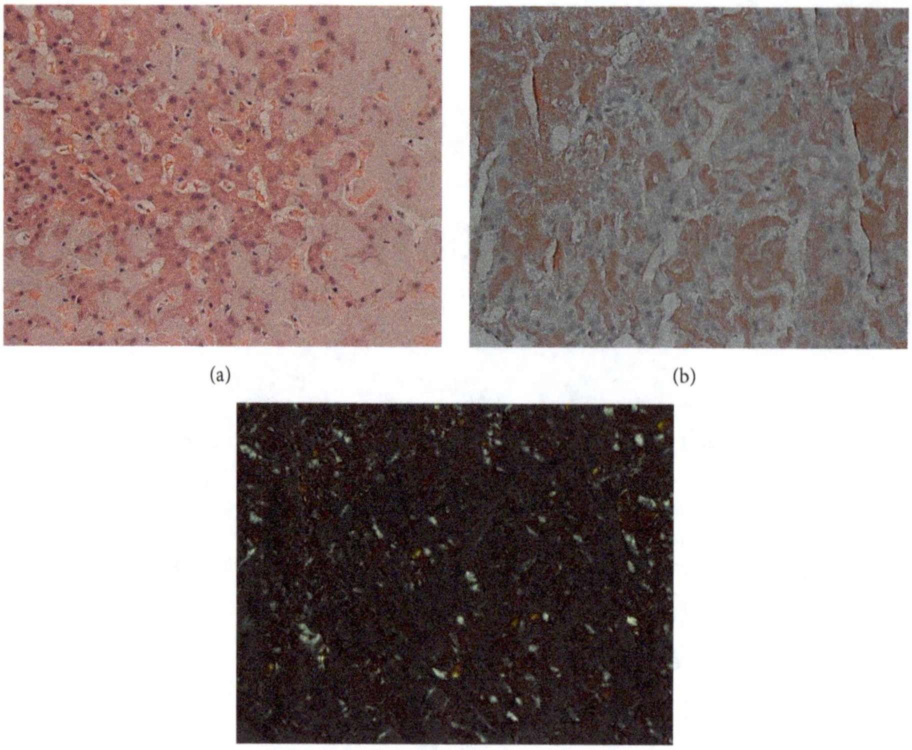

Figure 1: Case 1. Liver biopsy showing architectural distortion with extensive extracellular deposition of eosinophilic material ((a) H&E, ×200), which stains Congo red ((b) Congo red, ×200) and shows green birefringence under polarized light ((c) Congo red, ×200).

birefringence under polarized light (Figure 1), characteristic of hepatic amyloidosis.

The patient was referred to the Boston University Amyloid Treatment and Research Program for further management. Work-up revealed a kappa free light chain level of 890 mg/L (normal limits: 3.3–19.4 mg/L) and kappa to lambda free light chain ratio of 270 (normal limits: 5.7–26.3). A bone marrow biopsy was performed and revealed 90 percent plasma cells with kappa predominance of light chain immunoglobulins as well as amyloid deposits, consistent with multiple myeloma. 24-hour urine collection revealed 2.065 g of protein. Troponin I was noted to be 0.028 ng/mL and BNP was noted to be 207 pg/mL. An echocardiogram was performed and revealed an ejection fraction of 66 percent, an intraventricular septal diameter of 13 mm, and normal diastolic function. He was found to have restrictive pulmonary function tests and a chest CT revealing multifocal intralobular septal thickening and patchy nondependent ground glass opacities consistent with diffuse amyloidosis of his lungs.

Ultimately, the patient was diagnosed with AL amyloidosis with associated multiple myeloma with early cardiac, renal, pulmonary, liver, and soft tissue involvement. He underwent 4 cycles of Bortezomib (Velcade) and Dexamethasone and 2 cycles of Revlimid and Dexamethasone with 38 percent reduction of his serum free light chains after three months of treatment, consistent with a very good partial response (VGPR). At this time he also noted improvement of his activity and decreased fatigue. In preparation for an autologous stem cell transplant, he was then switched to weekly CyBorD (Cyclophosphamide 300 mg/m^2, Bortezomib 1.5 mg/m^2, and 20 mg Dexamethasone) therapy. Unfortunately, the patient passed away approximately 1 month after the initiation of CyBorD therapy of undocumented reasons. He survived 8 months after his initial diagnosis of amyloidosis.

3. Case 2

A 61-year-old man with past medical history of non-insulin dependent diabetes, coronary artery disease, heart failure with preserved ejection fraction, and proteinuria presented with a 3-year history of unintentional weight loss of 14 pounds. He also reported symptoms of early satiety, decreased appetite, fatigue, and dyspnea with exertion. He denied any abdominal pain, night sweats, or fevers. Physical examination revealed a thin man (BMI 19) with hepatomegaly. Laboratory results revealed microcytic anemia with hemoglobin level of 12.8 (MCV 77.7) and an alkaline phosphatase level of 166. Transaminase and bilirubin levels were within normal limits.

A liver ultrasound showed fatty infiltration or fibrosis of the liver. Subsequent MRI of his abdomen revealed hepatomegaly and small branch intraductal papillary mucinous neoplasm (IPMN) of the pancreas. EGD and colonoscopy

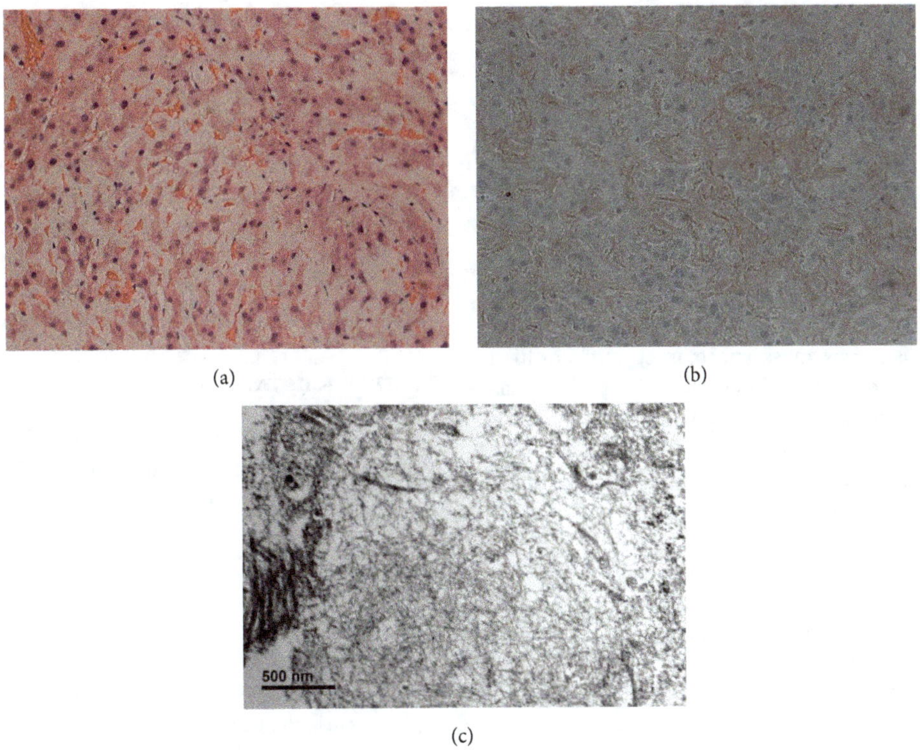

FIGURE 2: Case 2. Liver biopsy showing architectural distortion with extensive extracellular deposition of amorphous eosinophilic material ((a) H&E, ×200), which stains Congo red ((b) Congo red, ×200). Electron microscopy shows randomly oriented 8 nm diameter ultrastructural fibrils in the extracellular perisinusoidal spaces (c).

were significant for Barrett's Esophagus and *Helicobacter pylori* for which he received medical treatment. His alkaline phosphatase levels were persistently elevated within follow-up visits. His viral hepatitis, ANA, anti-mitochondrial antibody, and liver/kidney/microsomal antibody levels were within normal limits. He initially had a high retinyl palmitate vitamin A level of 0.36 mg/L (normal <0.10) from chronic consumption of vitamin A with suspicion of drug-induced liver injury from elevated vitamin A levels; however his levels resolved after suspending vitamin A consumption.

An endoscopic ultrasound (EUS) with fine needle biopsy of his liver was performed. The hepatic tissue stained with Congo red and electron microscopy revealed ultrastructural fibrils consistent with amyloidosis (Figure 2). Serum protein electrophoresis (SPE) revealed no apparent monoclonal gammopathy; however, urine protein electrophoresis (UPE) revealed a monoclonal peak in the gamma region. Urine IFE revealed a free lambda light chain. A serum free light chain assay revealed 20.1 kappa light chains (normal: 3.3–19.4) and 88.6 lambda light chains (normal: 5.7–26.3). Bone biopsy revealed monoclonal plasmacytosis of 15–20% with lambda light chain restriction. Troponin T was <0.01. Ntpro BNP measured 927. A cardiac MRI was conducted and was negative for infiltrative myocardial pathology and did not suggest amyloid. Cardiac muscle biopsy was negative for amyloid. Patient was initiated on CyBorD weekly therapy. He received 5 treatments of CyBorD therapy without reduction in his serum free light chains or improvement in his alkaline phosphatase levels. He suffered from cardiac arrest and passed away four months after his original diagnosis.

4. Discussion

Although the presentation of hepatic AL amyloidosis has been previously described [4], literature reporting the management and outcomes of these cases is lacking, likely secondary to the rarity and poor prognosis of this disease. Two biopsy-proven liver amyloidosis cases in our institution over the past 10 years were reported here with similar presentations to a previously reported cohort of hepatic amyloidosis patients described by Park et al. [4]. In that cohort of 98 patients, most patients presented with vague, nonspecific symptoms such as weight loss and fatigue, were noted to have hepatomegaly on physical examination, and had elevated alkaline phosphatase levels on presentation [4]. Both of our cases had unintentional weight loss, hepatomegaly, and elevated alkaline phosphatase levels.

Despite receiving treatment regimens consistent with National Comprehensive Cancer Network (NCCN) guidelines [5], the two cases presented here had poor outcomes, surviving only eight and four months after diagnosis for Cases 1 and 2, respectively. Several reasons may explain these outcomes. First, primary hepatic amyloidosis typically presents with advanced disease and is known to have a dismal prognosis with a median survival of only 8.5 months [4]. Both patients had multiple comorbidities that likely contributed to their poor outcomes with cardiac, renal, and pulmonary involvement in Case 1 and coexisting heart failure and proteinuria in Case 2. Second, given the rarity and poor prognosis of hepatic amyloidosis, prompt referral to amyloidosis centers of excellence may have benefited these patients. While Case 1 was referred to the Boston Medical Center's Amyloidosis Program, an established center of excellence, Case 2 received treatment without referral to a designated specialty center. Recent AL amyloidosis management algorithms propose that patients be referred to specialty centers for comprehensive work-up and patient-tailored therapy [6, 7]. Specific testing such as mass spectrometry to confirm amyloid protein composition and genetic testing which has implications on therapy selection can be conducted at these centers to tailor therapy regimens and improve outcomes [8, 9]. Third, careful selection of therapy with close monitoring should occur during the treatment of hepatic amyloidosis cases. In both cases, each patient ultimately was treated with CyBorD therapy, which has been shown to be effective in AL amyloidosis patients with 55 percent of patients projected to survive at 3 years [10]. Unfortunately, both patients in this report died approximately one month after the initiation of CyBorD therapy, raising the possibility of an adverse effect of the CyBorD therapy. In a study by Palladini et al., where AL amyloidosis patients were treated with CyBorD therapy, ten percent of their cohort suffered from severe adverse events, with the most common event being worsening heart failure [10]. Additionally, four of the 230 AL amyloidosis patients treated in that cohort died of sudden cardiac death as was the case in Case 2 of this report [10]. Cyclophosphamide and Bortezomib, primary components of the CyBorD regimen, are both liver-metabolized drugs that could be implicated if these poor outcomes were attributable to adverse effects. Cyclophosphamide, an antineoplastic alkylating agent, has been known to have cardiotoxic side effects such as tachyarrhythmias, complete A-V block, and congestive heart failure with acute symptoms usually presenting 1-2 weeks after administration [11, 12]. Similarly, although described rarely, Bortezomib-induced cardiotoxicity has also been reported in the literature [13]. While Case 1 was noted to have a very good partial response (VGPR) from initial chemotherapy, Case 2 did not respond to therapy despite five treatments with CyBorD therapy. In this disease with poor prognosis, frequent assessment of response to therapy is critical and therapy should immediately be switched if there is no response. In this case, alternative regimens such as high-dose melphalan which is shown to be effective in AL amyloidosis could have been implemented [14]. While we report two poor outcomes of hepatic amyloidosis, it is also worth noting that both patients did not survive long enough to receive stem cell transplant which has been shown to have good outcomes in patients presenting before advanced congestive heart failure [15]. Overall, the poor outcomes of hepatic amyloidosis reported here highlight the importance of prompt diagnosis and comprehensive management of this difficult-to-manage disease. Further investigation and prognostication for primarily liver AL amyloidosis are warranted to improve outcomes for this patient population.

5. Conclusion

Amyloidosis of the liver is a rare disease entity that often presents with vague, nonspecific findings and has a poor prognosis. Prompt diagnosis and management are required to improve outcomes for this patient population. Further investigation and research are needed to elucidate the risks and effectiveness of hepatic amyloidosis treatment regimens.

Acknowledgments

The authors thank Drs. Sui Zee and Jela Bandovic at the Department of Pathology, Stony Brook University Hospital, for their assistance providing pathology used in this case report.

References

[1] J. D. Sipe, M. D. Benson, J. N. Buxbaum et al., "Amyloid fibril protein nomenclature: 2012 recommendations from the Nomenclature Committee of the International Society of Amyloidosis," *Amyloid*, vol. 19, no. 4, pp. 167–170, 2012.

[2] G. Merlini and V. Bellotti, "Molecular mechanisms of amyloidosis," *The New England Journal of Medicine*, vol. 349, no. 6, pp. 583–596, 2003.

[3] A. D. Cohen and R. L. Comenzo, "Systemic light-chain amyloidosis: advances in diagnosis, prognosis, and therapy," *ASH Education Book*, vol. 2010, no. 1, pp. 287–294, 2010.

[4] M. A. Park, P. S. Mueller, R. A. Kyle, D. R. Larson, M. F. Plevak, and M. A. Gertz, "Primary (AL) hepatic amyloidosis: clinical features and natural history in 98 patients," *Medicine*, vol. 82, no. 5, pp. 291–298, 2003.

[5] National Comprehensive Cancer Network, *NCCN Clinical Practice Guidelines in Oncology: Systemic Light Chain Amyloidosis Version 1.2016*, National Comprehensive Cancer Network, 2016.

[6] G. Palladini and G. Merlini, "What is new in diagnosis and management of light chain amyloidosis?" *Blood*, vol. 128, no. 2, pp. 159–168, 2016.

[7] M. A. Gertz, "Immunoglobulin light chain amyloidosis: 2016 update on diagnosis, prognosis, and treatment," *American Journal of Hematology*, vol. 91, no. 9, pp. 947–956, 2016.

[8] T. Bochtler, U. Hegenbart, C. Kunz et al., "Gain of chromosome 1q21 is an independent adverse prognostic factor in light chain amyloidosis patients treated with melphalan/dexamethasone," *Amyloid*, vol. 21, no. 1, pp. 9–17, 2014.

[9] T. Bochtler, U. Hegenbart, C. Kunz et al., "Translocation t(11;14) is associated with adverse outcome in patients with newly diagnosed AL amyloidosis when treated with bortezomib-based regimens," *Journal of Clinical Oncology*, vol. 33, no. 12, pp. 1371–1378, 2015.

[10] G. Palladini, S. Sachchithanantham, P. Milani et al., "A European collaborative study of cyclophosphamide, bortezomib, and dexamethasone in upfront treatment of systemic AL amyloidosis," *Blood*, vol. 126, no. 5, pp. 612–615, 2015.

[11] E. Senkus and J. Jassem, "Cardiovascular effects of systemic cancer treatment," *Cancer Treatment Reviews*, vol. 37, no. 4, pp. 300–311, 2011.

[12] A. F. Reis-Mendes, E. Sousa, M. D. L. Bastos, and V. M. Costa, "The role of the metabolism of anticancer drugs in their induced-cardiotoxicity," *Current Drug Metabolism*, vol. 17, no. 1, pp. 75–90, 2016.

[13] S. Diwadkar, A. A. Patel, and M. G. Fradley, "Bortezomib-induced complete heart block and myocardial scar: the potential role of cardiac biomarkers in monitoring cardiotoxicity," *Case Reports in Cardiology*, vol. 2016, Article ID 3456287, 5 pages, 2016.

[14] M. Skinner, V. Sanchorawala, D. C. Seldin et al., "High-dose melphalan and autologous stem-cell transplantation in patients with AL amyloidosis: an 8-year study," *Annals of Internal Medicine*, vol. 140, no. 2, pp. 85–93, 2004.

[15] S. Madan, S. K. Kumar, A. Dispenzieri et al., "High-dose melphalan and peripheral blood stem cell transplantation for light-chain amyloidosis with cardiac involvement," *Blood*, vol. 119, no. 5, pp. 1117–1122, 2012.

Permissions

All chapters in this book were first published in CROM, by Hindawi Publishing Corporation; hereby published with permission under the Creative Commons Attribution License or equivalent. Every chapter published in this book has been scrutinized by our experts. Their significance has been extensively debated. The topics covered herein carry significant findings which will fuel the growth of the discipline. They may even be implemented as practical applications or may be referred to as a beginning point for another development.

The contributors of this book come from diverse backgrounds, making this book a truly international effort. This book will bring forth new frontiers with its revolutionizing research information and detailed analysis of the nascent developments around the world.

We would like to thank all the contributing authors for lending their expertise to make the book truly unique. They have played a crucial role in the development of this book. Without their invaluable contributions this book wouldn't have been possible. They have made vital efforts to compile up to date information on the varied aspects of this subject to make this book a valuable addition to the collection of many professionals and students.

This book was conceptualized with the vision of imparting up-to-date information and advanced data in this field. To ensure the same, a matchless editorial board was set up. Every individual on the board went through rigorous rounds of assessment to prove their worth. After which they invested a large part of their time researching and compiling the most relevant data for our readers.

The editorial board has been involved in producing this book since its inception. They have spent rigorous hours researching and exploring the diverse topics which have resulted in the successful publishing of this book. They have passed on their knowledge of decades through this book. To expedite this challenging task, the publisher supported the team at every step. A small team of assistant editors was also appointed to further simplify the editing procedure and attain best results for the readers.

Apart from the editorial board, the designing team has also invested a significant amount of their time in understanding the subject and creating the most relevant covers. They scrutinized every image to scout for the most suitable representation of the subject and create an appropriate cover for the book.

The publishing team has been an ardent support to the editorial, designing and production team. Their endless efforts to recruit the best for this project, has resulted in the accomplishment of this book. They are a veteran in the field of academics and their pool of knowledge is as vast as their experience in printing. Their expertise and guidance has proved useful at every step. Their uncompromising quality standards have made this book an exceptional effort. Their encouragement from time to time has been an inspiration for everyone.

The publisher and the editorial board hope that this book will prove to be a valuable piece of knowledge for researchers, students, practitioners and scholars across the globe.

List of Contributors

Alejandra C. Fuentes
Department of Internal Medicine, University of Florida, Gainesville, FL 32610, USA

Ellen Szwed, Cathy D. Spears, Long H. Dang and Nam H. Dang
Division of Hematology/Oncology, Department of Internal Medicine, University of Florida, Gainesville, FL 32610, USA

Sandeep Thaper
Florida Cancer Specialists and Research Institute, Leesburg, FL 34748,USA

Varun Sharma Tandra, KrishnaMohan Reddy Kotha, Moorthy Gadisetti Venkata Satyanarayana, Kali Varaprasad Vadlamani and Vyjayanthi Yerravalli
Department of Orthopaedics and Traumatology, Osmania Medical College, Osmania GeneralHospital, Afzalgunj, Hyderabad, Andhra Pradesh 500012, India

Liliana Vasquez, Mariela Tello, Ivan Maza and Monica Oscanoa
Department of Oncology and Radiotherapy, Rebagliati Hospital, Lima, Peru

Milagros Dueñas
Department of Genetics, Rebagliati Hospital, Lima, Peru

Haydee Castro
Department of Gynecology-Oncology, Rebagliati Hospital, Lima, Peru

Alan Latorre
Department of Pathology, Rebagliati Hospital, Lima, Peru

Mohamed H. Khattab, Ariel E. Marciscano, Michael Lim, Lawrence R. Kleinberg and Kristin J. Redmond
Department of Radiation Oncology & Molecular Radiation Sciences, Johns Hopkins University, 401 North Broadway, Suite 1440, Baltimore, MD 21231-5678, USA

Simon S. Lo
Department of Radiation Oncology, CaseWestern Reserve University, University Hospitals Seidman Cancer Center, Cleveland, OH 44106, USA

Michael Lim
Department ofNeurosurgery, Johns Hopkins University, 600 N. Wolfe Street, Phipps Room 123, Baltimore, MD 21287, USA

John J. Laterra
Department of Neurology/Neuro-Oncology, Johns Hopkins University, 601 N. Caroline Street, Baltimore, MD 21287, USA

Nishan Bingham and Christopher J. Anker
University of Vermont College of Medicine, 89 Beaumont Avenue, Burlington, VT 05405, USA

H. James Wallace III
Division of Radiation Oncology, University of Vermont Cancer Center, 111 Colchester Avenue, Mailstop 301SH2, Burlington, VT 05401, USA

Joanne Monterroso and Claire Verschraegen
Division of Hematology Oncology, University of Vermont Cancer Center, 89 Beaumont Avenue, Suite E-214, Burlington, VT 05405, USA

Brenda L. Waters
Department of Pathology and Laboratory Medicine, University of Vermont Medical Center, 111 Colchester Avenue Main Campus, East Pavilion, Burlington, VT 05401, USA

Kimberly A. Silverio
Department of Gynecologic Oncology, Helen Diller Family Comprehensive Cancer Center, University of California, San Francisco (UCSF), 550 16th Street, San Francisco, CA 94158, USA

Shyam A. Patel
Department of Medicine, Stanford University Medical Center, 300 Pasteur Drive, Stanford, CA 94305, USA

Vivekanand Sharma, Gajendra Anuragi, Suresh Singh, Pinakin Patel and Raj Govind Sharma
Division of Surgical Oncology, Department of Surgery, S.M.S. Medical College and Hospital, Jaipur, Rajasthan 302004, India

Arpita Jindal
Department of Pathology, S.M.S. Medical College and Hospital, Jaipur, Rajasthan 302004, India

Brandon T. Mullins
School of Medicine, University of North Carolina School of Medicine, 1033 Bondurant Hall, Chapel Hill, NC 27514, USA

Trevor Hackman
Division of Otolaryngology, University of North Carolina Hospitals, 101 Manning Drive, Chapel Hill, NC 27514, USA

A. B. Zarami
Department of Histopathology, University of Maiduguri Teaching Hospital, PMB 1414, Maiduguri, Borno State, Nigeria

N. A. Satumari and M. Ahmed
Department of Medical Laboratory Science, University of Maiduguri, PMB 1069, Maiduguri, Borno State, Nigeria

Michela Roberto, Maria Bassanelli, Silvana Giacinti, Anna Maria Aschelter and Paolo Marchetti
Department of Clinical and Molecular Medicine, Faculty of Medicine and Psychology "Sapienza", St. Andrea Hospital, Via di Grottarossa 1035-1030, 00189 Rome, Italy

Elsa Iannicelli
Department of Radiology, Faculty of Medicine and Psychology "Sapienza", St. Andrea Hospital, Via di Grottarossa 1035-1030, 00189 Rome, Italy

Chiara D'Antonio
Department of Medical and Surgical Sciences and Translational Medicine, Faculty of Medicine and Psychology "Sapienza", St. Andrea Hospital, Via di Grottarossa 1035-1030, 00189 Rome, Italy

Pamidimukkala Bramhananda Rao, Saptarshi Ghosh, P. Ravindra Kumar, Surendra Manam, Pradeep Karra and Vijay Krishna Jasti
Department of Radiotherapy, GSL Cancer Hospital, GSL Medical College, Rajahmundry, Andhra Pradesh 533105, India

Manisha Mohapatra
Department of Pathology, GSL Medical College, Rajahmundry, Andhra Pradesh 533296, India

N. Pramod Philip
Department of Radiology, GSL Medical College, Rajahmundry, Andhra Pradesh 533296, India

Lucas Novaes Teixeira, Victor Angelo Martins Montalli, Luiz Carlos Santana Teixeira, Fabrício Passador-Santos, Andresa Borges Soares and Vera Cavalcanti de Araújo
Department of Oral Pathology, São Leopoldo Mandic Institute and Research Center, Rua Jośe Rocha Junqueira 13, Ponte Preta, 13045-755 Campinas, SP, Brazil

Stephanie A. Terezakis
Department of Radiation Oncology and Molecular Radiation Sciences, Johns Hopkins Hospital, Baltimore, MD 21287, USA

Stephanie A. Terezakis, Sean L. Berry and Joachim Yahaloms
Department of Radiation Oncology, Memorial Sloan-Kettering Cancer Center, New York, NY 10065, USA

George C. Bohle III
Dental Service, Department of Surgery, Memorial Sloan-Kettering Cancer Center, New York, NY 10065, USA
College of Dentistry, University of Oklahoma, Oklahoma City, OK 73117, USA

Ying-Chun Lo
Department of Oncology, Johns Hopkins School of Medicine, Baltimore, MD 21287, USA
Department of Pathology, Yale-NewHaven Hospital, New Haven, CT 06510, USA

Jaleh Fallah, Maxwell Eyram Afari and Adam J. Olszewski
Department of Medicine, Memorial Hospital of Rhode Island, Pawtucket, RI 02860, USA

Jaleh Fallah, Maxwell Eyram Afari, Alfredo C. Cordova, Adam J. Olszewski and Taro Minami
The Warren Alpert Medical School of BrownUniversity, Pawtucket, RI 02860, USA

Alfredo C. Cordova
Department of Surgery, Memorial Hospital of Rhode Island, Pawtucket, RI 02860, USA

Taro Minami
Division of Pulmonary, Critical Care and Sleep Medicine, Memorial Hospital of Rhode Island, Pawtucket, RI 02860, USA

Geoffrey Alan Watson, Lorraine O'Neill, Ruth Law and Douglas Veale
St. Vincent's University Hospital, Dublin, Ireland

Geraldine McCarthy
Mater Misericordiae University Hospital, Dublin, Ireland

Glenda Ernst, Eduardo Borsini, Félix Vigovich, Alajandro Salvado and Martín Bosio
Hospital Británico de Buenos Aires, C1280AEB Buenos Aires, Argentina

Carla Torres
Hospital San Juan de Dios, Buenos Aires, Argentina

Daniel Downey
Hospital Espãnol, Buenos Aires, Argentina

Asako Yanagisawa, Takuma Hiroishi, Kohei Shikano, Noriko Hayama, Tetsuo Fujita, Hiroyuki Amano, Makoto Nakamura, Sukeyuki Nakamura and Hiroshi Tabeta
Department of Respiratory Medicine, Funabashi Municipal Medical Center, Chiba, Japan

Satoshi Hirano
Department of Medical Oncology, Funabashi Municipal Medical Center, Chiba, Japan

Shinichiro Shimizu
Department of Pathology, Funabashi Municipal Medical Center, Chiba, Japan

Diani Kartini, Maria K. Siswiandari, Gunawan Wibisana, Erwin D. Yulian, Ahmad Kurnia, Sonar S. Panigoro, Azdi Z. Albar and Muchlis Ramli
Oncology Division, Department of Surgery, Dr. Cipto Mangunkusumo General Hospital, Faculty of Medicine, Universitas Indonesia, Jakarta, Indonesia

Muhammad Husnain, Irbaz Bin Riaz and Amit Agarwal
Department of Medicine, University of Arizona, Tucson, AZ, USA

Sandra Kurtin, Nikki Barkett and Amit Agarwal
Banner University Medical Center Tucson, Department of Hematology Oncology, University of Arizona, Tucson, AZ, USA

Carolina Lara, Dalia Cuenca and Moisés Mercado
Department of Medicine, ABC Medical Center, Mexico City 01120, Mexico

Latife Salame and Moisés Mercado
Neurological Center, ABC Medical Center, Mexico City 01120, Mexico

Rafael Padilla-Longoria
Department of Surgical Oncology, Hospital Angeles de Interlomas, Huixquilucan 52763, Mexico

Ashley Albert, Robert Allbright and Srinivasan Vijayakumar
Department of Radiation Oncology, University of Mississippi Medical Center, Jackson, MS, USA

Todd Nichols and Edward Farley
Department of Radiology, University of Mississippi Medical Center, Jackson, MS, USA

Taku Mitome, Tadashi Tabei and Kazuki Kobayashi
Department of Urology, Yokosuka Kyosai Hospital, 1-16 Yonegahamadori, Yokosuka, Kanagawa, Japan

Yukio Tsuura
Department of Pathology, Yokosuka Kyousai Hospital, 1-16 Yonegahamadori, Yokosuka, Kanagawa, Japan

Andrew D. Liman and Vida A. Passero
Hematology and Oncology, VA Pittsburgh Healthcare System, University of Pittsburgh School of Medicine, Pittsburgh, PA 15240, USA

Agnes K. Liman
Laboratory and Pathology, VA Pittsburgh Healthcare System, University of Pittsburgh School of Medicine, Pittsburgh, PA 15240, USA

Jenna Shields
Pharmacy, VA Pittsburgh Healthcare System, Pittsburgh, PA 15240, USA

G. Chidananda-Murthy
Sri Venkateshwaraa Medical College Hospital & Research Centre, Department of Surgical Oncology, Puducherry, India

P. Babu
Sri Venkateshwaraa Medical College Hospital & Research Centre, Department of Plastic Surgery, Puducherry, India

J. Chandran
Sri Venkateshwaraa Medical College Hospital & Research Centre, Department of Pathology, Puducherry, India

G. Raja
Sri Venkateshwaraa Medical College Hospital & Research Centre, Department of Radiology, Puducherry, India

Sho Okimatsu, Hiroto Kamoda, Tsukasa Yonemoto, Shintaro Iwata and Takeshi Ishii
Division of Orthopedic Surgery, Chiba Cancer Center, Chiba 260-8717, Japan

Sho Okimatsu
Department of Orthopedic Surgery, Chiba University, Chiba 260-8677, Japan

Maxim Yankelevich, Sureyya Savasan and Roland Chu
Division of Hematology/Oncology, Department of Pediatrics, Children's Hospital of Michigan, Wayne State University, 3901 Beaubien Street, Detroit, MI 48201, USA

Igor Dolgopolov and George Mentkevich
Institute for Pediatric Oncology, N.N. Blokhin Russian Cancer Research Center, 24 Kashirskoye Shosse, Moscow 115478, Russia

Ifeoluwa Apanisile and Tamás Karosi
Department of Otolaryngology and Head and Neck Surgery, B-A-Z County Central Hospital and University Teaching Hospital, Miskolc, Hungary

Emily A. Kutzner
School of Medicine, Loma Linda University, 11175 Campus St., Loma Linda, CA 92350, USA

Joshua S. Park and Jared C. Inman
Department of Otolaryngology-Head and Neck Surgery, Loma Linda University Medical Center, 11234 Anderson St., Suite 2586A, Loma Linda, CA 92354, USA

Salman Zaheer
Department of Cardiothoracic Surgery, Loma Linda University Medical Center, 11234 Anderson St., Suite 1637, Loma Linda, CA 92354, USA

Filip Kohutek and Branislav Bystricky
Department of Oncology, Faculty Hospital Trencin, Trencin, Slovakia

Ladislav Badik
Department of Radiology, Faculty Hospital Trencin, Trencin, Slovakia

Pragathi Balakrishna
PGY3 Internal Medicine, Orange Park Medical Center, Orange Park, FL, USA

Augusto Villegas
Department of Hematology and Oncology, Orange Park Medical Center, Orange Park, FL, USA

María Facenda-Lorenzo, Alejandro Quijada-Fumero, Ana Laynez-Carnicero, Francisco J. Poncela-Mireles, and María Ramos-López
Servicio de Cardiología, Hospital Universitario de La Candelaria, Carretera del Rosario No. 145, 38010 Santa Cruz de Tenerife, Spain

Ana Sánchez-Quintana, Joaquín Breña-Atienza, Ana I. Cabello-Rodríguez and Francisco J. Poncela-Mireles
Hematology Service, University Hospital Nuestra Señora de La Candelaria, Santa Cruz de Tenerife, Tenerife, Canarias, Spain

Juan M. Llanos-Gómez
Radiology Service, University Hospital Nuestra Señora de La Candelaria, Santa Cruz de Tenerife, Tenerife, Canarias, Spain

Shinichi Harada, Keiki Nagaharu and Keiki Kawakami
Department of Hematology and Oncology, Suzuka General Hospital, Yamanohana 1275-53, Suzuka, Mie Prefecture 513-8630, Japan

Keiki Nagaharu and Toshiro Mizuno
Department of Hematology and Oncology, Mie University Hospital, Edobashi 2-174, Tsu, Mie Prefecture 514-0001, Japan

Youichirou Baba and Tetsuya Murata
Department of Pathology, Suzuka General Hospital, Yamanohana 1275-53, Suzuka, Mie Prefecture 513-8630, Japan

Elisa Quiroz, Adam Hafeez, Ramy Mando and Zhou Yu
Department of Internal Medicine, Beaumont Health, Royal Oak, MI, USA

Feroze Momin
Department of Hematology and Oncology, Beaumont Health, Royal Oak, MI, USA

Sven Jungmann, Nicolas Schönfeld, Torsten-Gerriet Blum, Christian Boch and Torsten T. Bauer
Department of Pneumology, Lungenklinik Heckeshorn, HELIOS Klinikum Emil von Behring, Berlin, Germany

Wolf-Dieter Ludwig
Drug Commission of the German Medical Association, Herbert-Lewin-Platz 1, Berlin, Germany

Claudia Großwendt
Department of Radiology, HELIOS Klinikum Emil von Behring, Berlin, Germany

Beate Rehbock
Diagnostic Radiology, -oracic Imaging, Bismarckstr 45-47, Berlin, Germany

Sergej Griff
Institute of Pathology, HELIOS Klinikum Emil von Behring, Berlin, Germany

Alexander Schmittel
Onkologie Seestrasse, Seestr. 64, 13347 Berlin, Germany

Smriti Panda, Chirom Amit Singh, Suresh C. Sharma and Pirabu Sakthivel
Department of Otolaryngology & Head & Neck Surgery, All India Institute of Medical Sciences, New Delhi, India

Madhu Rajeshwari
Department of Pathology, All India Institute of Medical Sciences, New Delhi, India

Carlos Eduardo Salazar-Mejía, Edio Llerena-Hernández, David Hernández-Barajas, Oscar Vidal-Gutiérrez, Adriana González-Gutiérrez, Rolando Jacob Martínez-Granados and Blanca Otilia Wimer-Castillo
Centro Universitario Contra el Cáncer, University Hospital "Dr. José Eleuterio González" and Faculty of Medicine, Universidad Autónoma de Nuevo León, Monterrey, Nuevo León, Mexico

Andrew D. Liman
Hematology and Oncology, VA PittsburghHealthcare System, University of Pittsburgh School ofMedicine, Pittsburgh, PA 15240, USA

Agnes K. Liman
Pathology, VA Pittsburgh Healthcare System, University of Pittsburgh School of Medicine, Pittsburgh, PA 15240, USA

Jenna Shields
Pharmacy, VA Pittsburgh Healthcare System, Pittsburgh, PA 15240, USA

Becky Englert
Hematology and Oncology, VA Pittsburgh Healthcare System, Pittsburgh, PA 15240, USA

Rashmikant Shah
Radiology, VA Pittsburgh Healthcare System, University of Pittsburgh School of Medicine, Pittsburgh, PA 15240, USA

EugeneWong, Lawrence J. Oh, Kazi Nahar, Adrian Lee and Stephen Clarke
Royal North Shore Hospital, Reserve Road, St Leonards, NSW2065, Australia

Ibrahim Azar, Saghi Esfandiarifard, Pedram Sinai and Ali Wazir
Department of Internal Medicine, Albany Medical Center, 47 New Scotland Ave., Albany, NY 12208, USA

Llewellyn Foulke
Department of Pathology, Albany Medical Center, 47 New Scotland Ave., Albany, NY 12208, USA

Syed Mehdi
Division of Hematology and Oncology, Department of Internal Medicine, Stratton Veterans Affairs Medical Center, 113 Holland Ave., Albany, NY 12208, USA

Daniel E. Ezekwudo, Bolanle Gbadamosi, Zhou Yu, Michael Stender and Ishmael Jaiyesimi
Department of Hematology and Oncology, Oakland University William Beaumont School of Medicine, William Beaumont Hospital, 3601 W. 13 Mile Rd., Royal Oak, MI 48073, USA

Tolulope Ifabiyi, Mitual Amin and Kenneth Shaheen
Oakland University William Beaumont School of Medicine, 3601 W. 13 Mile Rd., Royal Oak, MI 48073, USA

Kristle Haberichter and Mitual Amin
Department of Pathology and Laboratory Medicine, Oakland University William Beaumont School of Medicine, William Beaumont Hospital, 3601 W. 13 Mile Rd., Royal Oak, MI 48073, USA

R. A. Amir
Imam Abdulrahman Bin Faisal University, Dhahran, Saudi Arabia

Rola S. Rabah and S. S. Sheikh
Pathology Services Division, Johns Hopkins Aramco Healthcare, Dhahran, Saudi Arabia

Daniela Sciancalepore, Azzurra Sportelli, Angelo Vacca and Roberto Ria
Department of Biomedical Sciences and Human Oncology, Section of Internal Medicine and Clinical Oncology, University of Bari, Bari, Italy

Sergio Musci
Cardiology Unit, San Paolo Hospital, Contrada Caposcardicchio, Bari, Italy

Maria Rosaria Fracella and Grazia D'Alesio
Radiology Unit, San Paolo Hospital, Contrada Caposcardicchio, Bari, Italy

Giuseppe Ingravallo
Department of Pathology, University of Bari, Bari, Italy

Kathryn Fleming, James McGuinness, Hilary Glen and Pavlina Spiliopoulou
Beatson West of Scotland Cancer Centre (BWoSCC), Glasgow, UK

David Kipgen
Queen Elizabeth University Hospital, Glasgow, UK

Pavlina Spiliopoulou
Imperial College London, Hammersmith Hospital, London, UK

Ralph Kamel and Sanjay Jain
Saint Joseph University, Beirut, Lebanon

Talal Seoud
American University of Beirut, Beirut, Lebanon

Teniola Oluwadamilola
Morehouse School of Medicine, Atlanta, GA 30310, USA

Michael Karass
New York Medical College, Valhalla, NY 10595, USA

Emily Grossniklaus, Gabriela Oprea-Ilies and Daniel A. Goldstein
Emory University, Atlanta, GA 30322, USA

Brandon Yim
Department of Medicine, Stony Brook University Hospital, Stony Brook, NY, USA

Elizabeth Kertowidjojo
Department of Pathology, Stony Brook University Hospital, Stony Brook, NY, USA

Yue Zhang
Division of Hematology and Oncology, Department of Medicine, Stony Brook University Hospital, Stony Brook, NY, USA

Pruthvi Patel
Division of Gastroenterology, Department of Medicine, Stony Brook University Hospital, Stony Brook, NY, USA

Index

www.ingramcontent.com/pod-product-compliance
Lightning Source LLC
LaVergne TN
LVHW060940220926
848485LV00015B/1145